Ethical and Clinical Complexities in the Treatment of Schizophrenia

Ethical and Clinical Complexities in the Treatment of Schizophrenia

Liberty or Life

Edited by

Katherine Warburton
University of California, Davis

Stephen M. Stahl
University of California, Riverside

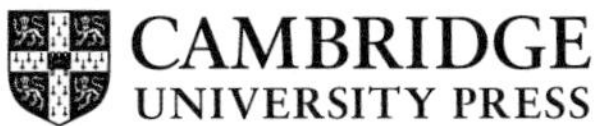

CAMBRIDGE
UNIVERSITY PRESS

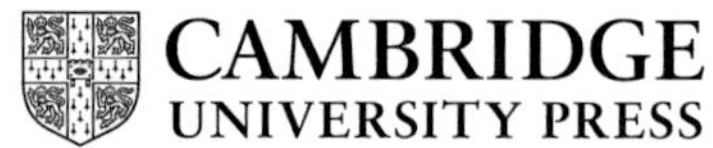

Shaftesbury Road, Cambridge CB2 8EA, United Kingdom

One Liberty Plaza, 20th Floor, New York, NY 10006, USA

477 Williamstown Road, Port Melbourne, VIC 3207, Australia

314–321, 3rd Floor, Plot 3, Splendor Forum, Jasola District Centre,
New Delhi – 110025, India

Cambridge University Press is part of Cambridge University Press & Assessment,
a department of the University of Cambridge.

We share the University's mission to contribute to society through the pursuit of
education, learning and research at the highest international levels of excellence.

www.cambridge.org
Information on this title: www.cambridge.org/9781009587754

DOI: 10.1017/9781009587747

First published 2026

A catalogue record for this publication is available from the British Library

*A Cataloging-in-Publication data record for this book is available from the
Library of Congress*

ISBN 978-1-009-58775-4 Paperback

Contents

Part III Neuroethics

Contributors

Xavier Amador
University of Utah School of Medicine, Salt Lake City, UT and LEAP Institute, Peconic, New York, NY, USA

Jacob M. Appel
Academy for Medicine & the Humanities, Icahn School of Medicine at Mount Sinai and Mount Sinai Health System, New York, NY, USA

Ai-Li W. Arias
University of California, Irvine, and University of California, Riverside, CA, USA

Craigen Armstrong
Inmate Mental Health Assistant

Justin Barry-Walsh
Fixated Threat Assessment Centre New Zealand, Te Whatu Ora Aotearoa, Wellington, New Zealand

Jhilam Biswas
Department of Psychiatry, Massachusetts General Hospital and Brigham and Women's Hospital, Boston, MA, USA

Rennie Burke
Contra Costa Regional Medical Center, Martinez, CA, USA

Felice F. Carabellese
Faculty of Medicine and Psychology, University of Rome "Sapienza," Rome, Italy

Alberto Carrara
Faculty of Philosophy and Neurobioethics Research Group (GdN), Pontifical Athenaeum Regina Apostolorum (APRA), Rome and Faculty of Psychology, European University of Rome (UER), Rome, Italy

Takesha Cooper
Department of Psychiatry and Behavioral Sciences, University of Nevada, Reno School of Medicine and Renown Health, Reno, NV, USA

Christoph U. Correll
Zucker Hillside Hospital, Glen Oaks, NY; Donald and Barbara Zucker School of Medicine at Hofstra/Northwell, Hempstead, NY, USA; Charité – Universitätsmedizin Berlin; German Center for Mental Health (DZPG), Berlin; and Einstein Center for Population Diversity (ECPD), Berlin, Germany

Michael A. Cummings
University of California, Irvine and University of California, Riverside, CA, USA

Mary Davoren
Trinity College Dublin, Dublin, Ireland; University of Bari "Aldo Moro," Bari; and University of Rome "Sapienza," Rome, Italy

Melinda DiCiro,
Forensic Services Division, California Department of State Hospitals, Sacramento, CA, USA

Christine E. Dri
Brain and Cognitive Discovery Foundation, Toronto, ON, Canada

Mathieu Dufour
Department of Psychiatry and Addictions, University of Montreal, Montreal, QC, Canada

Alexander Dvorak
Forensic Therapeutic Centre (FTZ) Göllersdorf, Vienna, Austria

Andrew Ellis
Justice Health NSW, University of New South Wales, Kensington, Australia

Sean E. Evans
Clinical Operations Division, California Department of State Hospitals, Sacramento, CA, USA

Ambarin Faizi
Clinical Operations Division, California Department of State Hospitals, Sacramento, CA, USA

List of Contributors

Nicole Fielding
Canadian Mental Health Association, Toronto, ON, Canada

Jon A. Gates
Neuroscience Education Institute, Malvern, PA, USA

John Gray
Schizophrenia Society British Columbia Provincial Board, Vancouver, BC, Canada

Philip D. Harvey
Department of Psychiatry and Behavioral Sciences, University of Miami Miller School of Medicine, Miami, FL, USA

Jahon Jabali
Arbor Scientia, Carlsbad, CA, USA

Harry G. Kennedy
Trinity College Dublin, Dublin, Ireland; Aarhus University, Aarhus, Denmark; and University of Bari "Aldo Moro," Bari, Italy

Sophia Kocher
Wilson Center for Science and Justice, Duke University School of Law and Duke University School of Medicine, Durham, NC, USA

Nina M. Labovich
Attorney New York, New York, United States of America

J. Steven Lamberti
University of Rochester Medical Center, Rochester, NY, USA

Kirsty MacDonald
Justice Health NSW, University of New South Wales, Kensington, Australia

Bernardo Martinez
Inmate Mental Health Assistant

Anthony Matzke
Inmate Mental Health Assistant

Elinore F. McCance-Katz
Warren Alpert School of Medicine, Brown University, Providence, RI and Able Americans, National Center for Public Policy Research, Washington, DC, USA

Barbara E. McDermott
Department of Psychiatry and Behavioral Sciences, University of California, Davis, Sacramento, CA, USA

Roger S. McIntyre
Departments of Psychiatry and Pharmacology and Toxicology, University of Toronto, ON, Canada

Jonathan M. Meyer
University of California, San Diego, CA, USA

Gerben Meynen
Willem Pompe Institute for Criminal Law and Criminology and Utrecht Centre for Accountability and Liability Law (UCALL), Faculty of Law, Economics and Governance, Utrecht University, The Netherlands

Kerry Morrison
Heart Forward LA, Hollywood, CA, USA

Debbi Ann Morrissette
Neuroscience Education Institute, Malvern, PA, USA

Esther Nauta
Willem Pompe Institute for Criminal Law and Criminology and Utrecht Centre for Accountability and Liability Law (UCALL), Faculty of Law, Economics and Governance, Utrecht University, The Netherlands

David Nelson
Inmate Mental Health Assistant

Lia Parente
Faculty of Medicine and Psychology, University of Rome "Sapienza", Rome and Section of Criminology and Forensic Psychiatry, University of Bari "Aldo Moro," Bari, Italy

Lyndal C. Petit
Department of Psychiatry, University of Ottawa, Ottawa, ON, Canada

Benjamin Rose
Clinical Operations Division, California Department of State Hospitals, Sacramento, CA, USA

Dain Sanderson
Inmate Mental Health Assistant

Charles L. Scott
Department of Psychiatry and Behavioral
Sciences, University of California, Davis, Sacramento,
CA, USA

Melanie Scott
Community Forensic Partnerships Division,
California Department of State Hospitals,
Sacramento, CA, USA

Karen Shin
Department of Psychiatry, University of Toronto,
Toronto, ON, Canada

Stephen M. Stahl
University of California, San Diego, CA, USA and
University of Cambridge, Cambridge, UK

Sean Sterling
Forensic Services Division, California Department of
State Hospitals, Sacramento, CA, USA

Thomas Stompe
Forensic Therapeutic Centre (FTZ) Göllersdorf,
Vienna, Austria

Joan M. Striebel
Semel Institute for Neuroscience and Human Behavior,
University of California, Los Angeles, CA, USA

Marvin Swartz
Department of Psychiatry and Behavioral Sciences,
Duke School of Medicine and Wilson Center for
Science and Justice, Duke University School of Law,
Duke University, Durham, NC, USA

Patrick Swoboda
Forensic Therapeutic Centre (FTZ) Göllersdorf,
Vienna, Austria

Katherine Warburton
California Department of State Hospitals, Sacramento
and Department of Psychiatry and Behavioral
Sciences, Division of Psychiatry and the Law,
University of California, Davis, Sacramento, CA, USA

Robert L. Weisman
University of Rochester Medical Center, Rochester,
NY, USA

Bethany Yeiser
CURESZ Foundation, Fairfield,
OH, USA

Liyang Yin
Brain and Cognitive Discovery Foundation, Toronto,
ON, Canada

Preface

Jordon was a beautiful kid, inside and out. Born and raised in an impoverished inner city, he had a family that loved him, a pure heart, and a physical appearance so attractive that he startled people. He was always taking care of stray animals and protecting the vulnerable kids in his neighborhood. It was no surprise, then, that when he saw a young woman being kidnapped by a known gang member who was involved in human trafficking, he immediately acted. He chased down the car, pulled the driver out, and knocked him to the ground, and then he took control of the vehicle. He reassured the young woman in the passenger seat that she was safe now. Just in time, he noticed another gang member trailing close behind. He pressed on the gas, leading them on a high-speed chase through busy city traffic. That's the last thing he remembered.

At his trial for aggravated assault, carjacking, and kidnapping, the young woman from the car corroborated some of Jordon's story. He did pull the driver out of the car and take off with her in the passenger seat. He repeatedly reassured her that she would be fine. But the driver of the vehicle was not a gang member; he was her boyfriend. And there was no car chasing them.

Jordon's family were devastated. Their beautiful, sweet boy had been acting strangely for months. He had started sleeping with a knife under his bed and had accused his older brother of being in a violent local gang. Some nights he would not come home. Other nights he would stay in his room, talking to himself. His parents took him to the emergency room (ER) six times, waiting hours to be seen. A couple of times he simply didn't wait. On the few occasions when social workers saw Jordon, they turned him away because he wasn't making acute threats of physical harm to either himself or others. One social worker suggested to Jordon's family that they call the police the next time he was out of control. But his parents knew what happened when you called the police in their neighborhood, so they ruled that option out. The social worker gave this standard form of advice to all worried parents, because these kids rarely evidenced the type of behavior that rose to the level requiring involuntary treatment. She hated to admit it, but she was always a little relieved when her hospital could turn these mental health cases away, because there was nowhere to send those youth who did require involuntary care. The local inpatient psychiatric hospital had closed years before, and city's few crisis beds were always full.

At trial, it didn't matter that Jordon's loving family had informed police that he'd been acting strangely paranoid. It didn't matter that hospital records documented his ER visits. It didn't matter that the woman from the car testified that Jordon had repeatedly told her she'd be safe, or that he'd seemed to think he was protecting her. His public defender took a deal; she was overworked, didn't have the time or budget to launch an insanity phase in the trial, and needed to clear her cases. When the district attorney offered a light sentence, she took it and moved on to her next case. Public defenders in that district often were too inundated by clients and injustice to get attached.

In prison, Jordon learned to keep his inner life to himself. His behavior was bizarre. Guards noticed him carrying out strange rituals with his food in his cell. He stayed up all night talking to himself. But he wasn't a problem inmate, so when he declined attention from the prison's limited mental health services, he received no further care. As long as he wasn't threatening himself or others, he didn't rise to the level of requiring involuntary treatment. The overwhelmed prison intake therapist was always a little relieved when nonviolent patients like Jordon refused treatment; after all, the inmate had the legal right to refuse. The prison didn't have enough psychiatrists to treat everyone, and falling behind on timely assessments negatively impacted their performance reports – hence the relief when prisoners refused treatment.

Jordon didn't make any friends in prison, so no one noticed when his paranoia worsened. He'd been refusing contact with his family because he was convinced the same neighborhood gang had taken control of their bodies. He began to suspect that the gang had infiltrated the correctional officers, too. He could tell from their hand gestures that they were signaling to him that his time on Earth was limited. They didn't reveal how they would kill him, but he knew it was coming. So, when the officers opened his cell one night, alarmed by his screaming, he seized the moment. He fought for his life, seriously wounding one of the guards before they pepper-sprayed him, forced him to the ground, and restrained him.

As Jordon sat in solitary confinement, he was at last cleared for mental health services. Since he'd hurt an officer, he now met the threshold for involuntary treatment. A psychiatrist started him on antipsychotic medication, and the paranoia quickly faded. With that, Jordon began to have a reality-based understanding of the situation he was in. He also was able to comprehend that he'd picked up serious additional charges during the interaction with the correctional officers and was now facing life in prison. For several days in solitary, he sobbed inconsolably, alone in his cell, unable to eat or sleep. Jordon was alternately overwhelmed with fear, shame, grief, and hopelessness. Sometimes he experienced all these feelings at once, and these were the moments he couldn't tolerate. He needed to do something. He started to plan. He watched the guards until he knew which ones did rounds and which ones didn't. When he knew it was the right time, he hung himself in his cell.

This is Jordon's story. But it is also the story of schizophrenia.

The Story of Schizophrenia
Liberty or Life

Katherine Warburton and Stephen M. Stahl

Why We Created This Book

KW

John C. was a remarkably nice person. He would greet me every morning after my mile-long journey through parking lots, sally ports, and many locked doors. I tended to arrive at my unit at around the same time, and when I approached the final locked door I would see his smiling face in the small square window. As soon as I stepped onto the unit he would exclaim, "Good Morning Doctor!" He would then update me about his prior evening, before politely inquiring as to how I was. One morning he complimented my pants, asking, "Did you make those yourself?" (I never wore them again.) Despite my young age, he had a strong maternal transference to me – not atypical for a long-term therapeutic relationship. It only gave me brief pause that he'd killed his mother several years earlier by cutting open her stomach and pulling out her internal organs. I wasn't worried because John C. had schizophrenia, which was now well controlled with medication, so the risk of him hurting me or anyone else was quite low – as long as he stayed on his medication.

Originally, I wanted to be a rural family doctor in the osteopathic tradition: a humane, holistic, cradle-to-grave kind of doctor in the Maine woods where I grew up. When I got my third-year rotation schedule in medical school and saw that my requisite psychiatry rotation was at the state forensic hospital, I was terrified. Images from old movies coursed through my mind. I went to the dean and strongly requested an outpatient setting, arguing that as a family doctor I would need skills more consistent with outpatient practice. As with everything at my traditional osteopathic medical school, the answer was: "Suck it up, do it, and stop complaining."

The state hospital infrastructure turned out to be everything I'd feared: decrepit buildings, razor wire fences, and a definite vibe that some very bad things had happened on these grounds. I hadn't felt so uncomfortable since my surgery rotation, in which some rough hazing from the scrub nurses had me throwing up behind the parking garage every morning. But something unusual happened when I walked through those two locked doors and onto my assigned unit: I sensed an unmistakable surge of empathy and kindness coming from the myriad patients wandering the day hall. A very large and tall woman approached me. She'd shaved off her eyebrows and painted them back on with hot pink nail polish. She wore her hair in a bleached blond afro, and her makeup heavily encircled her eyes. In other words, she looked bizarre. Being a relatively small person and knowing that this woman had to have been locked in this "back ward" for something quite violent, I should have felt fear or anxiety in her looming presence. But she immediately put me at ease with a kind smile, before stating, "Oh, you must be the new girl. I can tell you come from the light. We will take good care of you here."

Intrigued, I spent the morning reading through volumes of her records. You could do that on a state hospital rotation, during which you were assigned to a back ward. None of these patients were going anywhere, so the workload was light. I found out that the tall woman's name was Gretchen, and she'd shot her husband and children at close range while they'd slept. All she would say about it after that was that she'd saved their souls.

I found myself captivated by the stories of these patients. I also felt like I'd found my home. There is something about the disease of schizophrenia that strips away any pretense, any superficiality, and renders a person profoundly authentic. As an introvert, small talk and social artifice exhausted me. Spending the day sharing space with 45 people who were struggling to maintain their grasp on reality, sliding back and forth between delusions ("I'm the female Jesus, here to save you") and unit life ("What time is sick call today, my allergies are acting up?") left little room for the unessential of human interaction. And my need to feel needed, to find meaning by helping, was immediately satisfied. Within a week of starting that rotation, I went to the dean to rearrange my fourth-year schedule. I was going to be a psychiatrist.

Five years later, I was nearing the end of my residency in adult psychiatry, and the work remained fascinating. Reading Freud and being able to detect defense mechanisms felt like a form of magic. Learning about neurobiology was challenging but satisfying. I had a dog-eared first-edition copy of Stahl's *Essential Psychopharmacology* that I'd purchased during that first psychiatry rotation. Stahl was already very famous in my circles; he had an uncanny ability to take the most complicated and poorly understood area of the human body – the brain – and break it down with simple language and cartoon drawings to make it understandable. I'd read this book cover to cover many times. What I failed to appreciate then was that I was coming of age as a psychiatrist at a breakthrough moment in neuroscience. In my lifetime, people like Dr. Stahl had developed medications that actually worked to combat the deterioration in perception experienced by many of these patients. It was remarkable to see someone pull back from the edge of reality and at last be able to function simply after taking a small pill.

I had enjoyed my entire residency: working overnight in the ER and assessing those patients who had finally dragged themselves in from within the deep hole of depression; working in my therapy clinic once a week with the worried well and watching them take better control of their own lives; and doing outpatient medication management. But my favorite times were on the locked psychiatric units, helping my fellow human beings escape the torture of persecutory delusional systems, coaxing them back to reality with medication and compassion. These were my people, this was my calling, so I attended a conference of public psychiatrists and sat in on a lecture about schizophrenia. I thought we'd be talking about the newest therapies, but instead the presenter looked out at us and gravely intoned, "If you are a resident thinking about working with patients who have schizophrenia, you'd better go do a forensic fellowship because they are locking them all up." She then presented alarming statistics about these increasing rates of incarceration and arrest.

The term "forensic psychiatrist" brought to my mind Jodie Foster, fava beans, and a nice Chianti, and not much more. I'd rotated through a forensic hospital in another state as a medical student, but I'd never put it together that most of the patients in that state hospital had been confined there after committing a violent crime. This focus on patients with criminal legal involvement was what rendered the hospital "forensic." After conducting further research I learned that forensic psychiatry related to the practice and science of my profession at any point where it intersected with the law. Most state hospitals now are largely forensic in nature due to the increasing numbers of people with schizophrenia becoming entangled in the criminal legal system.

During the forensic fellowship that followed my residency, I studied the two primary legal pathways that many people with schizophrenia ended up traversing. The first is implemented before someone is convicted of a crime if they are too delusional or disorganized to stand trial after an arrest. These individuals are deemed Incompetent to Stand Trial (IST) and generally end up in state hospitals for treatment. People found IST are returned to court when their psychosis is under control. The second pathway is implemented after trial. Some states call it "Not Guilty by Reason of Insanity," others "Guilty Except Insane." In any case, this is a legal mechanism to divert people away from prison and into a state hospital if they can prove they were so delusional at the time of the crime that they did not know what they were doing, or did not know that it was wrong.

I was spending a day a week at a very large state hospital interacting with people who were on both legal pathways, and their stories were both bizarre and fascinating. I'd seen complicated schizophrenia before, but nothing on this scale. I decided that if I wanted to be a competent doctor for this population, I would need to be able to work with these most difficult and complicated cases, so I took a job there. I was assigned to a back ward of patients who had been found Not Guilty by Reason of Insanity. I had 36 patients and the luxury of plenty of time to get to know them and understand their long histories of hospitalization. One of my patients had been locked in that hospital longer than I'd been alive.

I loved my work, and my patients – with one exception. I really didn't care for Ellen M., probably because she would scream obscenities at me while referring to me, inexplicably, as Vivian. She was trapped in a delusional system, and she believed herself to be a prison warden. She thought I was a particularly naughty inmate. And by the time I got to sorting through her case files, I realized she was woefully undertreated. She hadn't had a medication change in the 10 years she'd been at the hospital because her previous doctor had believed her psychosis was due to a neurological condition. From a case review, however, it was clear she had a classic paranoid schizophrenia. Her paranoid delusions caused her to fear that aliens had infested the Earth and were waging an apocalyptic battle between good and evil. She believed that she herself was a warrior, advised by unseen generals. So, when these generals ordered her to run a red light into a crowd of people, she'd complied.

I started titrating Ellen up on a standard antipsychotic called Risperdal and moved on to the next case. Sometime later, she sheepishly approached me.

"Hello, excuse me, are you my social worker?" she asked.

"No, Ms. M., I am your doctor," I told her, then gestured to the clinician standing next to me. "But Penny here is your social worker."

"Thank you so much," Ellen answered politely. "Penny, can you please help me? I'm not sure what I'm doing here in the hospital, but I'd really like to call my husband and children to let them know where I am."

Penny and I stared at each other in shock. Ellen was clear as a bell, with no sign of any remaining psychosis. After 10 years of being trapped in an alternative reality, Ellen emerged as the kind, funny, and delightful woman she'd been prior to the development of the disease. A particular highlight of my career was the family meeting where I witnessed Ellen's two now-grown children emotionally reunite with the mother who'd been absent from their lives for well over a decade. I'd had my first "awakening" experience with these new-generation medications, and I now knew beyond a doubt that, under the right circumstances, they could be miraculous.

As I worked my way through the cases of all 36 patients on my ward, it was also becoming clearer to me that all of them would have escaped the fate of long-term state institutionalization if they'd received treatment earlier in the disease. Before their crimes, their records indicated that they all had loved ones who had been trying to get them into care. The kicker: They were invariably so delusional that they did not realize they were ill. In colloquial terms we refer to this as a "lack of insight." This also goes by a fancy Greek word: "anosognosia." Anosognosia roughly translates to "without disease knowledge." It is extremely common for people with schizophrenia to refuse treatment because they don't believe they are ill. Still, it came as a shock to recognize that every single one of my patients had been experiencing anosognosia at the time of their crimes.

Take Joe P. He himself was a licensed mental health professional, as were all his siblings. He was a middle-aged man from a close-knit, affluent family when he developed a psychotic depression, which can cause symptoms identical to schizophrenia. His family, some of whom were doctorate-level experts in this disease, repeatedly sought help for him. And every time they were turned away because, convinced that he did not have a mental illness, Joe refused treatment. Instead, he believed that imposters had invaded the bodies of his loved ones, and with each day that passed without treatment he grew more paranoid. He lost his job, and he lost his home. His father took Joe in despite his son's growing agitation and suspicions. One night, Joe beat him to death with a sledgehammer. The only way to save his father – to free him to reemerge, Joe had reasoned – was to beat the imposter to death. Joe was found Not Guilty by Reason of Insanity and quickly responded to the same medication as Ellen. That was the easy part. The hard part was helping him through his horror and grief at what he had done while he was out of his mind. His family forgave him and understood, but they railed against a system that had refused to treat Joe against his will. That system, they believed, was responsible for the murder. We tried to discharge Joe back to the community; he was no longer a danger. But the judge made it clear that he would never order a community release given the notoriety of the crime. I began to have questions about such a system that values autonomy so highly yet allows people to get so sick that they are institutionalized for life.

How did this come to be, I wondered? In that moment I became a student of the history of mental illness in general, and psychiatry in particular. An illustrious history it is not. Suffice it to say that because the brain was so poorly understood, the experimental treatments that fill the historical record are horrifying, among them induced insulin comas and frontal lobotomies. A patient on my locked psychiatric unit, Jorge C., was a survivor of that era. Jorge was an elderly man and the first patient to greet me when I started on the unit.

I'd barely stepped inside when he ran up and screamed, "Fuckyoufuckyoufuckyoufuckyou" in my face until a psych tech redirected him back to his room. I followed him, and I was overwhelmed by the smell of urine. The lack of sanitary conditions alarmed me, but the tech – who adored Jorge, and vice versa – explained that Jorge would store his urine in his room despite all staff efforts and interventions to prevent him from doing so. I'd never seen a patient present like this before. And when I got around to looking through his chart later that day it became clear why: In the 1960s Jorge had undergone experimental psychosurgery.

Jorge's ill-fated operation occurred in the mid-twentieth century, when state institutions were riddled with experimental, ineffective treatments, abysmal funding, and astonishing overcrowding. Human beings were involuntarily committed with no clear due process or thoughtful consideration. People were locked up for everything from sexually transmitted diseases to alcoholism to tuberculosis. A process called "deinstitutionalization" began in response to these horrific conditions, and such individuals were released to the community. Many scholars attribute a poorly planned process of deinstitutionalization with the later increases in homelessness and criminal legal involvement experienced by people with schizophrenia.

Several years after that back ward of 36 patients captured my heart, I'd been promoted to be the clinical leader of a large forensic hospital system with seven institutions, 6,500 patients, hundreds of doctors, and thousands of clinical staff. I had no idea what to expect, but I can tell you that low on my list of expectations was Stephen M. Stahl, MD, PhD, deciding that he wanted to come in and help. It seemed like a good idea: I would try to manage what had to be an enormous ego and, in turn, be able to leverage his expertise in psychopharmacology. He requested a weekly meeting with me, which seemed reasonable. These meetings would inspire and sustain me throughout a decade. Our first conversation began with a bang.

"You may not realize this, but I'm going to be mentoring you," he told me in a hypomanic but matter-of-fact manner. "You're pretty smart, and you seem to have some good ideas, but no one understands what the hell you're talking about half the time. You need to organize your thoughts. You need to ground your thoughts in the existing literature. You need to write them down; that's the only way you will be able to slow your brain down. And you need to stop apologizing for being ambitious, stop apologizing for being a young woman in your position, dammit. You are in that role because you earned it, and until you own that, you will not be effective. You need to lean in!"

For over a decade, Dr. Stahl and I worked through the problems facing our hospitals. We did it by using the methodology he'd laid out for me: mastering the literature, developing our own studies, and conferring with other states and countries. In time, the daily challenges we faced were eclipsed by an overwhelming increase in the number of patients with schizophrenia that county jails were sending us as IST. We engaged our research partners and sought to figure out the reasons for these increases in arrests of people with active psychosis. These were people with schizophrenia like John, Ellen, and Joe. But, we learned, they were only showing up at our doors after *years* of untreated disease. The overwhelming majority were homeless. Most had been incarcerated many times before. They had extensive underlying untreated medical problems. The trend of criminalization that I first heard about at that public psychiatry conference and saw on my own unit was getting worse – horribly worse.

It didn't help that the hospitals couldn't handle this influx. That meant that individuals with serious mental illness were trapped in county jails on long waiting lists to get into state hospitals. These waits got substantially longer during the COVID-19 pandemic, when we had to cease admissions during lockdowns. Judges and jail officials were understandably frustrated. As was I. As I sorted through the paperwork of the people on our waiting list, what I read broke my heart. Many had been arrested on felony charges for actions that spoke to untreated disease and pure survival: homeless people taking refuge in abandoned buildings or starting fires to stay warm; paranoid people throwing rocks through windows; starving people stealing food. And they were locked away in jails, untreated and at highest risk for a deadly virus that preyed on individuals with the types of medical conditions most people with schizophrenia experience.

As we dug deeper, it became clear that the massive challenges facing forensic state hospitals were not the fault of the hospitals; they were the result of large-scale policy failure. As we chewed on the bitter reality of the increasing incarceration, homelessness, and trauma experienced by our ballooning hospital population, the answers seemed obvious. But existing policy and legal structures guiding mental health treatment were nonsensical and entrenched. My Friday calls with Dr. Stahl turned into ranting sessions. Why hadn't certain laws passed? Why was funding being held up? We came up with grandiose ideas, ranging from forming a political action committee to beseeching the pope to help us.

I got myself onto state and federal committees, where we blandly discussed anemic and tangential attempts to fix the system. At the end of these meetings, members of the public were invited to comment. Like clockwork, the parents of people with schizophrenia stepped up, begging for help, because their children were incarcerated, untreated, and/or homeless, tortured by delusions and refusing help.

One day, I attended a public meeting for California's CARE Court, implementing a new law designed to compel care for people with schizophrenia who were at risk for homelessness and incarceration. During the comments from the public, a mother called in to speak. At her urging, her daughter had checked in to a homeless shelter. She was experiencing delusions and, as a result, had begun yelling, so the shelter had kicked her out. She'd taken a blanket and walked into the night, settling down to sleep in the dirt and refuse on an empty lot next door. The following morning, the unsuspecting driver of a delivery truck ran over her head, killing her. I found myself crying uncontrollably while listening to this story, one so similar to others I'd heard before.

I had heard so many horror stories by this point in my career, but this one got to me. I think it was the raw pain in the mother's voice. That Friday morning, at my rant session with Dr. Stahl, after asking how policymakers, advocates, and elected officials could be so unwilling to change the system, it finally dawned on us: People simply didn't understand this disease. They didn't understand that it was no different from Alzheimer's disease in terms of a person's inability to make decisions for themselves. The horrible history of psychiatric abuses, combined with the relative newness of promising scientific advances, had left gaping holes where misunderstanding, propaganda, politics, and ideology took root to prevent change.

Someone, we decided, needed to tell the story of schizophrenia. And who better than us?

SMS

My career can be described through three paradigm shifts, the final one relating to this book and our current project. My journey into psychiatry began with a first paradigm shift, namely entering psychiatry only after a detour into neurology, until I realized that with my MD–PhD in pharmacology that medications were much more effective in psychiatric disorders than in most neurological disorders, and that the future held more promise for new innovations in psychopharmacology treatments than in neurology. The decades since the beginning of my career have proven this to be true. Thus, I pivoted to psychiatry and developed my career in the midst of the serotonin selective reuptake inhibitor (SSRI) and atypical antipsychotic era, first as an academic with a lab and a research ward for schizophrenia at Stanford, then with a stint overseas to work for a brain research institute funded by the pharmaceutical industry in the UK, targeting brain disorders for new drug development, and finally back to the USA as a research professor at the University of California, San Diego.

The second paradigm shift occurred after years of doing psychopharmacology research, both basic and clinical, when I realized that it was a very long slog to "invent/discover" new drug treatments that were, in fact, usually just marginal improvements over what already existed, whereas teaching practitioners to close the gap between ideal psychiatric practice and actual practice, utilizing current drugs optimally, would potentially impact the field much more than many new "copycat" drugs. Thus, my era as a textbook author and international lecturer/symposium organizer began. This was and continues to be very gratifying, but I also experienced a blazing glimpse of the obvious: namely, that no matter how ideally drugs for psychosis were prescribed, "they didn't work if you didn't take them." Hard to believe!

I came to realize that there were radically different problems in the treatment of psychosis at the two ends of the spectrum of severity of this illness. On one end of the spectrum were the sickest of the sick, many of those in forensic hospitals like those described by Dr. Warburton, with a lifetime of nontreatment, intermittent treatment, and undertreatment. It struck me that this was analogous to what would have happened if I were in the field of oncology and the system in that field worked the same way as in my field: namely, that no one got effective cancer treatment until the terminal stage of the disease. Because schizophrenia is a progressive illness involving neurodegeneration of gray matter, especially when not treated, this would mean that untreated psychosis, once such an individual has been criminalized and institutionalized, especially for decades, would result in patients presenting in the late stages of psychosis. And indeed these patients would get treatment, but there were no guidelines on how to treat them with the antipsychotics developed while studying moderately ill patients able to give consent to participate in such research! It dawned on me that these forensic patients at the severe end of the spectrum were in the "top 1% of the 1%." Not economically, certainly, but a bit of math on the back of an envelope told me that if California has a population of 40 million, and 1–2% (or about 700,000) have serious mental illness, and the population of state hospitals was 7,000, this meant that state hospitals housed a population severely skewed to the severe end of the spectrum, and we really did not have guidelines for how to treat them with antipsychotics, especially if they were treatment resistant and violent. Thus, I embarked on a project in the state hospital system that Dr. Warburton runs to capture the collective experience of the experts who had "practice-based evidence" rather that the "evidence-based practice" that dominated my academic life. We developed and published guidelines for treatment resistance, violence, and how to dose guided by plasma antipsychotic drug levels, and we increased the number of experts in the use of clozapine and long-acting injectable antipsychotics. And, lo and behold, despite greatly improving the outcomes of these patients, I watched as hospitals began to overflow with patients at the other end of the spectrum.

These were patients in the earlier stages of their illness, homeless, receiving no treatment, getting arrested for their illness on the streets, and IST for their charges. They didn't lack effective and available treatments but rather did not want treatment, not recognizing that they were ill or that such treatments would work. The system allowed patients unable to make health care decisions for themselves due to illness – who had anosognosia and a lack of insight into their illness – to refuse treatment, all supposedly because of their rights and for liberty's sake. Of course, a patient with Alzheimer's disease eating out of a dumpster and wandering the streets would be rapidly taken into care no matter how much they protested, but for some reason the system decides

that schizophrenia is different. This propelled me to join Dr. Warburton in the third paradigm shift of my career: namely, one toward the implementation of policies that allow humane treatment of psychosis before a patient enters the forensic/criminal justice system.

I specifically came to realize that the system allowing patients to live horrible, unhoused, exploited lives without treatment was based largely on outdated – or frankly wrong – information. The concepts that there is no such thing as schizophrenia and, furthermore, that antipsychotics don't work are prime examples. Liberty over life was a recurring value justifying these tragic outcomes. To counter this nonsense, as a psychiatrist who understood well the exploitation of such patients in asylums of the past, I recognized that we needed help in assessing the dilemma of treating patients who did not want treatment because they did not know that they were sick. So, I consulted a distinguished neuroethicist, the Vatican priest Father Alberto Carrara, dean of the school of neuroethics at the Vatican University of Rome, about the ethics of treatment and nontreatment. After Dr. Warburton and I took him to see the fate of patients with schizophrenia in the USA, to Skid Row in Los Angeles to see homeless psychotic patients in tents eating out of dumpsters, and to a notorious jail housing thousands of psychotic individuals under arrest basically because of their psychotic symptoms, he began to ponder the question of how to consider these issues within a neuroethical framework. He finally figured out that in an untreated psychotic state, the patient has lost a certain amount of freedom, including the freedom to make rational health care decisions. In a stunning statement summing this all up, he found that what was happening was "abandonment dressed up as autonomy." Wow.

So, off we go – to help implement the treatment of psychosis across the spectrum, and especially to get psychotic individuals into housing with treatment that includes programs that provide their lives with meaning. The individuals writing the chapters in this book are all fellow warriors in this fight for justice and humane treatment – such as we have seen in Europe, especially in Italy – and we all know we can do this. The tools are all there, the housing can be found, the medications do work – we just need to put it all together! Our goal is nothing short of revolutionizing the treatment of psychosis in America! Please join us.

What Is the Neurobiology of Schizophrenia?

Michael A. Cummings, Ai-Li W. Arias, and Stephen M. Stahl

Schizophrenia spectrum disorders are a cluster of psychotic brain diseases that afflict approximately 0.4% to nearly 2.0% of persons in various worldwide populations.[1,2] In 2019, the direct and indirect annual costs of schizophrenia were estimated at $343.2 billion in the United States alone.[3] Moreover, in addition to a substantial economic burden on society as a whole, the schizophrenia spectrum disorders impose a variety of devastating personal and familial burdens, including but not limited to social isolation, disruption of education, unemployment, homelessness, intrafamilial violence, entanglement in the legal system, incarceration, increased injury and illness, and a shortened life span.[4,5] Given the costly and disastrous effects of the schizophrenia spectrum disorders, Emil Kraepelin, who first characterized these psychotic disorders, described them as dementia praecox or early dementia.[6] In the remainder of this review, we will consider the neurobiology underlying a cluster of brain diseases that can be conceptualized under an umbrella as a group of developmental dementias with similar core pathologies but heterogeneous variations in clinical detail.

The human genome was first published in 2001.[7] Since then, researchers have been working to identify protein-coding genes. The number of such genes is presently estimated at between 19,000 and 20,000.[8] Within the human genome, some 270 gene loci have been associated with schizophrenia spectrum disorders, with 108 risk genes being identified as single nucleotide polymorphisms.[9] The most obvious genetic associations have been with genetic variations in the major histocompatibility complex. Besides polymorphisms, structural variants in the form of copy number variants, such as microdeletions and microduplications, have a very high impact in a subset of patients. These variations are mainly microdeletions on 1q21.1, 2p16.3, 3q29, 15q13.3, and 16p11.2, as well as a large deletion on 22q11.21 and a microduplication on 16p11.2.[10] Importantly, many of the genes and gene

loci implicated in schizophrenia are involved in areas such as cell differentiation, cell regulation, cell maturation, cell migration, orientation of cells, the structure of cell receptors, cell adhesion, and, in the case of neurons, development of neural networks.[11,12] Additionally, those gene foci that are part of the histocompatibility complex play critical roles in immune identity and control of inflammatory processes.[8,13,14]

Although schizophrenia spectrum disorders are heavily genetically determined, it is thought that about 20% of the risk for overt illness is determined by environmental factors such as maternal stress during pregnancy, in utero infection exposure, childhood illnesses, childhood adversity, and childhood or adolescent exposure to drugs such as methamphetamine or cannabis.[1,15] Many of these environmental risk factors may influence the occurrence and phenotypic development of schizophrenia via epigenetic processes, such as gene promotion or inhibition of other genes using small peptides or short ribonucleic acid (RNA) sequences, methylation of deoxyribonucleic acid (DNA), or modulation of the acetylation of histone (protein involved in the winding and unwinding of DNA strands for copying).[16,17] Moreover, while no gene therapies currently exist for schizophrenia spectrum disorders, interventions in selected environmental risk factors hold promise for altering the phenotypic presentation of schizophrenia, as well as risk of overt illness in both present and future generations.[18,19]

The human central nervous system begins as a simple tube formed from neural crest cells. This relatively simple structure, however, then undergoes a complex and elegant series of steps to become the brain and spinal cord.[20] The brain is formed by overfolding of the cephalad portion of the neural tube with glial cells laying down the structural form of the brain and providing trails of chemical markers for motile neuroblasts to follow to their cortical and subcortical positions.[21] During the second trimester of pregnancy, neuroblasts (immature motile forms of later neurons) undergo rapid mitosis deep in the forming brain near the lateral ventricles. These neuroblasts then crawl to their later positions following neurotrophic markers and organize themselves into orderly neural assemblies.[20] They then form neural networks by sprouting axons and dendrites. Initially, the number of connections is 2 to 5 times greater than the connections present in the mature brain. That is, exposure to the environment and the process of learning selects those pathways that will be reinforced and those that will be allowed to atrophy as the brain matures.[22–24] The primary visual cortex is the first to mature at about 1 year of age, while the last areas to mature are the frontal and temporal lobes at between 18 to 25 years of age. Thus, the roughly 100 billion neurons of the central nervous system, along with their associated astrocytes, oligodendrogliocytes, and microglia, as well as other cell types, become the adult brain and spinal cord.[21,24,25]

In contrast, brain development and maturation in schizophrenia spectrum disorders is clearly abnormal. To begin, many of the neuroblasts produced during the second trimester of pregnancy fail to reach their correct positions, instead being found in postmortem studies isolated deep within the white matter of the brain.[26,27] Then, across childhood and adolescence individuals in the premorbid phase of schizophrenia exhibit excessive loss of neurons and synaptic connections, such that by the onset of overt psychosis some one-third to one-half exhibit clear atrophic changes and enlargement of the lateral ventricles on brain imaging.[28,29] Ventricular enlargement, reflecting loss of brain tissue in schizophrenia, is illustrated below (Figure 2.1).

Following the onset of overt illness, loss of brain mass continues and appears to be correlated with the duration of untreated illness and the number of psychotic exacerbations.[1,29,30] At least a portion of the brain tissue loss associated with psychotic exacerbations or longer durations of untreated active psychosis appears to be mediated by inflammatory processes, including activation of microglia and invasion of the brain by macrophages.[14,31,32] Interestingly, treatment of high-risk children (i.e., having two parents with schizophrenia spectrum disorders) with low-dose antipsychotic medications may reduce the rate of conversion to overt illness in adolescence.[33] Nevertheless, it should be noted that some subsequent studies have failed to find evidence that antipsychotic treatment during the premorbid phase of schizophrenia is protective with respect to later development of overt schizophrenia.[34] Better established appear to be observations that consistent antipsychotic treatment

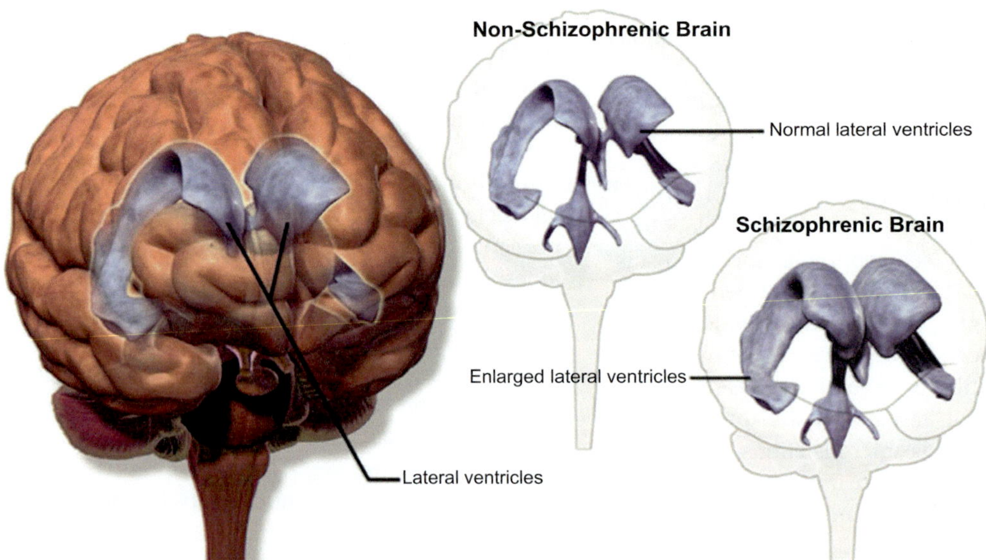

Figure 2.1 Ventricular enlargement/brain atrophy. openbooks.lib.msu.edu (open access).

(e.g., with long-acting injectables [LAIs]) slows but does not reverse the deterioration of the brain in schizophrenia spectrum disorders.[35–37]

Clinically, the signs and symptoms of schizophrenia have been divided into positive, negative, and cognitive deficit domains.[1,38] Positive signs and symptoms include hallucinations/illusions, delusional ideation, illogical thoughts and behavior, hyperactivity/agitation, and thought disorder.[1,38] Negative signs and symptoms include apathy, lethargy, abulia, avolition, and social withdrawal.[39] Cognitive deficits in schizophrenia spectrum disorders include deficits in attention, concentration, memory organization and recall, language processing, and executive functions such as self-awareness and social judgment.[38, 40] In addition to the developmental abnormalities and atrophic brain changes described earlier in this article, two neuromodulatory molecules, that is, dopamine and serotonin, appear to play important functional roles in schizophrenia spectrum disorders.[41,42] Below, we consider three neural networks with respect to the positive, negative, and cognitive domains of schizophrenia.

Positive signs and symptoms appear to arise in part from excessive dopamine stimulation of mesostriatal projections to temporal lobe association cortices and related structures (formerly termed the mesolimbic pathway).[41,43] This excessive stimulation of limbic D_2 dopamine receptors, in turn, appears to arise from a failure of inhibition by gamma aminobutyric (GABA) interneurons in the frontal cortex and failure of M_4 acetylcholine receptors on the cell bodies of the relevant mesostriatal dopamine neurons.[41,44] This is illustrated as follows (Figure 2.2).

Excessive serotonin (5-hydroxytryptamine) stimulation of $5HT_{2A}$ receptors may add to positive psychotic signs and symptoms, especially visual hallucinations, in schizophrenia.[41,45] This is illustrated as follows (Figure 2.3).

Finally, it appears that in addition to previously described developmental pathologies and atrophic changes, inadequate stimulation of frontal lobe D_1 and D_3 dopamine receptors contributes to the negative symptoms and cognitive impairments of schizophrenia spectrum disorders, including anosognosia (unawareness of illness).[41,46] This is illustrated as follows (Figure 2.4).

Importantly, all antipsychotic medications appear capable of ameliorating psychotic symptoms, with the

Integrative Hub Mesostriatal Hyperdopaminergia

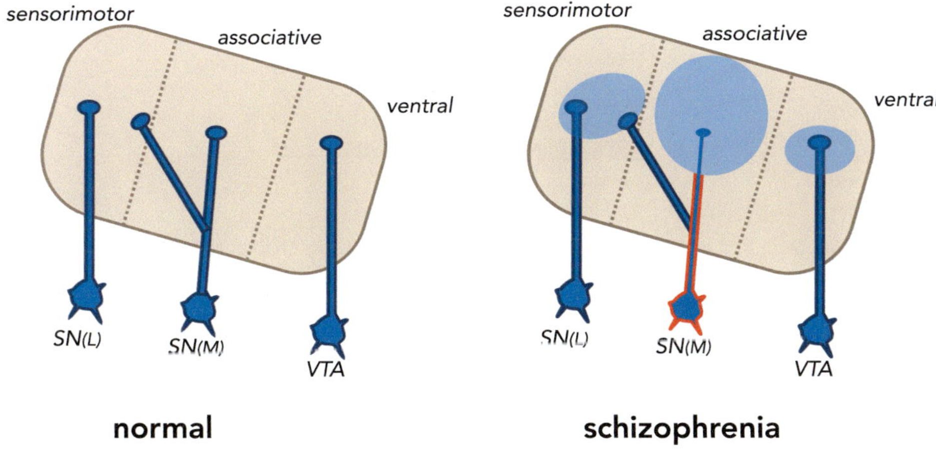

Figure 2.2 Mesostriatal dopaminergic hyperactivity. Stahl, S. Stahl's Essential Psychopharmacology, 5th Edition, Chapter 4, p. 93.

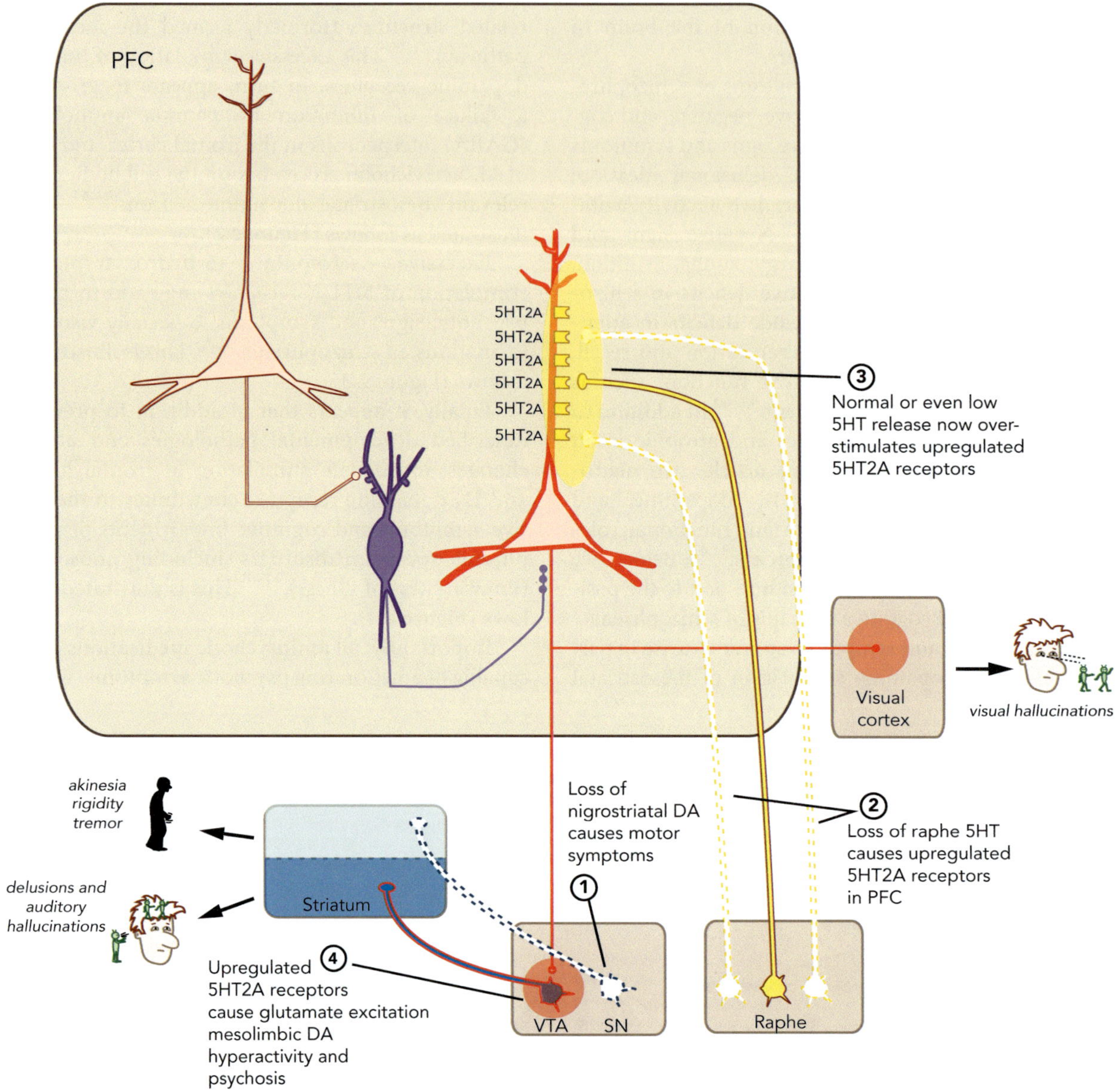

Figure 2.3 5HT$_{2A}$ serotonergic hyperactivity. Stahl, S. Stahl's Essential Psychopharmacology, 5th Edition, Chapter 4, p. 136.

largest effects being on positive signs and symptoms.[47] In particular, LAIs appear superior in preventing relapse and, thereby, illness progression, morbidity, and mortality.[35,48] In the near future, a new class of antipsychotics likely starting with xanomeline/trospium may be able to presynaptically modulate dopamine release in mesostriatal projections by targeting the M$_4$ acetylcholine auto-receptor.[44] Among the antipsychotics, clozapine remains the "gold standard" of treatment in several areas, that is, management of treatment-resistant illness, reduction of violence, reduction of suicide risk, and enhancement of cognitive executive functions.[49,50] Clozapine also appears to be unique in that it likely acts by exerting effects upstream of the mesostriatal dopamine neurons by improving glutamate signal transduction.[51,52]

Summary: Schizophrenia spectrum disorders are a group of related psychotic developmental

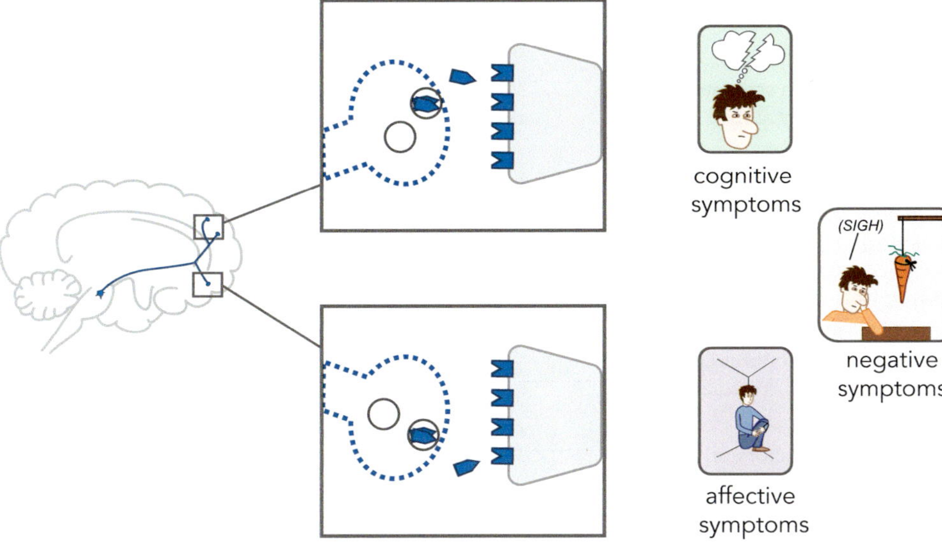

Figure 2.4 Mesocortical dopaminergic hypoactivity.
Stahl, S. Stahl's Essential Psychopharmacology, 5th Edition, Chapter 4, p. 95.

dementias (dementia praecox) characterized by positive, negative, and cognitive signs and symptoms usually beginning in adolescence or early adulthood. Illness is mediated by a combination of developmental and atrophic changes in brain structure and defects in the signal transductions of glutamate, gamma amino butyric acid (GABA), acetylcholine, dopamine, and serotonin. Importantly, defects in neurotransmitter signal transduction provide targets for pharmacotherapy with antipsychotic medications. Critically, failure to provide consistent antipsychotic treatment early in the course of illness (e.g., with LAIs) promotes atrophic brain pathology and deterioration of the illness course. Finally, while all antipsychotic medications can ameliorate acute signs and symptoms, clozapine shows superior efficacy in treating the positive, negative, and cognitive signs and symptoms of the schizophrenia spectrum disorders, as well as treatment resistance, violence, and suicide.

References

1. Kahn RS, Sommer IE, Murray RM, et al. Schizophrenia. *Nat Rev Dis Primers.* 2015;**1**:15067.

2. McGrath J, Saha S, Chant D, Welham J. Schizophrenia: a concise overview of incidence, prevalence, and mortality. *Epidemiol Rev.* 2008;**30**:67–76.

3. Kadakia A, Catillon M, Fan Q, et al. The economic burden of schizophrenia in the United States. *J Clin Psychiatry.* 2022;**83**(6):22M14458.

4. Gibb S, Brewer N, Bowden N. Social impacts and costs of schizophrenia: a national cohort study using New Zealand linked administrative data. *New Zealand Med J.* 2021;**134**:66–83.

5. Kennedy JL, Altar CA, Taylor DL, Degtiar I, Hornberger JC. The social and economic burden of treatment-resistant schizophrenia: a systematic literature review. *Int Clin Psychopharmacol.* 2014;**29**:63–76.

6. Kendler KS. The development of Kraepelin's concept of dementia praecox: a close reading of relevant texts. *JAMA Psychiatry.* 2020;**77**:1181–1187.

7. Green ED, Watson JD, Collins FS. Human genome project: twenty-five years of big biology. *Nature.* 2015;**526**:29–31.

8. Amaral P, Carbonell-Sala S, De La Vega FM, et al. The status of the human gene catalogue. *Nature.* 2023;**622**:41–47.

9. Legge SE, Santoro ML, Periyasamy S, et al. Genetic architecture of schizophrenia: a review of major advancements. *Psychol Med.* 2021;**51**:2168–2177.

10. Rujescu D. Search for risk genes in schizophrenia. *Der Nervenarzt.* 2017;**88**: 751–754.

11. Stauffer EM, Bethlehem RAI, Dorfschmidt L, et al. The genetic relationships between

brain structure and schizophrenia. *Nat Commun.* 2023;**14**:7820.

12. Owen MJ, Legge SE, Rees E, Walters JTR, O'Donovan MC. Genomic findings in schizophrenia and their implications. *Mol Psychiatry.* 2023;**28**:3638–3647.

13. Debnath M, Cannon DM, Venkatasubramanian G. Variation in the major histocompatibility complex [MHC] gene family in schizophrenia: associations and functional implications. *Prog Neuropsychopharmacol Biol Psychiatry.* 2013;**42**:49–62.

14. Khandaker GM, Cousins L, Deakin J, et al. Inflammation and immunity in schizophrenia: implications for pathophysiology and treatment. *Lancet Psychiatry.* 2015;**2**:258–270.

15. Stilo SA, Murray RM. Non-genetic factors in schizophrenia. *Curr Psychiatry Rep.* 2019;**21**:100.

16. Richetto J, Meyer U. Epigenetic modifications in schizophrenia and related disorders: molecular scars of environmental exposures and source of phenotypic variability. *Biol Psychiatry.* 2021;**89**:215–226.

17. Srivastava A, Dada O, Qian J, et al. Epigenetics of schizophrenia. *Psychiatry Res.* 2021;**305**:114218.

18. Xavier MJ, Roman SD, Aitken RJ, Nixon B. Transgenerational inheritance: how impacts to the epigenetic and genetic information of parents affect offspring health. *Human Reprod Update.* 2019;**25**:518–540.

19. Svrakic DM, Zorumski CF, Svrakic NM, Zwir I, Cloninger CR. Risk architecture of schizophrenia: the role of epigenetics. *Curr Opin Psychiatry.* 2013;**26**:188–195.

20. Lu Z, Zhang M, Lee J, et al. Tracking cell-type-specific temporal dynamics in human and mouse brains. *Cell.* 2023;**186**:4345–4364.e24.

21. Hendriks D, Pagliaro A, Andreatta F, et al. Human fetal brain self-organizes into long-term expanding organoids. *Cell.* 2024;**187**:712–732.e38.

22. Dambska M, Laure-Kamionowska M. Myelination as a parameter of normal and retarded brain maturation. *Brain Dev.* 1990;**12**:214–220.

23. Holzer L, Halfon O, Thoua V. La maturation cérébrale à l'adolescence [Adolescent brain maturation]. *Archives de pediatrie: organe officiel de la Societe francaise de pediatrie.* 2011;**18**:579–588.

24. Forde NJ, Ronan L, Zwiers MP, et al. Healthy cortical development through adolescence and early adulthood. *Brain Struct Funct.* 2017;**222**:3653–3663.

25. Walhovd KB, Tamnes CK, Fjell AM. Brain structural maturation and the foundations of cognitive behavioral development. *Curr Opin Neurol.* 2014;**27**:176–184.

26. Connor CM, Crawford BC, Akbarian S. White matter neuron alterations in schizophrenia and related disorders. *Int J Dev Neurosci.* 2011;**29**:325–334.

27. Wu Q, Liu J, Fang A, et al. The dynamics of neuronal migration. *Adv Exp Med Biol.* 2014;**800**:25–36.

28. Chung Y, Cannon TD. Brain imaging during the transition from psychosis prodrome to schizophrenia. *J Nerv Ment Dis.* 2015;**203**:336–341.

29. Haukvik UK, Hartberg CB, Agartz I. Schizophrenia–what does structural MRI show? *Tidsskrift for den Norske laegeforening : tidsskrift for praktisk medicin, ny raekke.* 2013;**133**:850–853.

30. Kubota M, van Haren NE, Haijma SV, et al. Association of IQ changes and progressive brain changes in patients with schizophrenia. *JAMA Psychiatry.* 2015;**72**:803–812.

31. Cai HQ, Catts VS, Webster MJ, et al. Increased macrophages and changed brain endothelial cell gene expression in the frontal cortex of people with schizophrenia displaying inflammation. *Mol Psychiatry.* 2020;**25**: 761–775.

32. Zhu Y, Webster MJ, Murphy CE, et al. Distinct phenotypes of inflammation associated macrophages and microglia in the prefrontal cortex schizophrenia compared to controls. *Front Neurosci.* 2022;**16**:858989.

33. Yung AR, Nelson B. Young people at ultra high risk for psychosis: research from the PACE clinic. *Revista brasileira de psiquiatria (Sao Paulo, Brazil : 1999).* 2011;**33**(Suppl 2):s143–s160.

34. Zhang T, Xu L, Tang X, et al. Real-world effectiveness of antipsychotic treatment in psychosis prevention in a 3-year cohort of 517 individuals at clinical high risk from the SHARP (ShangHai At Risk for Psychosis). *Aust N Z J Psychiatry.* 2020;**54**:696–706.

35. Horvitz-Lennon M, Predmore Z, Orr P, et al. The predicted long-term benefits of ensuring timely treatment and medication adherence in early schizophrenia. *Adm Policy Ment Health.* 2020;**47**:357–365.

36. Hunsberger J, Austin DR, Henter ID, Chen G. The neurotrophic and neuroprotective effects of psychotropic agents. *Dialogues Clin Neurosci.* 2009;**11**:333–348.

37. Lawrie SM. Do antipsychotic drugs shrink the brain? Probably not. *J Psychopharmacol (Oxford, England).* 2022;**36**:425–427.

38. McCutcheon RA, Reis Marques T, Howes OD. Schizophrenia-an overview. *JAMA Psychiatry.* 2020;**77**:201–210.

39. Marder SR, Kirkpatrick B. Defining and measuring negative symptoms of schizophrenia in clinical trials. *Eur Neuropsychopharmacol.* 2014;**24**: 737–743.

40. Javitt DC. Cognitive impairment associated with schizophrenia: from pathophysiology to treatment. *Annu Rev Pharmacol Toxicol.* 2023; **63**: 119–141.

41. Stahl SM. Beyond the dopamine hypothesis of schizophrenia to three neural networks of psychosis: dopamine, serotonin, and glutamate. *CNS Spectr.* 2018;23:187–191.

42. Cumming P, Abi-Dargham A, Gründer G. Molecular imaging of schizophrenia: neurochemical findings in a heterogeneous and evolving disorder. *Behav Brain Res.* 2021;**398**:113004.

43. Howes OD, Shatalina E. Integrating the neurodevelopmental and dopamine hypotheses of schizophrenia and the role of cortical excitation-inhibition balance. *Biol Psychiatry.* 2022;92:501–513.

44. Foster DJ, Bryant ZK, Conn PJ. Targeting muscarinic receptors to treat schizophrenia. *Behav Brain Res.* 2021;**405**:113201.

45. Preller KH, Burt JB, Ji JL, et al. Changes in global and thalamic brain connectivity in LSD-induced altered states of consciousness are attributable to the 5-HT2A receptor. *eLife.* 2018;7: E35082.

46. Howes OD, Kapur S. The dopamine hypothesis of schizophrenia: version III–the final common pathway. *Schizophr Bull.* 2009;35:549–562.

47. Sabe M, Pillinger T, Kaiser S, et al. Half a century of research on antipsychotics and schizophrenia: a scientometric study of hotspots, nodes, bursts, and trends. *Neurosci Biobehav Rev.* 2022;**136**:104608.

48. Taipale H, Mittendorfer-Rutz E, Alexanderson K, et al. Antipsychotics and mortality in a nationwide cohort of 29,823 patients with schizophrenia. *Schizophrenia Res.* 2018;**197**:274–280.

49. Meltzer HY, McGurk SR. The effects of clozapine, risperidone, and olanzapine on cognitive function in schizophrenia. *Schizophr Bull.* 1999;25:233–255.

50. Stahl SM. Clozapine: is now the time for more clinicians to adopt this orphan? *CNS Spectr.* 2014;19:279–281.

51. Nucifora FC, Woznica E, Lee BJ, Cascella N, Sawa A. Treatment resistant schizophrenia: clinical, biological, and therapeutic perspectives. *Neurobiol Dis.* 2019;**131**:104257.

52. McQueen G, Sendt KV, Gillespie A, et al. Changes in brain glutamate on switching to clozapine in treatment-resistant schizophrenia. *Schizophr Bull.* 2021;**47**:662–671.

What Is Schizophrenia?

Symptomatology

Joan M. Striebel

Schizophrenia is clinically heterogeneous: patient cases

Marta is a 65-year-old woman with schizophrenia. She suffered her first psychotic break at age 25 and has had multiple hospitalizations over the years. Her primary delusion is centered on the belief that she is a psychiatrist. She believes that medications she had taken in the past allowed the Central Intelligence Agency (CIA) to gain control of her mind and that the CIA sends people "mindreaders" to follow her. She refutes the diagnosis of schizophrenia and declines treatment. She's been arrested multiple times for vandalism, terrorist threats, and assault. Although she's been intermittently homeless, most recently, she was living at a motel, hit another guest whom she believed was sent by the CIA, and was arrested. In jail, correctional officers notice that she wears her clothes inside out, talks to herself, and when she talks to them, what she says doesn't make sense.

DeShawn is a 23-year-old man with schizophrenia. He played sports in school, earned average grades, and had a large circle of friends. In high school, he began smoking cannabis and slowly withdrew from all activities. He suffered his first psychotic break at age 19 and was hospitalized for three months. While hospitalized, he felt so hopeless about the diagnosis of schizophrenia that he tried to hang himself in the bathroom. He attempted suicide again shortly after he was discharged. After spending several years recovering, he returned to community college. While his parents are thrilled with his progress, they worry that he spends so much time in his room, seldom talks with them, and has few friends. They miss the energetic, outgoing young man that he used to be and wonder if there's a medication or something they can do to bring him back.

Marta and DeShawn illustrate the substantial variation in how individuals experience schizophrenia.

The clinical complexity of the disorder manifests in different symptom domains, associated symptoms, comorbidities, disease trajectories, and in treatment response. The variation in the presentation and course of the illness was recognized when schizophrenia was first described over 150 years ago.

The two patient cases illustrate the core schizophrenia symptom clusters (Table 3.1). The diagnosis of schizophrenia is based on a combination of distinctive symptoms of sufficient duration and severity in the absence of other possible causes, e.g., substance use, medical or neurological illnesses, or other psychiatric illnesses. The diagnostic criteria for schizophrenia are outlined in the two diagnostic classification systems currently used in clinical practice—the Diagnostic Statistical Manual of Mental Disorders, Fifth Edition, Text Revision (DSM-5-TR) and the International Classification of Diseases, 11th Revision (ICD-11) (Table 3.2). A key difference between the two systems is the DSM-5-TR's inclusion of functional deficits as a criterion. This inclusion acknowledges the importance of neurocognitive and social cognitive impairments, symptoms that are largely responsible for the magnitude of disability in schizophrenia.[1-5]

Table 3.1 Schizophrenia symptoms and comorbidities

Primary symptoms	Accessory symptoms	Comorbidities
Positive symptoms	Mood disturbances	Substance use
Negative symptoms	Anxiety	Suicide
Disorganization	Violence	–
Neurocognitive deficits	–	–
Social cognition deficits	–	–

Table 3.2 Comparison of DSM-5-TR and ICD-11 diagnostic criteria for schizophrenia

Subject of comparison	DSM–5-TR classification	ICD–11 classification
Name of chapter	Schizophrenia spectrum and other psychotic disorders	Schizophrenia and other primary psychiatric disorders
Nomenclature	Schizophrenia F20.9	Schizophrenia 6A20
Main symptoms	• Delusions • Hallucinations • Disorganized speech (e.g., frequent derailment or incoherence)	• Persistent delusions • Persistent hallucinations • Disorganized thinking (formal thought disorder) • Experiences of influence, passivity, or control
Diagnostic criteria	At least one main symptom is present for a significant portion of time during a 1-month period (or less if successfully treated).	At least one main symptom must be present (by the individual's report or through observation by the clinician or other informants) most of the time for a period of 1 month or more.
Additional symptoms	• Grossly disorganized or catatonic behavior • Negative symptoms (i.e., diminished emotional expression or avolition)	• Negative symptoms • Grossly disorganized behaviour that impedes goal-directed activity • Psychomotor disturbances such as catatonic restlessness or agitation, posturing, waxy flexibility, negativism, mutism, or stupor
Diagnostic criteria	If only one main symptom is present, at least one additional symptom is required.	If only one main symptom is present, at least one additional symptom is required.
Functionality criteria	For a significant portion of the time since the onset of the disturbance, level of functioning in one or more major areas, such as work, interpersonal relations, or self-care, is markedly below the level achieved prior to the onset (or when the onset is in childhood or adolescence, there is failure to achieve expected level of interpersonal, academic, or occupational functioning).	–
Duration	Continuous signs of the disturbance persist for at least 6 months. This 6-month period must include at least 1 month of symptoms and may include periods of prodromal or residual symptoms. During these prodromal or residual periods, the signs of the disturbance may be manifested by only negative symptoms or by two or more symptoms present in an attenuated form (e.g., odd beliefs, unusual perceptual experiences).	Symptoms must be present most of the time for a period of 1 month or more.
Exclusions	• Schizoaffective disorder, depressive disorder, or bipolar disorder with psychotic features • The disturbance is not attributable to the physiological effects of a substance (e.g., a drug of abuse, a medication) or another medical condition. • If there is a history of autism spectrum disorder or a communication disorder of childhood onset, the additional diagnosis of schizophrenia is made only if prominent delusions or hallucinations, in addition to the other required symptoms of schizophrenia, are also present for at least 1 month (or less if successfully treated).	• Schizotypal disorder • Schizophrenic reaction • Acute and transient psychotic disorder • The symptoms are not a manifestation of another health condition (e.g., a brain tumor) and are not due to the effect of a substance or medication on the central nervous system (e.g., corticosteroids), including withdrawal (e.g., alcohol withdrawal).

Natural history of schizophrenia

For many individuals, schizophrenia follows a typical course that can be divided into four phases: premorbid, prodromal, psychotic, and chronic/residual (Figure 3.1).

Premorbid stage

Children who go on to develop schizophrenia later in life are not prospectively distinguishable from their peers. If any abnormalities are present, they are subtle and nonspecific. Given schizophrenia's

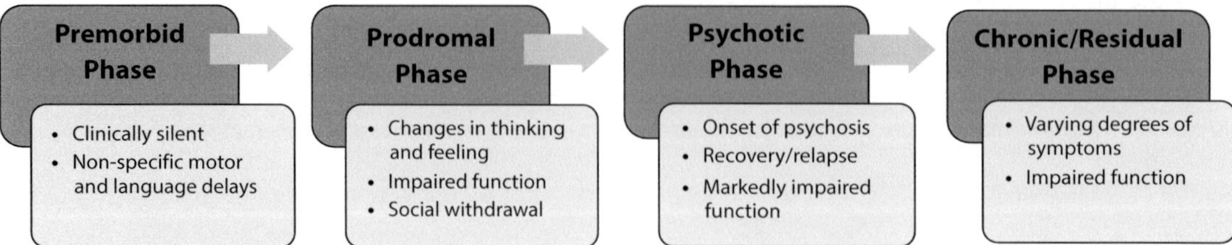

Figure 3.1 The natural history of schizophrenia.

neurodevelopmental origin, abnormalities in brain development manifest as early intellectual [6-8] and neuromotor abnormalities.[9] Academic underachievement is often observed in elementary school and onwards in children who later develop schizophrenia compared with peers who do not go on to develop schizophrenia.[10]

Prodromal stage

About 75-80% of people who develop schizophrenia experience a prodromal phase.[11] For most patients, this stage lasts years and typically occurs in adolescence or early adulthood. Depressive symptoms are typically the first to emerge and appear on average 52 months prior to the first hospitalization.[11] Other changes in thinking and feeling include anxiety, sleep disruption, and difficulties concentrating. Social withdrawal, role failure resulting in academic/occupational problems, and a decline in self-care are common. As the prodrome progresses, attenuated psychotic symptoms may develop. These include perceptual changes (colors may seem brighter or distorted, increased sensitivity to sounds), paranoia, uneasiness, preoccupation with certain ideas, and ideas of reference.

Psychotic stage

This stage begins with the onset of frank psychosis, which may emerge abruptly over a period of days to weeks or insidiously over months or longer. The onset for men is in the early to mid-20s and for women in the late-20s or after age 40. Psychosis is characterized by the loss of touch with reality, altered perceptions, and can be profoundly distressing to the individual. Symptoms include hallucinations, delusions, and disorganized speech and behavior. The first psychotic episode is a crucial timepoint for intervention as patients tend to be more responsive to antipsychotics and psycho-

social treatment. Delays in treatment result in a longer duration of psychosis which is associated with poorer outcomes in a variety of domains including increased severity of symptoms and decreased likelihood of remission.[12-14]

Chronic/residual stage

There is considerable variation in the trajectory of the disease after the first psychotic episode, and many factors influence the course of the illness including genetics, gender, premorbid functioning, substance use, adherence to treatment, and physical health. After the first psychotic episode, about 20% of patients will recover as defined by clinical and social/functional recovery for at least one year.[15] Others experience recurring psychotic relapses. Frequent and/or severe relapses can result in clinical deterioration or disease progression, which leads to decreased responsiveness to treatment, inability to achieve full recovery, and greater degrees of disability.[16,17] Only one in seven patients experiences recovery when recovery is defined as a very good outcome in two domains— clinical and social/functional for at least two years.[18]

Primary symptoms of schizophrenia

Positive symptoms

Positive symptoms—hallucinations and delusions—refer to ideas, beliefs, and perceptions that *add to or distort* an individual's normal functioning.

A delusion is a false belief, judgment, or knowledge that is held despite evidence to the contrary. The decision to call a belief a delusion is made by an observer, not by the believer, since the believer holds the delusional belief with the same conviction as nondelusional beliefs. A delusion transforms an individual's basic experience of the world. For example, Marta's experience of the world is one of malevolence and persecution. Twelve delusional themes have been identified with persecutory delusions being the most common with a pooled point prevalence of 64.5% (60.6-68.3), followed by referential delusions 39.7% (34.5-45.3), grandiose delusions 28.2% (24.8-31.0), delusions of control 21.6% (17.8- 26.0), and religious delusions 18.3% (15.4-21.6).[19] It is not uncommon for patients to have multiple delusions.[20]

Hallucinations are false perceptions that occur spontaneously in any sensory modality (sight, hearing, smell, taste, touch). Auditory hallucinations are the most common type of hallucinations with a lifetime prevalence of up to 80%.[21] Auditory hallucinations can take the form of sounds (bells, screeches, screams) or voices (auditory verbal hallucinations, AVH). AVH can range from single words to conversations involving multiple different voices to voices giving commands. Visual hallucinations have been observed in up to 26% of patients, followed by tactile hallucinations, olfactory hallucinations, and gustatory hallucinations, which occur less frequently.[22-24] Visual hallucinations have been associated with more severe illness, suicide attempts, and with certain types of delusions.[22,25]

Hallucinations and delusions may emerge concomitantly, one may emerge before the other, or only one or the other may be present.[26] The formation and content are influenced by the social and cultural background of the patient.[27,28] Positive symptoms typically follow a remitting and relapsing course.[29-31] Persistent delusions and hallucinations can interfere with employment,[32] relationships, daily function, and increase the risk of violence.[33] Activity (as opposed to inactivity) and frequent social contacts are protective. Positive symptoms are the symptom cluster that responds best to currently available antipsychotic medications; however, the rate of response drops from 90% to 65% across the first two relapses.[34]

Negative symptoms

Symptoms that are consistent with a deficit or loss of function are called *negative symptoms* and are apparent in two domains: expression (blunted affect, alogia) and motivation (amotivation, asociality, anhedonia). Negative symptoms commonly emerge during the prodromal phase and are a risk factor for progression to psychosis.[35] In chronic schizophrenia, almost 60% of patients demonstrate at least one negative symptom with social withdrawal being the most common (45.8%), followed by emotional withdrawal (39.1%), poor rapport (35.8%), and blunted affect (33.1%).[36] Negative symptoms worsen with age and are poorly responsive to most currently available pharmacologic

treatments,[30,37] although potential treatments may be on the horizon.[38] Primary negative symptoms are directly related to the pathophysiology of the illness, while secondary negative symptoms are caused by antipsychotic side effects, comorbid depression, substance use, social deprivation, or as sequelae of positive symptoms.[39] Since secondary negative symptoms can be treated, disentangling them from primary negative symptoms is important.

As shown in Table 3.3, negative symptoms significantly impact an individual's ability to live independently, build relationships, and maintain employment. They are a key contributor to schizophrenia-related disability.[40-44]

Disorganization

Disorganization emerged as a symptom cluster when it separated from positive and negative symptoms in studies using factor analysis.[45-47] Since an individual's thought process cannot be known, it is inferred through communication or speech. Disorganized speech infers disorganization of the form of thoughts and reflects a cluster of related cognitive and linguistic disturbances.[48] This became known over time as a *formal thought disorder* to distinguish it from pathology involving the content of thought, i.e., delusions and ideas of reference. Ozbek and Alptekin (2022) define a formal thought disorder as " . . . any deficiency of organizing words, concepts, phrases, or ideas in a logical order to express a certain purpose."[49] Disorganization is commonly identified in speech that seems to slip off track or derails, is tangential, or is circumstantial.[45] More pathological forms of disorganization are incoherent speech, neologisms, clang association, thought blocking, and echolalia.

As an individual becomes increasingly psychotic, the degree of disorganization increases exponentially.[48] Disorganization is a prominent feature in first-episode patients, and it diminishes with treatment.[50] It affects approximately half of patients with schizophrenia.[51] As expected, there is a strong relationship between disorganization and all domains of neurocognitive functioning[41] and a significant, inverse relationship with social functioning.[52]

Cognition in schizophrenia

Cognition encompasses neurocognition and social cognition. Neurocognition refers to mental abilities such as attention, memory and learning, reasoning

Table 3.3 Negative symptoms, association with other impairments, and functional outcome

Domain	Characteristics[119,120]	Relationship to cognitive impairments and impact on functional outcomes
Expression		
Blunted affect	Components: 1. Decrease in facial expression and eye contact; 2. Decrease in expressive gestures and body language; 3. Decrease in vocal expression	Related to social cognitive domain of emotion processing, i.e., patients with flat affect show greater impairment in emotion processing[121] Reduced facial expression predicts less favorable social interactions[122,123] Reduced nonverbal behaviors are associated with poorer social outcomes[124]
Alogia (poverty of speech)	Decreased quantity of speech, reduced spontaneous speech, loss of conversational fluency, avoidance of communication	Related to cognitive domain of verbal fluency, i.e., as severity of alogia increases, verbal fluency decreases[125] Lower levels of inattention-alogia predicted competitive employment two years after acute exacerbation[126]
Motivation		
Amotivation/ avolition	Reduction in the desire to perform, initiate and maintain goal-directed activities such as work, studying, sports, and personal hygiene. Includes a subjective reduction in interests and desires and a behavioral reduction of self-initiated and purposeful acts	Mediates relationship between neurocognition and social cognition[41] Social amotivation is negatively correlated with employment at one and two years after acute exacerbation[126] Significant negative correlation with functional outcomes, e.g., interpersonal relations, social participation, recreation, self-reliance and execution, employment[44]
Asociality	Reduction in the frequency of social interactions, decreased interest in forming relationships with others. Loss of interest in intimate (sexual) relationships	Overlap with social cognition[68] Significant negative correlation with functional outcomes, e.g., interpersonal relations, social participation, recreation, self-reliance and execution, employment[44] Potentially linked to social disconnection which is associated with poorer physical health[68]
Anhedonia	Reduced ability to anticipate or experience pleasure across activity domains (e.g., social, physical, recreational, work/school). The anticipation of pleasure is more impaired than the ability to experience pleasure in the moment	Certain cognitive deficits are risk factors for anhedonia. Specifically, language deficits are a risk factor for anticipatory anhedonia, while delayed memory deficits are a risk factor for consummatory anhedonia[127] Over the course of the illness, physical anhedonia becomes more strongly associated with worse functional status[128]

and problem-solving. Social cognition includes processes involved with perceiving, processing, and regulating information about other people and ourselves. Deficits in neurocognition and social cognition result in difficulties in social, educational, and occupational spheres of life [1,2,4,5,32,53-55]

Neurocognition in schizophrenia

There is considerable cognitive heterogeneity among individuals with schizophrenia. Three cognitive subgroups have been identified: a group that is relatively cognitive intact with mild impairments (25% of sample), an intermediate group, and a group with severe and widespread deficits (44% of the sample).[56] The magnitude of the neurocognitive deficits can be significant with scores of 1–2 standard deviations below healthy controls across multiple domains.[57-59]

Evidence of neurocognitive impairments can be seen as early as childhood. Woodberry and colleagues (2008) found that years before the onset of psychotic symptoms, as a group, individuals with schizophrenia demonstrated mean IQ scores that were one-half standard deviation below those of healthy controls.[8] Deficits in attention, memory, executive functions, and processing speed have been observed in the premorbid stage.[60] Although data from shorter-term cohort studies suggests that cognition remains fairly stable after illness onset, Jonas and colleagues (2022) performed the largest long-term cohort study of cognition which showed that the trajectory of general cognitive ability is stable until 14 years prior to psychosis onset. Then, general cognitive ability declines from adolescence through the first psychotic episode and during the first two decades of the illness. At age 49,

Table 3.4 Profile of neurocognitive dysfunction in schizophrenia and real-world example using a patient case

Domain	Description of domain	Degree of impairment	Real-world example of functional impairment
Attention	Selective attention is the ability to focus on relevant stimuli and ignore irrelevant stimuli. Sustained attention is the ability to maintain a consistent focus.	Moderate[129]	While in class, DeShawn is distracted from the lecture by the rustling of papers and the sounds outside. Even at home where it is quiet, he has trouble maintaining a consistent focus on what he's reading.
Working memory	Verbal working memory is the ability to temporarily store verbal information in order to plan and carry out behavior. Visuospatial working memory is the ability to retain and process an object's identity and location in space.	Moderate to severe[130]	In biology lab, the professor gave instructions for how to prepare a microscope slide. DeShawn struggled to remember the sequence even after the lab tech repeated it. DeShawn has practiced labeling the parts of a cell multiple times, so he remembers where they are for the test.
Processing speed	Processing speed is the time that it takes to perceive information, process it, and formulate or enact a response.	Moderate to severe[131]	In his college algebra class, DeShawn is the last student to hand in his test and he did not have enough time to work through all the problems.
Executive functions	Executive functions are a set of interrelated, higher level cognitive processes, and abilities that allow planning and execution of goals and monitoring behavior. Core subcomponents are response inhibition and interference control, working memory, and cognitive flexibility	Moderate[132]	After school, DeShawn goes to the tutoring center for help with organizing the homework from his different classes, structuring his study time, and completing papers and projects on time.
Verbal fluency	Verbal fluency is the ability to move from thoughts to words and involves the capacity to access and organize vocabulary	Mild-Moderate[133]	DeShawn's small group collected differing viewpoints on a local water issue. Although DeShawn understood the project, when it came to interviewing members of the public, he struggled to formulate and ask the interview questions.

a second decline in cognitive abilities commences, well before that seen in healthy controls.[61,62] This earlier decline may be due in part to accelerated aging.[63]

Neurocognitive impairment is correlated with functional disability (Table 3.4) and is responsible for the indirect costs of the disease. Typical goals of adulthood – educational achievement, competitive employment, self-sufficiency, self-care – may not be attained by individuals with schizophrenia due to cognitive impairments and social deficits. For example, at any given time, as few as 10% of individuals with schizophrenia are employed.[64] Approximately 25–40% of people with schizophrenia live independently, and over 75% of this group is supported by disability compensation.[32] Only 31% of people with schizophrenia own a car.[65] Cognitive impairments interfere with patients' ability to manage chronic medical conditions and medications. Medical problems go untreated, and poor medication adherence increases the risk of a psychotic relapse.[32]

Social cognitive impairment

Approximately 75% of people with schizophrenia demonstrate at least mild impairments in social cognition.[66] Similar to neurocognitive deficits, there is considerable heterogeneity with most people experiencing mild–moderate deficits and one-third of patients suffering from severe impairments (Table 3.5). Severe impairments are associated with older age, fewer years of education, symptom burden, more neurocognitive impairment, and poorer function.[66,67] Social cognitive impairments are present well before the onset of the first psychotic break and remain stable over the course of the illness.[1,53,68]

Social cognition demonstrates an even stronger link to community functioning than does neurocognitive impairment and accounts for about 16% of the variance in functioning compared to 6% for neurocognitive functioning.[55] Deficits in mental state attribution, or the ability to infer the mental state of another, account for most of the variance. Social disability encompasses three areas: independent living,

Table 3.5 Social cognitive processes and real-world example of impairment using a patient case

Social cognitive process	Definition	Degree of impairment	Real-world example
Perception of social cues	Perceiving social cues contained in facial expressions, voices, and body movements allows appropriate responses that drive interpersonal interactions.	Significant[134]	At the motel where Marta lives, she observes the manager frowning as he enters the laundry room. Marta notices his pursed lips and wrinkled brow. Although he greets her with, "Good Morning, Marta!" his voice sounds irritable, and he is standing with his arms crossed over his chest. Marta interprets these social cues as indicating that the manager is angry with her.
Mental state attribution	Mental state attribution (MSA) is the ability to infer the mental state of others. Cognitive MSA is the capacity to interpret another person's beliefs. Affective MSA is the capacity to interpret another person's feelings	Significant impairment in both cognitive and affective MSA[134]	While Marta initially felt good to be greeted kindly, the feeling fades as she thinks about the manager's frown. Marta infers that the manager believes that she is vandalizing the laundry room. She interprets his facial expression and body language as irritation and frustration with her.
Attribution bias	Attribution bias or style reflects how people explain their actions, the intentions and actions of others, and events.	Consistent impairment has not been demonstrated[134,135]	Marta wonders if the manager's irritation with her is due to an episode months ago when a washer broke and flooded the laundry room.
Emotion processing	Emotion processing refers to an interrelated set of abilities that includes experiencing, understanding emotions, differentiating different emotions, and managing emotions.	Emotional experience is intact[53] Significant impairment in other aspects of emotion processing[134]	Marta initially felt good about the manager's greeting. Several hours later and as she ruminates about his frown, she becomes increasingly fearful that he is going to ask her to leave the motel.

education and employment, and interpersonal relationships. In terms of interpersonal relationships, friendship networks tend to be small (mean number of friends is 1.57) but when present, friendships are highly valued.[69] Although approximately one-third of patients never marry, those who do find marriage to be a source of support.[70] People with schizophrenia may experience social disconnection, which appears to be due to impairments in both social cognition as well as social motivation.[68] Social disconnection is associated with an increased risk of adverse health outcomes and all-cause mortality.

Accessory symptoms of schizophrenia

Mood disturbances

Depression is common in all phases of schizophrenia with factor analysis identifying it as a major symptom dimension. Over 40% of help-seeking individuals at high risk for developing psychosis fulfill criteria for a depressive disorder.[71] During the prodromal phase of the illness, over 60% of patients fulfilled criteria for a lifetime depressive disorder.[72] Nearly 50% of first-episode patients have clinically relevant levels of depressive symptoms, with 25% experiencing a full-depressive episode.[73] In chronic schizophrenia, higher rates of depression – up to 60% of patients – are seen during acute episodes[74] compared to a rate of 30% during periods of stability.[75,76]

Depression is linked to negative outcomes in schizophrenia. It is a major risk factor for suicide and is present in over 50% of patients who die by suicide.[77] Following a cohort of depressed patients with schizophrenia over three years, Conley and colleagues (2007) found that depressed patients were more likely to suffer a relapse of psychosis, use substances, be a safety concern (violent, arrested, victimized, suicidal), report poorer relationships and greater functional impairment, suffer from poorer health (mental, physical), and be less adherent with treatment.[78] Despite the high prevalence and association with negative outcomes, major depressive disorder in schizophrenia is underdiagnosed. Moreover, when diagnosed and treated with antidepressants, 44% of patients remain symptomatic.[76]

The diagnosis of depression in schizophrenia is not straightforward. First, there is a significant overlap between depressive symptoms and other symptom clusters. For example, anhedonia, apathy, and social withdrawal are negative symptoms and are seen in depression. Cognitive dysfunction is common to both depression and schizophrenia. Antipsychotic treatments and their effects on dopaminergic neurotransmission can produce drug-induced parkinsonism, which may be associated with anergia and emotional withdrawal or akathisia, which is associated with dysphoria. Patients who use illicit substances may experience dysphoria during substance withdrawal.

Anxiety

In parallel with what is observed for depression, anxiety symptoms and syndromes are common in all phases of schizophrenia with rates several-fold that seen in the general population. They contribute to negative outcomes[79,80] and are underrecognized.[81] In terms of prevalence, 38.5% of schizophrenia patients have at least one comorbid anxiety disorder with 14.9% fulfilling criteria for social anxiety disorder, 12.4% for post-traumatic stress disorder (PTSD), 12.2% for obsessive-compulsive disorder (OCD), and 10.9% for generalized anxiety disorder, followed by panic disorder and specific phobia.[82] Although the DSM-5-TR has reconceptualized PTSD as a trauma and stressor-related disorder as opposed to an anxiety disorder, it shares neurobiological features with anxiety disorders.[83]

Violence

Although most patients with schizophrenia do not engage in violent behavior, schizophrenia increases the risk for violence.[84-87] Short et al. (2013) used a case linkage design to compare patterns of violence between 4,168 schizophrenia patients and community controls. Of the schizophrenia sample, one in four patients had been charged with a criminal offense, and one in ten had been convicted, a rate higher than that seen in the community sample (10% of people charged, 2.4% convicted).[85] Substance use disorders (SUDs) increase risk; however, violence cannot be entirely attributed to substance use.[85,88] Women with schizophrenia are at greater risk of committing a violent act than men with schizophrenia.[84,85] Victims of violence are acquaintances (49.7%), followed by relatives (28.9%), and strangers (21.4%).[89] Among relatives, mothers of individuals with schizophrenia are the most common target of violent acts and threats.[90] Many factors have the potential to increase the risk of violence in schizophrenia. These include the catechol-O-methyltransferase genotype, developmental factors (childhood trauma, conduct disorders), antisocial personality disorder, substance use, neurocognitive impairment, treatment non-adherence, and certain positive symptoms such as persecutory delusions.[91,92]

Comorbidities in schizophrenia

Substance use

Substance use often pre-dates the first psychotic episode with half of first-episode patients fulfilling criteria for a co-occurring SUD.[93] Cannabis exerts a dose-dependent effect on the risk of developing a psychotic illness and accelerates illness onset by almost three years in regular users compared to non-users.[94,95] Methamphetamine appears to increase the risk of developing schizophrenia on par with cannabis.[96] In patients with an established illness, 50% have a lifetime history of a SUD, a rate five-times greater than that in the general population.[97,98] Alcohol is the most used substance, followed by cannabis, and then followed by other drugs.[99,100] At any timepoint in the illness, SUDs are associated with greater positive symptom severity, less treatment adherence, more aggression and violence, and poorer social functioning.[101] Several different hypotheses attempt to explain the high prevalence of SUDs in people with schizophrenia. These include the *primary addiction hypothesis*, which proposes that substance use and schizophrenia share abnormalities in striatal dopaminergic neurotransmission and the *two-hit model* in which substance use is an environmental stressor that precipitates the development of psychosis in vulnerable individuals.[100-103]

Suicide

Psychotic disorders have one of the highest rates of mortality among mental disorders.[104] Suicide is the greatest relative risk factor for mortality in people with schizophrenia.[105] Using linked national databases to follow approximately 76,000 people with schizophrenia for up to 20 years, Zaheer and colleagues (2020) found that 1 in 58 individuals died by suicide, with suicide typically occurring within 4 years

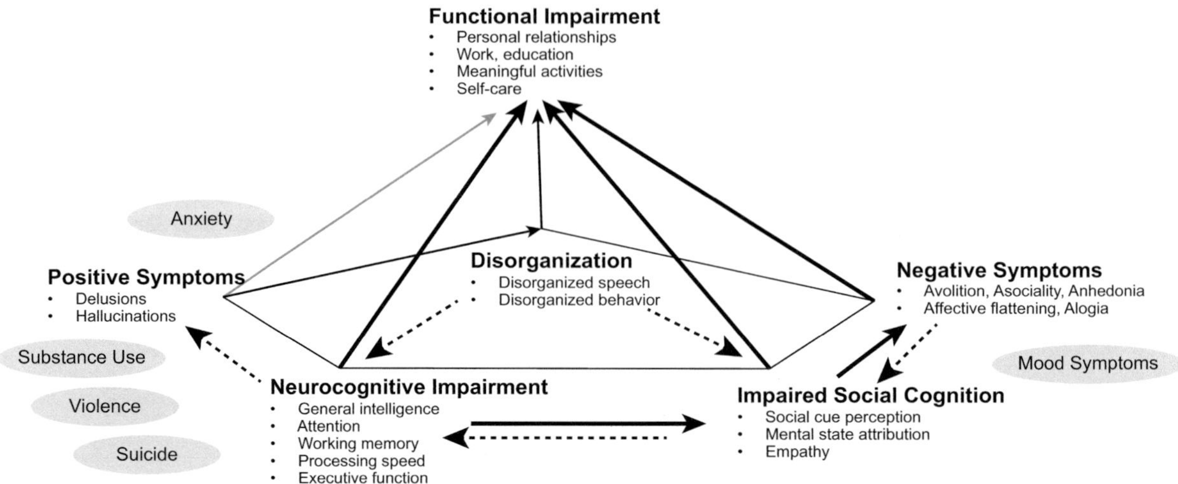

Figure 3.2 The relationship between core schizophrenia symptoms and functional impairment. Core symptoms affect each other to varying degrees. For example, there is a strong relationship between disorganization and all domains of neurocognitive functioning and an inverse relationship with social functioning. Negative symptoms are associated with deficits in empathy and the ability to infer emotions, impacting social cognition. Neurocognitive and social cognitive deficits along with negative symptoms have the greatest impact on functional outcome.

of the initial diagnosis.[106] Further, 25–50% of patients attempt suicide[107] for an overall increase of 50–100-fold compared to that of the general population.[108]

Popovic and colleagues (2014) performed a systematic review of 77 studies to identify risk factors for suicide with the most conclusive evidence base. Factors that were strongly associated with suicide in hospitalized patients and outpatients were depressed mood, history of suicide attempt(s), and the number of psychiatric hospitalizations. Other factors included hopelessness, younger age, close proximity to illness onset, and hospital admission (during admission or within one week of discharge). While male gender and substance use have been associated with suicide in the general population, the data in schizophrenia are mixed.[77] Command auditory hallucinations often command self-harm or suicide; however, the data have not shown them to be a consistent risk factor for suicide.[109] Nevertheless, this type of auditory verbal hallucination should prompt careful suicide risk assessment and safety planning. The primary protective factor against suicide is adherence to comprehensive treatment including pharmacotherapy and psychosocial treatments.[105,109,110]

Conclusion

The symptoms and signs of schizophrenia and schizophrenia spectrum disorders are well established.

The patient cases – Marta and DeShawn – illustrate the heterogeneity in the clinical presentation of schizophrenia, the disease trajectory, and in functional outcomes. While Marta's hallucinations, delusions, and disorganization or DeShawn's asociality and alogia are obvious, both patients suffer from neurocognitive and social cognitive impairments that impact their ability to engage in meaningful activities, manage independent living, and navigate productive interactions with others. Figure 3.2 illustrates the relationship between schizophrenia symptom clusters and functional impairments.

These patients' experience confirms that treatment of positive symptoms is the first step in improving function.[5,32,33,110,111] There is a clear relationship between Marta's persecutory delusions and violence. When her illness is optimally treated with antipsychotic medication, the conviction with which she holds delusional beliefs diminishes, her perception of others as malevolent dissipates, and violence risk decreases, outcomes described in the literature.[112-114] For DeShawn, pharmacologic treatment of positive symptoms after the first psychotic break resolved suicidality and prevented rehospitalization. Treatment at the time of the first psychotic episode is critical to improving symptomatic and functional recovery.[14,34,105,115-118] Psychiatric stability allowed DeShawn to resume his education. The next step in treatment is implementing psychosocial treatment for negative symptoms, neurocognitive symptoms, and social cognitive symptoms, with the goal of improving interpersonal relationships and facilitating academic and occupational success.

References

1. Bowie CR, Harvey PD. Cognitive deficits and functional outcome in schizophrenia. *Neuropsychiatr Dis Treat*. 2006;**2**(4):531–536.

2. Harvey PD, Bosia M, Cavallaro R, et al. Cognitive dysfunction in schizophrenia: an expert group paper on the current state of the art. *Schizophr Res Cogn*. 2022;**29**:100249.

3. McCutcheon RA, Reis Marques T, Howes OD. Schizophrenia: an overview. *JAMA Psychiatry*. 2020;**77**(2):201–210.

4. Green MF. What are the functional consequences of neurocognitive deficits in schizophrenia? *Am J Psychiatry*. 1996;**153**(3):321–330.

5. Harvey PD, Strassnig MT, Silberstein J. Prediction of disability in schizophrenia: symptoms, cognition, and self-assessment. *J Exp Psychopathol*. 2019;**10**(3):2043808719865693.

6. Kahn RS, Keefe RS. Schizophrenia is a cognitive illness: time for a change in focus. *JAMA Psychiatry*. 2013;**70**(10):1107–1112.

7. Mollon J, David AS, Zammit S, Lewis G, Reichenberg A. Course of cognitive development from infancy to early adulthood in the psychosis spectrum. *JAMA Psychiatry*. 2018;**75**(3):270–279.

8. Woodberry KA, Giuliano AJ, Seidman LJ. Premorbid IQ in schizophrenia: a meta-analytic review. *Am J Psychiatry*. 2008;**165**(5):579–587.

9. Filatova S, Koivumaa-Honkanen H, Hirvonen N, et al. Early motor developmental milestones and schizophrenia: a systematic review and meta-analysis. *Schizophr Res*. 2017;**188**:13–20.

10. Tempelaar WM, Termorshuizen F, MacCabe JH, Boks MP, Kahn RS. Educational achievement in psychiatric patients and their siblings: a register-based study in 30,000 individuals in the Netherlands. *Psychol Med*. 2017;**47**(4):776–784.

11. Häfner H, Löffler W, Maurer K, Hambrecht M, an der Heiden W. Depression, negative symptoms, social stagnation and social decline in the early course of schizophrenia. *Acta Psychiatr Scand*. 1999;**100**(2):105–118.

12. Marshall M, Lewis S, Lockwood A, et al. Association between duration of untreated psychosis and outcome in cohorts of first-episode patients: a systematic review. *Arch Gen Psychiatry*. 2005;**62**(9):975–983.

13. Penttilä M, Jääskeläinen E, Hirvonen N, Isohanni M, Miettunen J. Duration of untreated psychosis as predictor of long-term outcome in schizophrenia: systematic review and meta-analysis. *Br J Psychiatry*. 2014;**205**(2):88–94.

14. Perkins DO, Gu H, Boteva K, Lieberman JA. Relationship between duration of untreated psychosis and outcome in first-episode schizophrenia: a critical review and meta-analysis. *Am J Psychiatry*. 2005;**162**(10):1785–1804.

15. Hansen HG, Speyer H, Starzer M, et al. Clinical recovery among individuals with a first-episode schizophrenia an updated systematic review and meta-analysis. *Schizophr Bull*. 2022;**49**(2):297–308.

16. Emsley R, Chiliza B, Asmal L. The evidence for illness progression after relapse in schizophrenia. *Schizophr Res*. 2013;**148**(1–3):117–121.

17. Lin D, Joshi K, Keenan A, et al. Associations between relapses and psychosocial outcomes in patients with schizophrenia in real-world settings in the United States. *Front Psych*. 2021;**12**:695672.

18. Jääskeläinen E, Juola P, Hirvonen N, et al. A systematic review and meta-analysis of recovery in schizophrenia. *Schizophr Bull*. 2013;**39**(6):1296–1306.

19. Collin S, Rowse G, Martinez AP, Bentall RP. Delusions and the dilemmas of life: a systematic review and meta-analyses of the global literature on the prevalence of delusional themes in clinical groups. *Clin Psychol Rev*. 2023; **104**:102303.

20. Brakoulias V, Starcevic V. A cross-sectional survey of the frequency and characteristics of delusions in acute psychiatric wards. *Australas Psychiatry*. 2008;**16**(2):87–91.

21. McCarthy-Jones S, Smailes D, Corvin A, et al. Occurrence and co-occurrence of hallucinations by modality in schizophrenia-spectrum disorders. *Psychiatry Res*. 2017;**252**:154–160.

22. Chouinard VA, Shinn AK, Valeri L, et al. Visual hallucinations associated with multimodal hallucinations, suicide attempts and morbidity of illness in psychotic disorders. *Schizophr Res*. 2019;**208**:196–201.

23. Lewandowski KE, DePaola J, Camsari GB, Cohen BM, Ongür D. Tactile, olfactory, and gustatory hallucinations in psychotic disorders: a descriptive study. *Ann Acad Med Singap*. 2009;**38**(5):383–385.

24. Mueser KT, Bellack AS, Brady EU. Hallucinations in schizophrenia. *Acta Psychiatr Scand*. 1990;**82**(1):26–29.

25. Kreis I, Wold KF, Åsbø G, et al. The relationship between visual hallucinations, functioning, and suicidality over the course of illness: a 10-year

follow-up study in first-episode psychosis. *Schizophrenia*. 2024;**10**(1):30.

26. Compton MT, Potts AA, Wan CR, Ionescu DF. Which came first, delusions or hallucinations? An exploration of clinical differences among patients with first-episode psychosis based on patterns of emergence of positive symptoms. *Psychiatry Res*. 2012;**200**(2–3):702–707.

27. Ghanem M, Evangeli-Dawson C, Georgiades A. The role of culture on the phenomenology of hallucinations and delusions, explanatory models, and help-seeking attitudes: a narrative review. *Early Interv Psychiatr Serv*. 2023;**17** (9):843–863.

28. Lucas CJ, Sainsbury P, Collins JG. A social and clinical study of delusions in schizophrenia. *J Ment Sci*. 1962;**108**:747–758.

29. Addington J, Heinssen RK, Robinson DG, et al. Duration of untreated psychosis in community treatment settings in the United States. *Psychiatr Serv*. 2015;**66**(7):753–756.

30. Correll CU, Schooler NR. Negative symptoms in schizophrenia: a review and clinical guide for recognition, assessment, and treatment. *Neuropsychiatr Dis Treat*. 2020;**16**:519–534.

31. Rosen C, Harrow M, Humpston C, et al. 'An experience of meaning': a 20-year prospective analysis of delusional realities in schizophrenia and affective psychoses. *Front Psych*. 2022;**13**:940124.

32. Harvey PD, Heaton RK, Carpenter WT, Jr., et al. Functional impairment in people with schizophrenia: focus on employability and eligibility for disability compensation. *Schizophr Res*. 2012;**140** (1–3):1–8.

33. Swanson JW, Swartz MS, Van Dorn RA, et al. A national study of violent behavior in persons with schizophrenia. *Arch Gen Psychiatry*. 2006;**63**(5):490–499.

34. Lieberman JA, Alvir JM, Koreen A, et al. Psychobiologic correlates of treatment response in schizophrenia. *Neuropsychopharmacology*. 1996;**14**(3 Suppl):13s–21s.

35. Piskulic D, Addington J, Cadenhead KS, et al. Negative symptoms in individuals at clinical high risk of psychosis. *Psychiatry Res*. 2012;**196**(2):220–224.

36. Bobes J, Arango C, Garcia-Garcia M, Rejas J. Prevalence of negative symptoms in outpatients with schizophrenia spectrum disorders treated with antipsychotics in routine clinical practice: findings from the CLAMORS study. *J Clin Psychiatry*. 2010;**71** (3):280–286.

37. Crow TJ. The two-syndrome concept: origins and current status. *Schizophr Bull*. 1985;**11**(3):471–486.

38. Marder SR, Umbricht D. Negative symptoms in schizophrenia: newly emerging measurements, pathways, and treatments. *Schizophr Res*. 2023;**258**:71–77.

39. Kirschner M, Aleman A, Kaiser S. Secondary negative symptoms – a review of mechanisms, assessment and treatment. *Schizophr Res*. 2017; **186**:29–38.

40. Foussias G, Agid O, Fervaha G, Remington G. Negative symptoms of schizophrenia: clinical features, relevance to real world functioning and specificity versus other CNS disorders. *Eur Neuropsychopharmacol*. 2014; **24** (5):693–709.

41. Ventura J, Hellemann GS, Thames AD, Koellner V, Nuechterlein KH. Symptoms as mediators of the relationship between neurocognition and functional outcome in schizophrenia: a meta-analysis. *Schizophr Res*. 2009;**113**(2–3):189–199.

42. Ventura J, Subotnik KL, Gitlin MJ, et al. Negative symptoms and functioning during the first year after a recent onset of schizophrenia and 8 years later. *Schizophr Res*. 2015;**161**(2–3):407–413.

43. Strauss GP, Sandt AR, Catalano LT, Allen DN. Negative symptoms and depression predict lower psychological well-being in individuals with schizophrenia. *Compr Psychiatry*. 2012;**53** (8):1137–1144.

44. Okada H, Hirano D, Taniguchi T. Impact of negative symptom domains and other clinical characteristics on functional outcomes in patients with schizophrenia. *Schizophr Res Treat*. 2021;**2021**:8864352.

45. Andreasen NC, Grove WM. Thought, language, and communication in schizophrenia: diagnosis and prognosis. *Schizophr Bull*. 1986;**12**(3):348–359.

46. Bilder RM, Mukherjee S, Rieder RO, Pandurangi AK. Symptomatic and neuropsychological components of defect states. *Schizophr Bull*. 1985; **11**(3):409–419.

47. Blanchard JJ, Cohen AS. The structure of negative symptoms within schizophrenia: implications for assessment. *Schizophr Bull*. 2006;**32**(2):238–245.

48. Roche E, Creed L, MacMahon D, Brennan D, Clarke M. The epidemiology and associated phenomenology of formal thought disorder: a systematic review. *Schizophr Bull*. 2015;**41** (4):951–962.

49. Uzman Özbek S, Alptekin K. Thought disorder as a neglected dimension in schizophrenia. *Alpha Psychiatry*. 2022;**23**(1):5–11.

50. Pelizza L, Leuci E, Maestri D, et al. Disorganization in first episode schizophrenia: Treatment response and psychopathological findings from the 2-year follow-up of the "Parma early psychosis" program. *J Psychiatr Res*. 2021;**141**:293–300.

51. Breier A, Berg PH. The psychosis of schizophrenia: prevalence, response to atypical antipsychotics, and prediction of outcome. *Biol Psychiatry*. 1999;**46**(3):361–364.

52. Marggraf MP, Lysaker PH, Salyers MP, Minor KS. The link between formal thought disorder and social functioning in schizophrenia: A meta-analysis. *Eur Psychiatry*. 2020;**63**(1):e34.

53. Green MF, Horan WP, Lee J. Social cognition in schizophrenia. *Nat Rev Neurosci*. 2015;**16**(10):620–631.

54. Green MF, Kern RS, Braff DL, Mintz J. Neurocognitive deficits and functional outcome in schizophrenia: are we measuring the "right stuff"? *Schizophr Bull*. 2000;**26**(1):119–136.

55. Fett AK, Viechtbauer W, Dominguez MD, et al. The relationship between neurocognition and social cognition with functional outcomes in schizophrenia: a meta-analysis. *Neurosci Biobehav Rev*. 2011;**35**(3):573–588.

56. Carruthers SP, Van Rheenen TE, Gurvich C, Sumner PJ, Rossell SL. Characterising the structure of cognitive heterogeneity in schizophrenia spectrum disorders. A systematic review and narrative synthesis. *Neurosci Biobehav Rev*. 2019;**107**:252–278.

57. Heinrichs RW, Zakzanis KK. Neurocognitive deficit in schizophrenia: a quantitative review of the evidence. *Neuropsychology*. 1998;**12**(3): 426–445.

58. Keefe RS, Harvey PD. Cognitive impairment in schizophrenia. *Handb Exp Pharmacol*. 2012;**213**:11–37.

59. McCutcheon RA, Keefe RSE, McGuire PK. Cognitive impairment in schizophrenia: aetiology, pathophysiology, and treatment. *Mol Psychiatry*. 2023;**28**(5):1902–1918.

60. Sheffield JM, Karcher NR, Barch DM. Cognitive deficits in psychotic disorders: a lifespan perspective. *Neuropsychol Rev*. 2018;**28**(4):509–533.

61. Fett A-KJ, Velthorst E, Reichenberg A, et al. Long-term changes in cognitive functioning in individuals with psychotic disorders: findings from the Suffolk county mental health project. *JAMA Psychiatry*. 2020;**77**(4):387–396.

62. Jonas K, Lian W, Callahan J, et al. The course of general cognitive ability in individuals with psychotic disorders. *JAMA Psychiatry*. 2022;**79**(7): 659–666.

63. Seeman MV. Subjective overview of accelerated aging in schizophrenia. *Int J Environ Res Public Health*. 2022;**20**(1):737.

64. Marwaha S, Johnson S, Bebbington P, et al. Rates and correlates of employment in people with schizophrenia in the UK, France and Germany. *Br J Psychiatry*. 2007;**191**:30–37.

65. Steinert T, Veit F, Schmid P, Jacob Snellgrove B, Borbé R. Participating in mobility: people with schizophrenia driving motorized vehicles. *Psychiatry Res*. 2015;**228**(3):719–723.

66. Hajdúk M, Harvey PD, Penn DL, Pinkham AE. Social cognitive impairments in individuals with schizophrenia vary in severity. *J Psychiatr Res*. 2018;**104**:65–71.

67. Vaskinn A, Sundet K, Haatveit B. Social cognitive heterogeneity in schizophrenia: A cluster analysis. *Schizophr Res Cogn*. 2022;**30**:100264.

68. Green MF, Horan WP, Lee J, et al. Social disconnection in schizophrenia and the general community. *Schizophr Bull*. 2018;**44**(2):242–249.

69. Harley EW, Boardman J, Craig T. Friendship in people with schizophrenia: a survey. *Soc Psychiatry Psychiatr Epidemiol*. 2012;**47**(8):1291–1299.

70. Lyngdoh LAM, Antony S, Basavarajappa C, Kalyanasundaram JR, Ammapattian T. Marriage in persons with severe mental illness: a narrative review-based framework for a supported relationship. *J Family Med Prim Care*. 2023;**12**(12):3033–3041.

71. Fusar-Poli P, Borgwardt S, Bechdolf A, et al. The psychosis high-risk state: a comprehensive state-of-the-art review. *JAMA Psychiatry*. 2013;**70**(1): 107–120.

72. Rosen JL, Miller TJ, D'Andrea JT, McGlashan TH, Woods SW. Comorbid diagnoses in patients meeting criteria for the schizophrenia prodrome. *Schizophr Res*. 2006;**85**(1):124–131.

73. Herniman SE, Allott K, Phillips LJ, et al. Depressive psychopathology in first-episode schizophrenia spectrum disorders: a systematic review, meta-analysis and meta-regression. *Psychol Med*. 2019;**49**(15):2463–2474.

74. Upthegrove R, Marwaha S, Birchwood M. Depression and schizophrenia: cause, consequence, or trans-diagnostic issue? *Schizophr Bull*. 2017;**43**(2): 240–244.

75. Etchecopar-Etchart D, Korchia T, Loundou A, et al. Comorbid major depressive disorder in schizophrenia: a systematic review and meta-analysis. *Schizophr Bull*. 2021;**47**(2):298–308.

76. Fond G, Boyer L, Berna F, et al. Remission of depression in patients with schizophrenia and comorbid major depressive disorder: results from the FACE-SZ cohort. *Br J Psychiatry*. 2018;**213**(2):464–470.

77. Popovic D, Benabarre A, Crespo J, et al. Risk factors for suicide in schizophrenia: systematic review and clinical recommendations. *Acta Psychiatr Scand*. 2014;**130**(6):418–426.

78. Conley RR, Ascher-Svanum H, Zhu B, Faries DE, Kinon BJ. The burden of depressive symptoms in the long-term treatment of patients with schizophrenia. *Schizophr Res.* 2007;**90**(1–3):186–197.

79. Temmingh H, Stein DJ. Anxiety in patients with schizophrenia: epidemiology and management. *CNS Drugs.* 2015;**29**(10):819–832.

80. Buonocore M, Bosia M, Baraldi MA, et al. Exploring anxiety in schizophrenia: new light on a hidden figure. *Psychiatry Res.* 2018;**268**:312–316.

81. Wilk JE, West JC, Narrow WE, et al. Comorbidity patterns in routine psychiatric practice: is there evidence of underdetection and underdiagnosis? *Compr Psychiatry.* 2006;**47**(4):258–264.

82. Achim AM, Maziade M, Raymond É, et al. How prevalent are anxiety disorders in schizophrenia? A meta-analysis and critical review on a significant association. *Schizophr Bull.* 2011;**37**(4):811–821.

83. Williamson JB, Jaffee MS, Jorge RE. Posttraumatic stress disorder and anxiety-related conditions. *Continuum (Minneap Minn).* 2021;**27**(6):1738–1763.

84. Fazel S, Gulati G, Linsell L, Geddes JR, Grann M. Schizophrenia and violence: systematic review and meta-analysis. *PLoS Med.* 2009;**6**(8):e1000120.

85. Short T, Thomas S, Mullen P, Ogloff JR. Comparing violence in schizophrenia patients with and without comorbid substance-use disorders to community controls. *Acta Psychiatr Scand.* 2013;**128**(4):306–313.

86. Whiting D, Gulati G, Geddes JR, Dean K, Fazel S. Violence in schizophrenia: triangulating the evidence on perpetration risk. *World Psychiatry.* 2024;**23**(1):158–160.

87. Whiting D, Gulati G, Geddes JR, Fazel S. Association of schizophrenia spectrum disorders and violence perpetration in adults and adolescents from 15 countries: a systematic review and meta-analysis. *JAMA Psychiatry.* 2022;**79**(2):120–132.

88. Witt K, van Dorn R, Fazel S. Risk factors for violence in psychosis: systematic review and meta-regression analysis of 110 studies. *PLoS One.* 2013;**8**(2):e55942.

89. He Y, Gu Y, Yu M, et al. Research on interpersonal violence in schizophrenia: based on different victim types. *BMC Psychiatry.* 2022;**22**(1):172.

90. Estroff SE, Swanson JW, Lachicotte WS, Swartz M, Bolduc M. Risk reconsidered: targets of violence in the social networks of people with serious psychiatric disorders. *Soc Psychiatry Psychiatr Epidemiol.* 1998;**33**(Suppl 1):S95–101.

91. Jones G, Zammit S, Norton N, et al. Aggressive behaviour in patients with schizophrenia is associated with catechol-O-methyltransferase genotype. *Br J Psychiatry.* 2001;**179**:351–355.

92. Volavka J, Citrome L. Pathways to aggression in schizophrenia affect results of treatment. *Schizophr Bull.* 2011;**37**(5):921–929.

93. Brunette MF, Mueser KT, Babbin S, et al. Demographic and clinical correlates of substance use disorders in first episode psychosis. *Schizophr Res.* 2018;**194**:4–12.

94. Myles H, Myles N, Large M. Cannabis use in first episode psychosis: meta-analysis of prevalence, and the time course of initiation and continued use. *Aust N Z J Psychiatry.* 2016;**50**(3):208–219.

95. Myles N, Newall H, Nielssen O, Large M. The association between cannabis use and earlier age at onset of schizophrenia and other psychoses: meta-analysis of possible confounding factors. *Curr Pharm Des.* 2012;**18**(32):5055–5069.

96. Callaghan RC, Cunningham JK, Allebeck P, et al. Methamphetamine use and schizophrenia: a population-based cohort study in California. *Am J Psychiatry.* 2012;**169**(4):389–396.

97. Regier DA, Farmer ME, Rae DS, et al. Comorbidity of mental disorders with alcohol and other drug abuse: results from the epidemiologic catchment area (ECA) study. *JAMA.* 1990;**264**(19):2511–2518.

98. Sara GE, Burgess PM, Malhi GS, Whiteford HA, Hall WC. Stimulant and other substance use disorders in schizophrenia: prevalence, correlates and impacts in a population sample. *Aust N Z J Psychiatry.* 2014;**48**(11):1036–1047.

99. Martins SS, Gorelick DA. Conditional substance abuse and dependence by diagnosis of mood or anxiety disorder or schizophrenia in the U.S. population. *Drug Alcohol Depend.* 2011;**119**(1–2):28–36.

100. Volkow ND. Substance use disorders in schizophrenia—clinical implications of comorbidity. *Schizophr Bull.* 2009;**35**(3):469–472.

101. Ward HB, Nemeroff CB, Carpenter L, et al. Substance use disorders in schizophrenia: prevalence, etiology, biomarkers, and treatment. *Pers Med Psychiatry.* 2023;**39–40**:100106.

102. Bayer TA, Falkai P, Maier W. Genetic and non-genetic vulnerability factors in schizophrenia: the basis of the "two hit hypothesis". *J Psychiatr Res* 1999;**33**(6):543–548.

103. Chambers RA, Krystal JH, Self DW. A neurobiological basis for substance abuse comorbidity in schizophrenia. *Biol Psychiatry.* 2001;**50**(2):71–83.

104. Walker ER, McGee RE, Druss BG. Mortality in mental disorders and global disease burden implications: a systematic review and meta-analysis. *JAMA Psychiatry.* 2015;**72**(4):334–341.

105. Correll CU, Solmi M, Croatto G, et al. Mortality in people with schizophrenia: a systematic review and

meta-analysis of relative risk and aggravating or attenuating factors. *World Psychiatry.* 2022;**21**(2):248–271.

106. Zaheer J, Olfson M, Mallia E, et al. Predictors of suicide at time of diagnosis in schizophrenia spectrum disorder: a 20-year total population study in Ontario, Canada. *Schizophr Res.* 2020;**222**:382–388.

107. Meltzer HY. Treatment of suicidality in schizophrenia. *Ann N Y Acad Sci.* 2001;**932**:44–58; discussion 58–60.

108. Cassidy RM, Yang F, Kapczinski F, Passos IC. Risk factors for suicidality in patients with schizophrenia: a systematic review, meta-analysis, and meta-regression of 96 studies. *Schizophr Bull.* 2018;**44**(4):787–797.

109. Pompili M, Amador XF, Girardi P, et al. Suicide risk in schizophrenia: learning from the past to change the future. *Ann General Psychiatry.* 2007; **6**(1):10.

110. Sher L, Kahn RS. Suicide in schizophrenia: an educational overview. *Medicina (Kaunas).* 2019;**55**(7):361.

111. Helldin L, Kane JM, Karilampi U, Norlander T, Archer T. Remission in prognosis of functional outcome: a new dimension in the treatment of patients with psychotic disorders. *Schizophr Res.* 2007;**93**(1):160–168.

112. Sariaslan A, Leucht S, Zetterqvist J, Lichtenstein P, Fazel S. Associations between individual antipsychotics and the risk of arrests and convictions of violent and other crime: a nationwide within-individual study of 74 925 persons. *Psychol Med.* 2021;**52**(16):1–9.

113. Frogley C, Taylor D, Dickens G, Picchioni M. A systematic review of the evidence of clozapine's anti-aggressive effects. *Int J Neuropsychopharmacol.* 2012;**15**(9):1351–1371.

114. Faden J, Citrome L. A systematic review of clozapine for aggression and violence in patients with schizophrenia or schizoaffective disorder. *Schizophr Res.* 2024;**268**:265–281.

115. Kane JM, Correll CU. Pharmacologic treatment of schizophrenia. *Dialogues Clin Neurosci.* 2010;**12**(3):345–357.

116. Correll CU, Rubio JM, Kane JM. What is the risk-benefit ratio of long-term antipsychotic treatment in people with schizophrenia? *World Psychiatry.* 2018;**17**(2):149–160.

117. Taipale H, Mehtälä J, Tanskanen A, Tiihonen J. Comparative effectiveness of antipsychotic drugs for rehospitalization in schizophrenia: a nationwide study with 20-year follow-up. *Schizophr Bull.* 2018;**45**(6):1381–1387.

118. Tiihonen J, Tanskanen A, Taipale H. 20-year nationwide follow-up study on discontinuation of antipsychotic treatment in first-episode schizophrenia. *Am J Psychiatry.* 2018;**175**(8):765–773.

119. Kirkpatrick B, Fischer B. Subdomains within the negative symptoms of schizophrenia: commentary. *Schizophr Bull.* 2006;**32**(2):246–249.

120. Millan MJ, Fone K, Steckler T, Horan WP. Negative symptoms of schizophrenia: clinical characteristics, pathophysiological substrates, experimental models and prospects for improved treatment. *Eur Neuropsychopharmacol.* 2014;**24**(5):645–692.

121. Gur RE, Kohler CG, Ragland JD, et al. Flat affect in schizophrenia: relation to emotion processing and neurocognitive measures. *Schizophr Bull.* 2006; **32**(2):279–287.

122. Riehle M, Lincoln TM. Investigating the social costs of schizophrenia: Facial expressions in dyadic interactions of people with and without schizophrenia. *J Abnorm Psychol.* 2018;**127**(2):202–215.

123. Riehle M, Mehl S, Lincoln TM. The specific social costs of expressive negative symptoms in schizophrenia: reduced smiling predicts interactional outcome. *Acta Psychiatr Scand.* 2018;**138**(2):133–144.

124. Lavelle M, Healey PG, McCabe R. Nonverbal behavior during face-to-face social interaction in schizophrenia: a review. *J Nerv Ment Dis.* 2014;**202**(1):47–54.

125. Fervaha G, Takeuchi H, Foussias G, Agid O, Remington G. Using poverty of speech as a case study to explore the overlap between negative symptoms and cognitive dysfunction. *Schizophr Res.* 2016;**176**(2):411–416.

126. Mueser KT, Salyers MP, Mueser PR. A prospective analysis of work in schizophrenia. *Schizophr Bull.* 2001;**27**(2):281–296.

127. Yu L, Ni H, Wu Z, et al. Association of cognitive impairment with anhedonia in patients with schizophrenia. *Front Psych.* 2021;**12**:762216.

128. Herbener ES, Harrow M, Hill SK. Change in the relationship between anhedonia and functional deficits over a 20-year period in individuals with schizophrenia. *Schizophr Res.* 2005;**75**(1):97–105.

129. Caspi A, Reichenberg A, Weiser M, et al. Cognitive performance in schizophrenia patients assessed before and following the first psychotic episode. *Schizophr Res.* 2003;**65**(2–3):87–94.

130. McGurk SR, Coleman T, Harvey PD, et al. Working memory performance in poor outcome schizophrenia: relationship to age and executive functioning. *J Clin Exp Neuropsychol.* 2004;**26**(2):153–160.

131. Dickinson D, Ramsey ME, Gold JM. Overlooking the obvious: a meta-analytic comparison of digit symbol coding tasks and other cognitive measures in schizophrenia. *Arch Gen Psychiatry*. 2007;**64**(5):532–542.

132. Thai ML, Andreassen AK, Bliksted V. A meta-analysis of executive dysfunction in patients with schizophrenia: different degree of impairment in the ecological subdomains of the behavioural assessment of the dysexecutive syndrome. *Psychiatry Res*. 2019;272:230–236.

133. Kaneda Y, Sumiyoshi T, Keefe R, et al. Brief assessment of cognition in schizophrenia: validation of the Japanese version. *Psychiatry Clin Neurosci*. 2007;**61**(6):602–609.

134. Savla GN, Vella L, Armstrong CC, Penn DL, Twamley EW. Deficits in domains of social cognition in schizophrenia: a meta-analysis of the empirical evidence. *Schizophr Bull*. 2013;**39**(5):979–992.

135. Vaskinn A, Horan WP. Social cognition and schizophrenia: unresolved issues and new challenges in a maturing field of research. *Schizophr Bull*. 2020;**46**(3):464–470.

Assessment and Treatment of Anosognosia in Schizophrenia

Xavier Amador

The problem of poor insight into mental illness in patients with schizophrenia and related disorders has been widely studied over the past 30 years.[1,2] The clinicians, policymakers, family caregivers, and criminal justice professionals involved in the care and safety of persons suffering from these illnesses understand that the assessment of insight is meaningful if not critical for personal as well as public health and safety reasons. In fact, the research is unequivocal in this regard. Patients with poor insight into these disorders are more likely to be involuntarily hospitalized, to have more hospitalizations generally, poorer psychosocial functioning, and more episodes of aggression, and are far less engaged in treatment.[3] Indeed, lack of insight, also known as "anosognosia," is the top predictor of noncompliance with treatment[3] and the prevalence of poor insight is much higher than the other symptoms of these disorders, such as hallucinations.[1,4,5] In this chapter I discuss the prevalence of this problem, terminology (how we should talk about insight), etiology, assessment, and treatment of patients with this condition.

A brief word on terminology is necessary. "Insight" suggests the individual has knowledge of their illness that is buried outside of conscious awareness. With effective intervention there is a possibility that such a person will gain access to this information and hence gain insight. My colleagues and I have argued previously that we should not rush to judgment in this instance that poor insight is a coping strategy or psychological defense, and instead we should use conceptually neutral terms like "unawareness" or "lack of awareness" until there is more conclusive evidence regarding the etiology of this common symptom.[1]

When we look at the research on the etiology of unawareness of illness in these disorders, a new term becomes even more appropriate: "anosognosia." Among the most common symptoms of schizophrenia, unawareness of illness affects approximately 50% of all patients.[4,5] There is robust and ample evidence that this is a product of brain dysfunction and structural brain abnormalities rather than denial or poor insight.[3,6–10] As such, this symptom has a substantial impact on and relevance to clinical assessment and treatment. It also has relevance to discussions and debates around involuntary treatment options for persons suffering from serious mental illness (SMI). As this is a product of brain dysfunction and/or abnormalities, ethical considerations strongly suggests that when a person with SMI who does not believe they have SMI refuses treatment on that basis, we must provide a range of services and interventions in light of the associated lack of competency. Given the evidence, arguably the proper term to describe this symptom is "anosognosia," not "poor insight" or "denial." The term "anosognosia" was coined by the neurologist Joseph Babinski in 1914 to describe unawareness of neurological deficits following strokes, dementias, and other types of damage to the brain. The word "anosognosia" comes from the ancient Greek ἀ- (a-, "not, without"), νόσος (nósos, "disease"), and γνῶσις (gnôsis, "knowledge"). Phenomenologically, there should be no question or debate that unawareness of illness describes a patient who is without knowledge of their disease – in this case, schizophrenia. Regardless of the causes, use of the term "anosognosia" to describe the very high rate of lack of awareness of mental illness in schizophrenia is phenomenologically appropriate and long overdue.[11] For these reasons, henceforth, I will use the term "anosognosia" in place of "poor insight," except when necessary to describe assessments of this symptom that have relied on earlier terms.

Awareness of illness is commonly assessed in the context of the Mental Status Exam, a cornerstone assessment in psychiatry and psychology. Clinicians are required to rate the patient's "insight" as absent, moderate, or good. My research group at Columbia University and many others have proposed that "insight" cannot be assessed with a single item or question. Instead, it is better understood as being multidimensional, involving awareness of various aspects of schizophrenia and other psychotic disorders.[1,2,12] As a result, we developed the Scale to Assess Unawareness of Mental Disorder (SUMD) that assesses awareness of having an illness, awareness of the achieved positive effects of medication, awareness of the social consequences of illness, and awareness of symptoms and other dimensions, including attributions for symptoms that the patient recognizes.[13] The SUMD is among the most widely used instruments of its kind, having been translated into 18 languages by investigators worldwide. Its use clinically is far more limited.

Others have devised clinical research scales that similarly assess awareness of illness in a multidimensional manner, though some have conflated illness awareness with compliance, such as in the Insight and Treatment Attitudes Questionnaire.[14] Anthony S. David[12] defined the concept of "insight" as having at least three distinct dimensions: the recognition that one has a mental illness (awareness); the ability to relabel unusual mental events (delusions and hallucinations) as pathological (attribution); and the recognition of the need for treatment (action). Although many of the dimensions assessed in these studies have been fruitful as predictors of meaningful clinical factors, the common feature of assessing whether the patient recognizes that they have a mental illness is clearly the dimension with the most predictive validity with respect to engagement in treatment, reduced recidivism in the forensic setting, and improved psychosocial function. Similarly, awareness of how medication has improved one's quality of life (item 2 on the SUMD: "Awareness of response to medication"), regardless of whether the person believes they have an illness (item 1 on the SUMD: "Awareness of mental disorder"), has also shown predictive validity with respect to acceptance of and adherence to treatment. Consequently, for clinicians and forensic evaluators, these first two items of the SUMD, rated on a Likert scale, may offer the most useful information for treatment planning and forensic evaluation. Table 4.1 provides an overview of the scales that are most commonly used in this context.

It should be noted that some have argued that what is considered poor insight, or lack of awareness, is in fact just a disagreement between the patient and the doctor.[2] This argument is a fallacy because the

Table 4.1 Scales to assess unawareness of mental illness/poor insight in schizophrenia*

Instrument	Domains	No. of items
PANSS item G12 (lack of judgment and insight)	Unidimensional, but rating is based on: (1) nonrecognition of past or present psychiatric illness or symptoms; (2) denial of need for psychiatric hospitalization or treatment; (3) decisions characterized by poor anticipation of consequences and unrealistic short-term and long-range planning	1
ITAQ	(1) Recognition of mental illness; (2) need for hospitalization; (3) need to take medications	11
SAI, SAI-E	(1) Awareness and relabeling of symptoms; (2) awareness of illness; (3) treatment compliance	8 (original version), 12 (expanded version)
SUMD	(1) Insight into mental disorder; (2) insight into need for treatment; (3) insight into social consequences; (4) insight into presence of symptoms; (5) insight into attribution of symptoms	74
BIS	(1) Awareness of illness; (2) awareness of need for treatment; (3) relabeling of symptoms	8 (self-report)
BCIS	(1) Self-reflectiveness (expression of introspection and willingness to acknowledge fallibility); (2) self-certainty (certainty about beliefs or judgments)	15 (self-report)

Note: All instruments are intended to rate clinical insight, except for the BCIS, which is intended to measure cognitive insight.

*This table was originally published in Belvederi Murri and Amore (2019).[22]

PANSS = Positive and Negative Syndrome Scale; ITAQ = Insight and Treatment Attitudes Questionnaire; SAI-E = Schedule for the Assessment of Insight, expanded version; SUMD = Scale to Assess Unawareness of Mental Disorder; BIS = Birchwood Insight Scale; BCIS = Beck Cognitive Insight Schedule.

disagreement is not only with the doctor but also with family members, mental health court judges, police officers, and crisis workers, who can immediately recognize a SMI. The majority of these individuals are not relying on a doctor's diagnosis.

Knowing that anosognosia involves a core deficit in knowledge stemming from brain dysfunction, how are we to help the patient who is at risk for noncompliance, repeated hospitalizations, criminalization, poor psychosocial functioning, and other negative outcomes associated with this symptom? One such strategy involves the LEAP communication program. The acronym LEAP stands for Listening (actively and reflectively), Empathizing (strategically with normalization of the emotions expressed), Agreeing (finding areas of agreement), and Partnering (working together on those goals that have been agreed upon). This approach also involves three additional communication tools with the acronym DOA: respectfully Delaying contrary hurtful opinions (e.g., "I will answer your question about whether I think you have a mental illness. Before I do, can you tell me more about how you ended up in jail and I will tell you after?"); Opining with humility (e.g., "I am sorry I have this view as I think it may anger you, I could be wrong, I hope we don't have to argue about it because there's much we agree on. Yes, I think you are suffering from a mental illness."); and Apologizing for acts and statements that were hurtful to the patient. The goal of DOA is to preserve the alliance and trust that is being built through respectful, validating, and nonjudgmental communication. In a double-blind placebo-controlled study, LEAP was found to increase compliance with long-acting injectable antipsychotic medications and to increase positive attitudes about treatment while not improving scores on the SUMD.[15] Other research has found LEAP to increase medication compliance and improve the quality of relationships with patients.[16,17] As of this writing, I am not aware of any other interventions aimed at improving outcomes in patients with anosognosia for SMI.

LEAP grew out of a funded research study of a short-term inpatient psychotherapy intervention devised by Dr. Aaron T. Beck and myself.[18] As such, LEAP is based in part on cognitive behavioral therapy (CBT), but it also draws heavily on aspects of motivational interviewing and Rogerian client-centered therapy. Unlike these three approaches, LEAP does not employ psychoeducation, as the patient with anosognosia typically rejects and is angered by attempts to teach them that they have schizophrenia or another

psychotic disorder. Instead, it relies on creating an alliance imbued with respect, trust, and a complete lack of judgment. In short, the relationship is the path to treatment acceptance and adherence, not insight or knowledge. Indeed, research indicates that even when treatment response to antipsychotics is achieved, the majority of patients with anosognosia continue to be unaware of having an illness.[19] On a personal note, this was my experience with my older brother, Henry Amador. As I wrote in the book *I Am Not Sick, I Don't Need Help! How to Help Someone with Mental Illness Accept Treatment*,[18] despite accepting a long-acting antipsychotic given by injection for nearly 20 years, when asked if he had schizophrenia, Henry replied, "No! You know I don't have that!" When I then asked him why he had accepted the injections for so many years, he said, "I do it for you." There is much more that could be said regarding how my use of LEAP encouraged my brother to accept treatment for an illness he was certain he did not have, but the headline is sufficient for the purposes of the present chapter: He was in treatment because of a trusting relationship and not because he had "insight" or awareness of having any illness.

In the USA, there is no national standard for compulsory treatments. Each state and territory has its own standard. That said, they all center on two to three prongs: (1) imminent harm to self; (2) imminent harm to others; and (3) grave disability as a result of a mental illness. With respect to protecting lives, there are two problems with these standards. The requirement that the harm be imminent does not safeguard anyone. An individual can have paranoid delusions and command hallucinations telling them to kill their mother, but when the police or crisis team evaluate them, they might say that they have no such plan. Since the danger of harm is evaluated as not imminent, this individual would be left alone with their mother. Then, later that night, they feel compelled to act on the voices and delusions, and do so. Or consider the same scenario but with the psychotic symptoms focused on self-harm, and the person dies from suicide soon after the crisis intervention has failed them. I have seen this kind of scenario all too often. And what exactly is "grave disability"? At its extreme, when the patient is malnourished and/or medically compromised, involuntary treatment becomes possible. But what of the person with schizophrenia who has not left their room for weeks or months, drapes closed and lights off, defecating on the floor, and only eating food left outside their door by a concerned family member? Often, I have seen crisis interventions that have failed to transport such people to the hospital. But doesn't such a person and those that are not imminently planning to harm themselves and others have a right to personal liberty? Many have argued that they do. I understand that position. I believe that it nonetheless is arrived at through either a lack of knowledge about or appreciation for the nature of these brain disorders, specifically how symptoms of psychosis can steal a person's capacity to make intelligent, knowing, and voluntary decisions about their safety and that of others.

If a patient with Alzheimer's disease wanders from their assisted living facility into the streets, we send out a "Silver Alert," resulting in the person being transported back to that facility or to a hospital against their will. Most people understand that in this instance the person lacks the cognitive capacity to make an intelligent, knowing, and voluntary decision about their own safety and welfare. Because people with schizophrenia and related disorders do not always suffer from severe disorientation and memory loss, like we see in advanced Alzheimer's disease and other dementias, their intact abilities are confused with the ability to make intelligent, knowing, and voluntary decisions about their safety and that of others. We focus on and overgeneralize their statements that they are okay, that nothing is wrong, and that it has all been a big misunderstanding. If – like half of all people with these disorders – the person has anosognosia, they often convincingly deny that they have any mental health disorder whatsoever, and that whoever called the crisis team or police are the ones who are overreacting and "crazy." If, in this scenario, the person has paranoid delusions that compel them to run and hide, foregoing food and shelter, or to purchase a gun to kill their delusionally imagined persecutors but have not yet suffered malnutrition or made a specific assassination plan, they typically cannot be hospitalized involuntarily. Indeed, such a person would meet most criteria for involuntary hospitalization only after the harm had been done – sometimes irreversible harm. On the other hand, when someone with schizophrenia has been stabilized using antipsychotic medication and the life-threatening (to self or others) delusions have abated, as they might still have anosognosia they will usually decide to stop the medication that the illness has convinced them they derive no benefit from.[3] Wouldn't this person and public safety benefit substantially from assisted outpatient involuntary treatment?

It is important to note that individuals with schizophrenia are generally no more violent than the rest of the population; however, their rate of violence does increase when they are symptomatic, which is typically the case when they are not in pharmacological treatment.[20]

Some patients and patient advocacy groups adamantly oppose compulsory treatments. I have personally spoken to many such individuals and groups, and I am struck by the absence of anosognosia in their cases. Their concerns are understandable in the context of someone who is able to be aware of their illness and the potentially beneficial effects of treatment – in other words, understandable in someone *without* anosognosia. In the USA and elsewhere, we have a history of violating civil liberties when mental impairment leads to self-harm or violence toward others. This violation is indeed paternalistic, and it represents (typically in my experience) a demonstration of the harm that occurs when a person is left free to succumb to their brain disorders. My own experience with involuntary treatments is that, at their heart, they are motivated by compassion and an appreciation of the harm that withholding treatment would cause rather than an exercise of power for its own sake.

One final thought on the question of involuntary treatments: According to Department of Justice statistics, approximately 2.5 million individuals are incarcerated in the USA: 20–25% of those individuals have a diagnosed SMI.[21] My personal experience is that I have seen persons with untreated schizophrenia in our jails and prisons when arguably they should be in hospital, as the crimes they have been charged with, or convicted of, were solely the product of their untreated mental illness (usually not rising to the very high standard of insanity). In my opinion, the criminalization of persons with untreated schizophrenia is a product of inadequate mental health care and criminal justice systems not offering engagement strategies like that discussed earlier (i.e., LEAP) and/or involuntary treatments, both of which can divert the individual with SMI from jail/prison to mental health care and hospitalization.

Summary

In this chapter, I discussed the prevalence of the problem of poor insight, that terminology should recognize the neurological basis of most cases (i.e., use the term "anosognosia" instead of "poor insight"), and the etiology and treatment of patients with this condition. This latter topic included a discussion of involuntary treatments. An argument was made for engagement strategies that persuade patients with anosognosia to accept treatment despite their being certain that they do not have a SMI. One such strategy, LEAP, was described, which avoids psychoeducation entirely and instead focuses on those problems that the patient with anosognosia can see and acknowledge. Sometimes the problems are an FBI conspiracy or aliens, and the clinician's goal is to validate, not agree with, the patient's experience so that the person feels heard, understood, and trusting. In the context of this kind of relationship, though not based on logic, the suggestion/offer of treatment is more likely to be accepted. The goals of the individual are the motivators for accepting treatment, not an understanding that they have a SMI.

References

1. Amador XF, Strauss DH, Yale SA, Gorman JM (1991) Awareness of illness in schizophrenia. *Schizophrenia Bulletin*, **17**(1):113–132.

2. David AS (2020) Insight and psychosis: the next 30 years. *The British Journal of Psychiatry*, **217**:521–523.

3. American Psychiatric Association (2022) *Diagnostic and Statistical Manual for Mental Disorders*, 5th edition, Text Revision edition. American Psychiatric Association Press.

4. Carpenter WT Jr., Strauss JS, Bartko JJ (1973) Flexible system for the diagnosis of schizophrenia. Report from the World Health Organization International Pilot Study of Schizophrenia. *Science*, **182**:1275–1278.

5. Wilson WH, Ban TA, Guy W (1986) Flexible system criteria in chronic schizophrenia. *Comprehensive Psychiatry*, **27**:259–265.

6. Morgan KD, David AS (2004) Neuropsychological studies of insight in patients with psychotic disorders, in Amador XF, David AS (eds.), *Insight and Psychosis: Awareness of Illness in Schizophrenia and Related Disorders*, 2nd edition. Oxford University Press.

7. Flashman LA, Roth RM (2004) Neural correlates of unawareness of illness in psychosis, in Amador XF, David AS (eds), *Insight and Psychosis: Awareness of Illness in Schizophrenia and Related Disorders*, 2nd edition. Oxford University Press.

8. van der Meer L, de Vos AE, Stiekema AP, et al. (2013) Insight in schizophrenia: Involvement of self-reflection networks? *Schizophrenia Bulletin*, **39**(6):1288–1295.

9. Aleman A, Agrawal N, Morgan K, David AS (2006) Insight in psychosis and neuropsychological function: A meta-analysis. *British Journal of Psychiatry*, **189**:204–212.

10. Kasapis C, Amador XF, Yale SA, Gorman JM (1996) Neuropsychological and defensive aspects of poor insight and depression in schizophrenia. *Schizophrenia Research*, **18**(2–3):117–118.

11. Amador XF (2023) Denial of anosognosia in schizophrenia. *Clinical Insights, Schizophrenia Research*, **252**:242–243.

12. David AS (1990) Insight and psychosis. *British Journal of Psychiatry*, **156**:798–808.

13. Amador XF, Strauss DH, Yale SA, et al. (1993) Assessment of insight in psychosis. *American Journal of Psychiatry*, **150**(6):873–879.

14. McEvoy JP, Apperson LJ, Appelbaum PS, et al. (1989) *Insight and Treatment Attitudes Questionnaire (ITAQ)* [Database record]. APA PsycTests.

15. Paillot C, Goetz R, Amador XF (2009) Double blind, randomized, controlled study of a psychotherapy designed to improve motivation for change, insight into schizophrenia and adherence to medication. *Schizophrenia Bulletin*, **35**:55076.

16. Holt G, Speicher H, Amador X (2023) *Assessing the Efficacy of a Program Designed to Engage Patients with Poor Insight Into Illness* [Presentation]. American Psychological Association.

17. Lasser R, Schooler N, Kujawa M, et al. (2009) A new psychosocial tool for gaining patient understanding and acceptance of long-acting injectable antipsychotic therapy. *Psychiatry*, **6**(4):22–27.

18. Amador X (2022) *I Am Not Sick, I Don't Need Help! How to Help Someone with Mental Illness Accept Treatment*. Vida Press.

19. McEvoy JP, Apperson LJ, Applebaum PS, et al. (1989) Insight in schizophrenia: Its relationship to acute psychopathology. *Journal of Nervous and Mental Disorders*, **177**:43–47.

20. Torrey EF (2011) Stigma and violence: Isn't it time to connect the dots? *Schizophrenia Bulletin*, **37**(5):892–896.

21. Department of Justice (DOJ), Bureau of Justice Statistics (2024) Publications list. https://bjs.ojp.gov/library/publications/list

22. Belvederi Murri M, Amore M (2019) The multiple dimensions of insight in schizophrenia-spectrum disorders. *Schizophrenia Bulletin*, **45**(2):277–283.

Chapter 5

Anosognosia in Schizophrenia

Benjamin Rose and Philip D. Harvey

Introduction

As described in a thorough review of the history of anosognosia,[1] the neurologist Babinski coined the term anosognosia in 1914. The word comes from "a" without, "nosos" disease, and "gnosis" knowledge, or without knowledge of the disease. While getting most of the credit, Babinski was not the only researcher to study this lack of awareness, which is present in neurological and neuropsychiatric conditions. Before Babinski, the concept was defined by another neuropsychiatrist, Gabriel Anton in 1899, who considered this lack of awareness as potentially distinct from the underlying neurological condition. A few years before Anton, Dejerine, Van Monakow, and Vialet systematically described the lack of awareness of disease in certain neurological conditions. Two thousand years earlier, the philosopher Seneca, sending a letter to Lucilius, had described anosognosia and captured the separation of impairment (possible brain blindness originating from a stroke) and the lack of awareness of the impairments.

> *This foolish woman suddenly lost her sight ... Incredible as it may appear ... she does not know she is blind.*
> -Seneca

Since the early 20th century, anosognosia, or "without knowledge of disease" has been recognized as an important component of serious mental illness. Despite the recognition of the importance of anosognosia in schizophrenia, little new knowledge was obtained throughout the first half of the 20th century. During this time the lack of treatment for psychotic symptoms made differentiation of symptoms and insight challenging. After the introduction of antipsychotic treatments in the 1950s, a shift started in the 1970s, when the World Health Organization concluded that "lack of insight," unawareness of the implausibility of psychotic experiences, was a feature that was the most common sign of the illness.[2, 3] A few years later, there was a significant growth in interest and publications related to defining anosognosia, relabeled as insight[4] or unawareness,[5] targeting clinical correlates[6] and prognostic implications,[7] and trying to help patients with poor insight.[8]

Definitions of insight have progressed over the last 30 years and current thought includes the concepts of cognitive insight,[9] neurocognitive insight,[10] and clinical insight.[4] Cognitive insight refers to an attitudinal structure involving limits in self-reflectiveness and self-certainty, which can lead to underestimations of potential. Neurocognitive insight indexes a patient's understanding of their functioning in various neurocognitive domains compared with objective performance. Clinical insight is the awareness that one may have a mental illness, acknowledging the reality of experiences, and acceptance of the need for treatment for the illness. Impairment in insight across domains is common in patients with schizophrenia, with estimates ranging from 50% to 98% of individuals with schizophrenia not aware that they have a mental illness.[11–13] The defining features of poor awareness in schizophrenia are multidomain inaccuracies in a patient's self-assessment, with notable impacts on multiple elements of functional outcome.

In addition to accuracy failures in self-assessment, directional patterns of mis-estimations have been seen in schizophrenia. The tendency to overestimate abilities or underestimate task difficulty is common in schizophrenia.[14] Bias can occur because of the failure to adequately consider externally originating information, meaning that patients with schizophrenia might miss or discount important information from the world around them.[15] Finally, there can be difficulties in discriminating between self and other generated information.[16] Confusion on whether something is happening internally or externally clouds a patient's ability to accurately assess what is real. This neurological impairment has enough scientific support that it is now included in the Diagnostic and Statistical Manual of Mental Disorders (DSM-5), which lists a "lack of insight or awareness of their disorder" as an associated feature supporting the diagnosis. This feature of schizophrenia is correlated with a host of downstream impacts, including challenges in treatment adherence,[17] increased severity of symptoms,[18] greater everyday disability,[19] reduced response to cognitive training interventions,[20] and increased likelihood of more intensive interventions to sustain community residence.[21]

> *To know that one knows what one knows, and to know that one doesn't know what one doesn't know, there lies true wisdom. – Confucius (ca. 551–479 B.C.E.)*

Awareness of illness spans far beyond the recognition that psychotic symptoms are not real experiences. There are other issues in the self-assessment of features of schizophrenia, including cognitive impairments, functional disability, and altered emotional functioning. A concept that has been introduced to describe these challenges in awareness is Introspective Accuracy (IA)[22]: the ability to judge skills, experiences, moods, and successfulness of performance accurately. Challenges in IA can be measured in terms of immediate, momentary judgments (e.g., "Was that answer correct?" "How many words did I remember?")[23] or global self-assessments (e.g., "How good am I at work, social functioning or self-care?").[24] Global Self Assessments also commonly have an anticipatory component, such as: "How well could you do X, Y, or Z?"[25] Such assessments are challenging for anyone,[26] because accurate anticipation of future performance requires recollection of past performance, including the nature of the previous task, its difficulty, and perceived level of success, and comparison of the current task with prior tasks. Even minimal errors in any of these elements of judgments can skew the accuracy of estimates of functional capabilities. In people with schizophrenia, the lack of experience with functional tasks[27] and low rates of achievement of milestones[28] can easily lead to biases based on lack of information.

When an incorrect self-assessment (error in IA) occurs, the second important factor is the direction of the inaccurate response. Referred to as Introspective Bias (IB), it is commonly reported that people with schizophrenia manifest a predominant positive IB[29] as a product of the tendency to underestimate difficulty or overestimate abilities.[30] Both IA and IB are not unique to individuals with schizophrenia, as healthy individuals also struggle with having an accurate perception of their skills and abilities, with a similarly predominant positive IB seen on the part of average or poorer performers.[31] While this response bias causes functional challenges for all individuals, these biases are often pernicious for individuals with schizophrenia, in large part because of high levels of confidence in both momentary self-assessments of performance[30,32–34] and global judgments of abilities.[35,36]

This high level of confidence in self-assessment is related to the tendencies of individuals with schizophrenia to commonly make judgments based on less information than healthy controls.[37] This "jumping to conclusions" bias is comprised of failures to consider possible sources of information and rapidly come to judgments before healthy people would be willing. In addition to overestimation and rapid decisions, schizophrenia patients also show a "resistance to disconfirmation."[38] Even mildly discrepant feedback can lead healthy people to recalibrate their decisions,[39] at least temporarily. When given external feedback suggesting misestimation or inaccuracy, schizophrenia patients show reduced ability to adjust performance, accuracy assessments, and confidence in self-assessments.[40]

There is a basic information-processing bias that underlies this process, in that schizophrenia patients show a bias to prioritize decisions based on internally generated, as compared with externally provided, information. Coltheart and Davies[41] demonstrated that patients with schizophrenia discounted new, externally originating information that was not congruent with existing information that they believed. When evaluating the reason for this discounting, Moritz et al. [42] suggested that external information is ignored because of challenges in problem-solving and prioritization. An additional possibility is more fundamental. Harvey et al. [43] showed that people with schizophrenia manifested a greater recall benefit for self-generated, as compared with externally originating, information compared with healthy individuals. Further, a well-supported hypothesis, "hyperfocusing" suggests that people with schizophrenia manifest a reduced ability to consider all elements of a complex situation because of reductions in their overall information-processing capacity.[44] Thus, when having to select information to process, they tend to focus on a limited set of more easily processed data. The universe of more easily processed information includes a predominance of self-generated information and long-held beliefs and opinions, requiring less cognitive capacity and effort to retrieve and utilize in decision-making.

Neurological origins of anosognosia in schizophrenia

Flashman et al.[45] noted neuroanatomical and neuro-psychological similarities between anosognosia in neurological conditions and a lack of insight in schizophrenia. In neurological conditions, lesions in the frontal and right parietal lobe were observed in patients with anosognosia, and within schizophrenia, patients with poor insight have been shown to do poorly in neuropsychological assessment measures that test the frontal and parietal lobes.[46–48] Shad et al.[49] concluded that there is a similarity between anosognosia in neurological conditions and insight deficits in schizophrenia.

Neuropsychological tests have limits for identifying regionalized deficits in schizophrenia because of the background challenges of global performance deficits inducing deficits across tests of many different domains in neurological patients.[50] To develop an integrated perspective on insight and structural and functional factors, researchers have used Voxel-Based Morphometry (VBM) to image the brain and fMRI studies to measure brain activation in schizophrenia patients across levels of insight. Structural neuroimaging has shown abnormalities in several areas of the brain for patients with schizophrenia and insight difficulties, but primarily in the prefrontal and insular cortices.[51] Interestingly, in healthy people[52] self-assessment ability is correlated with better functioning in both of these regions, as well as the right rostrolateral prefrontal cortex (RRPFC). Altered functioning in these areas could reduce a person's ability to process and maintain external information (i.e., working memory) while making decisions regarding its source and importance (i.e., executive functioning).

Finally, researchers have considered differences in brain activation associated with IA performance using fMRI. One study in this area was conducted by Pinkham et al.[53] In this study, participants with schizophrenia and healthy controls were imaged while they performed social cognitive tests, with and without the requirement to concurrently make an accurate judgment regarding their performance. In previous studies of momentary IA judgments, two critical frontal lobe regions, the RRPFC and dorso-anterior cingulate cortex (DACC), were found to be

implicated in performance. Three levels of evidence implicating regional brain dysfunction and unawareness came out of the study. First, when compared with healthy controls, individuals with schizophrenia showed reduced activation of the RRPFC and DACC while performing the self-assessment test. Second, in healthy individuals, but not participants with schizophrenia, the level of activation of these brain regions predicted the quality of performance on the self-assessment task. Third, and critical for real-world functional implications, in participants with schizophrenia, despite the general failure to activate the brain regions during self-assessment, greater activation of the RRPFC and DACC during self-assessment were associated with independently generated ratings of social functioning. Thus, the findings regarding alterations in functioning in critical brain regions translate to real-world social functioning, which has been shown to be strongly correlated with social cognitive IA deficits and a positive IB when errors are made in social cognitive judgments.

Clinical correlates and manifestations of IA

Challenges in IA and directional biases in IB are found for both momentary and global decision-making regarding the correctness of cognitive and functional performance and emotional processing. We advance the novel, but clearly empirically supported idea that many responses that are designated as self-assessments of immediate performance or global abilities, are actually not. In many different decisional domains responses should originate from the decision-making processes, described above, regarding recollection of past performance and comparison of the current task with prior tasks; the observable data suggests that this is not common. There is also clear evidence that participants with schizophrenia may apply different decision rules and standards for evidence compared with what would be considered normative.

Clinical insight and treatment failures

Psychotropic medications are the first-line treatment for patients with schizophrenia. To be effective, patients must obtain the medication, take the medication as directed, and be regularly monitored by a mental health professional. Prescription medication schedules include patients taking pills daily or less frequent injectable depot medication. Effectively treating a serious mental illness is complicated, even for a motivated recipient. A lack of insight adds additional difficulty.

There are several domains where reduced insight can reduce adherence to medication regimens and impact general orientation toward treatment. Table 5.1 describes adherence challenges and likely origins. Reduced adherence has several consequences, including full relapse of psychotic symptoms or a chronic state of partial medication response. As described below, breakthrough psychotic symptoms appear to covary with a number of other challenges in insight and awareness, with the causal direction not exactly clear. However, there are significant risks to CNS integrity associated with non-adherence, relapse, and chronic psychotic symptoms. In a review of 13 meta-analyses and 25,657 patients, Howes et al.[54] reported "highly suggestive" evidence that untreated psychosis leads to more severe positive symptoms, more severe negative symptoms, and lower chance of remission. Zoghbi et al.[55] also reviewed 83 studies that looked at the neuroanatomy of untreated psychosis and concluded that while there was not sufficient evidence of global neurological impairment, specific brain structures like the temporal lobe could be vulnerable to adverse impacts of early untreated psychosis. A classic study, pre-dating the availability of clozapine in the United States, shows these same adverse impacts in chronic patients. Davis et al.[56] reported that chronic

treatment-refractory patients showed evidence of 4-year longitudinal ventricular enlargement, particularly left-sided, compared with similarly treated chronic patients whose symptoms responded to treatment. These data underscore the importance of medication treatment and adherence to stave off avoidable neurological deterioration associated with untreated symptoms.

Self-generated information and quality of test performance

In a study that sought to specifically elucidate the nature and consequences of reliance on externally provided versus self-generated information, Tercero et al.[35] used a modified version of the Wisconsin Card Sorting Task (WCST) that included a meta-cognitive component. Participants were asked to sort 64 cards, generate an immediate accuracy judgment after each sort, and then rate their confidence in each accuracy judgment. They were then provided feedback as in the standard administration of the WCST. Participants with schizophrenia underperformed participants with bipolar disorder on sorting, while both equivalently overestimated the accuracy of their sorting performance on a momentary basis. Participants with schizophrenia were more confident in the correctness of their sorts on a momentary, sort-by-sort basis, and their confidence did not change after receiving feedback regarding sorting errors,[57] while participants with bipolar disorder manifested confidence ratings that tracked performance feedback. However, the fundamental difference between the groups is that participants with schizophrenia based their overall judgments regarding task performance solely on their own accuracy decisions, with no correlation between feedback received (tracking the actual accuracy of their responses) and global judgments. Participants with bipolar disorder provided global judgments of their performance that were highly correlated with performance feedback.

WCST performance on the part of participants with schizophrenia was negatively influenced by reliance on recollection of self-generated information. This response pattern was also marked by the exceptional accuracy of participants with schizophrenia in recalling their self-generated responses while showing no evidence of considering the feedback they received. In this case, recalling only self-generated information rendered feedback irrelevant. The commonly

Table 5.1 Elements of poor adherence to treatment and possible causes

Adherence challenge	Possible origin
Not self-administering medication	Lack of perceived need for treatment
Not attending psychiatric appointments	Lack of perceived need for treatment
Failing to refill medication	Organizational/executive functioning challenges leading to poor planning
Incorrectly self-administering medication	Lack of understanding of the actual effects of medication/executive functioning
	Challenges leading to poor organization
Not taking care of physical health	Lack of understanding/sedentary behavior associated with avolition

observed lack of correlation between true performance and judgments of performance in participants with schizophrenia seems not to reflect random responses. Instead, it appears to be the result of applying very well-remembered information (Trial x trial responses) to the wrong purpose: recalling and using external information about performance to generate a global competence assessment.

Momentary monitoring failures and psychotic symptoms

In a study of immediate self-assessment of cognitive performance, study participants completed an ecological momentary assessment (EMA) study with 90 surveys over 30 days. Each survey had queries about several different illness features, including the momentary occurrence and severity of psychotic symptoms. At the endpoint, a cognitive assessment was performed and participants with schizophrenia underperformed participants with bipolar disorder on five different neuropsychological tests.[23] Participants were asked to make quantitative judgments about their performance immediately after they completed each of the five tests. On an absolute basis, misestimation errors had an effect size of Cohen's $d = 0.85$ for both samples, although the directional nature of IB was different. Participants with schizophrenia overestimated their performance when they made an incorrect decision and participants with bipolar disorder underestimated. Introspective inaccuracy in schizophrenia was significantly correlated with the frequency of momentary psychotic symptoms, consistent with earlier theories of the origins of delusions as being challenges in self-assessment. However, there was no correlation between momentary psychotic symptoms and test performance, suggesting that psychosis has a greater impact on evaluating the quality of performance than on cognitive performance itself.

Positive symptoms and impossible self-assessments

In a related challenge, people with schizophrenia may generate reports of engagement in activities that are impossible, because the requisite congruence between reports of performing the activities and their actual observed behavior are incompatible. For example, in the study mentioned above, participants with schizophrenia who were alone for over 90% of 90 EMA surveys over 30 days reported that they were more capable of engaging in activities that cannot be performed at home, including taking public transportation, in-person banking, and in-store shopping, compared with participants who were more commonly away from home with others.[58] Interestingly the same participants who were alone were found to be more commonly experiencing psychotic symptoms on a momentary basis. Thus, the boundary between decision rules about behavior (e.g., "Did I do it?" vs. "Could I do it?") overlaps with psychotic experiences related to the lack of clinical insight. We suggest that self-reports of competence are actually ideas that originated from the same processes that lead to the development of other delusions. These impossible reports may reflect being confused about whether or not previous events actually occurred. Reporting engagement in away-from-home activities while continuously at home is not qualitatively different than reporting attempts at persecution by others that never occurred. Another source of impossible reports is described below, the application of uniquely, and idiosyncratically, applied decision rules where the boundary between recollection of actual performance and self-assessments of competence disappears.

Are there uniquely and individually applied rules of evidence?

The process of endorsement of high competence in activities that are never performed may also originate from uniquely applied decision rules combined with response biases. These "home-alone" participants could not be making a self-assessment based on recollection of experiences (i.e., success, task completion, repetition of strategies) associated with a history of performance. We have previously hypothesized that these participants are reporting on their belief that they could perform the tasks, even if they never do, and are providing an honest report on their perceived competence and not a recollection-based report of their previous behavior. Thus, a positive IB would lead to reports of engaging in activities that never occurred, wherein participants believe that they could succeed if they were given the opportunity or were somehow required to do the task.

A related phenomenon occurs with self-reports of medication adherence. There is a common, yet unusual, phenomenon related to awareness of and reports of medication adherence. People with schizophrenia may report that they are self-administering

Table 5.2 Model of "alternative reality" in reports of engagement in activities

Statement	Underlying logic
If I have medication at home, that means I am taking my medication	Medication adherence is redefined as medication possession because I could take it if I wanted to
If I think that I know how to take the bus, even if I have never done it, I am successful in taking the bus	Subjective knowledge is redefined as real-world performance
I have the skills to be working at least part-time (even though the participant has never worked)	I know lots of people who are working, and I am as good at work skills as them
I do not want to take drugs anymore; so that means that I stopped taking them	Positive intent is a synonym for actions

their medication when they have medication on hand but are not taking it, even when they are being tested for medication adherence. These findings suggest that they might have different definitions of what "taking medication" means, with responses based on medication possession rather than medication self-administration. Thus, the report of high levels of medication adherence would be subjectively supported by 100% medication possession, even if self-administration was negligible. Table 5.2 provides a heuristic model of altered decision-making as applied to oneself in a situation where implausible endorsements are generated. Consistent with jumping to conclusions regarding task-based decisions, available evidence regarding behaviors in functional situations seems to be only partially evaluated before the generation of reports of engaging in the activity. Thus, consistent with hyperfocusing, liberal acceptance bias, and a preference for self-generated information, reports of competence in engaging in activities seem to be made without considering information regarding prior performance. A self-assessment of competence, likely overestimated because of lack of experience, is reported as equivalent to success while engaging in the activity.

Poorer functioning associated with IA and IB

IA correlates with cognitive deficits and has been found in multiple studies to correlate with neurocognitive impairments.[59] IA errors alone do not necessarily lead to disability nor is an IA error necessarily dysfunctional. Normal range uncertainty about the quality of performance of activities can lead to thoroughness in task completion and giving a task "the once over" such as in proofreading or reviewing a shopping list, which can lead to better functioning. In such a case, the individuals might very well be responding to a mild but adaptive negative IB: "I am not sure that I have done the job thoroughly."

IB may lead to multiple motivational challenges that have the potential to impact functioning differently depending on the direction of the bias. A positive IB, the belief that one is more competent than one actually is, can lead to reduced interest in rehabilitation-focused interventions and missing out on opportunities to learn new skills, obtain employment, or live independently. "I don't need any help; I could get a job if I wanted to."

Negative IB can suppress efforts to undertake tasks that are in fact possible to accomplish. IB, in either direction, does not seem to be related to poorer momentary performance on formal cognitive assessments across multiple studies.[60] However, the lifelong experience of lower intelligence or academic ability seems to be predictive of overconfidence in healthy adults[31] and this may also apply to people with schizophrenia.[59,60]

Treatment of self-assessment challenges

Different treatments may be required for IA and IB. In theory, computerized cognitive training could improve neurocognition and thereby reduce misestimation, which may improve IA and reduce opportunities for the influence of IB. Response bias may be addressed by social cognitive interventions and metacognitive training. Further, a host of cognitive behavior therapies and metacognitive therapies target IB in its various forms[8], with strategies not dissimilar to those applied to treatment-resistant delusional beliefs. Describing these interventions is beyond our scope, but these interventions are widely available and utilize a theoretical framework focusing on teaching the participant to recognize the possibility of IA and then addressing the dominant tendency toward positive IB.

Successful treatment of psychotic symptoms can lead to changes in clinical insight. It is very common for individuals whose psychosis has been remitted or even reduced through antipsychotic treatments to state that they no longer believe that their psychotic experiences were real. Improvement in psychotic symptoms has been reported to precede improvements in insight and participants with remission of psychosis at 6 months show improvements in awareness that continue to accelerate for up to 12 months.[61] Information is harder to obtain regarding the time course of relapse, including the timing of medication discontinuation, changes in insight, and relapse. Studies have suggested that poor therapeutic alliance, negative attitudes toward medication, and substance use may lead to medication discontinuation, which then leads to changes in symptoms, which then leads to reduced insight.[17] Further, in those studies, poor treatment response and never developing insight in response to clinical changes are also risk factors for relapse. Newly developing digital strategies may both be able to untangle the sequence of events leading up to relapse as well as provide intervention strategies.[62]

Social-cognitive deficits as a treatment target

Social-cognitive deficits are another target for treatment. Attributional bias is common in patients with paranoia.[63] These biases often lead to patients inferring negative intentions to others and sometimes feeling the need to engage in various actions based on goals of self-preservation. Positive IB was found to be correlated with both poor performance on social-cognitive tests[19,30,33,64] and poorer social outcomes.[65] The connection between these two impaired domains, social cognition, and social outcomes, can be related to patients overestimating the extent to which they understand other people's intentions and interest in them. If social competence is poor, but an individual thinks that it is excellent, or even perfect, then that person might have an increased likelihood of negative interactions with others based on misperceptions, leading to confusion. Such a combination of overconfidence in abilities and misperception of others' interest in them is likely one cause of stalking behavior on the part of people with schizophrenia.[66]

As described above, participants with schizophrenia manifesting anosognosia show deficits in the strategies they use to gather information, the amount of information that they gather, and the rapidity of decision-making, all of which also can lead to impairments in the processes referred to as a theory of mind.[67] These social-cognitive deficits have a substantial functional impact on patients as described above and can lead both to negative interactions, including violence[68] and self-selected social avoidance[69] based on failed attempts to interact.

Treatment of social-cognitive deficits has commonly focused on interaction-focused training. Social Cognition Interaction Training or SCIT[70] is a group treatment aimed at improving social-cognitive processes for patients with psychotic disorders. SCIT looks to improve common social-cognitive problems seen in schizophrenia: emotion perception, theory of mind, hostile attribution bias, and jumping to conclusions with elevated confidence levels in their beliefs. SCIT uses principles of neurocognitive remediation with Cognitive Behavioral Therapy techniques to address these deficits and biases. Multiple studies have shown that SCIT is portable across cultures and settings. Within a forensic environment,[71] patients receiving active treatment showed statistically significant improvements in the theory of mind, emotion perception, hostile attribution bias, cognitive flexibility, social functioning, intolerance of ambiguity, and a reduction of aggressive incidents in the SCIT group compared with the control group which received coping skills training. Conversely, Dark et al.[72] completed a randomized controlled trial that gave SCIT to patients with schizophrenia with a "befriending" group as a control. Results showed no difference in measures of social cognition. Dark et al. noted that in their community intervention, they believed that one of the difficulties was session adherence which was lower than previously published studies. An inpatient environment might be a more appropriate place for SCIT as treatment adherence can be more closely regulated. In addition, that study did not address whether patients were adherent to their psychotropic medications and did not use any standardized measures of symptoms. It is unclear the impact that psychiatric symptoms have on the patient's ability to engage with the material in the treatment group.

Treatments for social-cognitive deficits have been shown to be effective in improving domains of social cognition,[73] but a follow-up meta-analysis suggested that improvements in social functioning are not uniformly found.[74] Social cognition treatments require that a patient has at least a rudimentary awareness of their disorder. Again, in an inpatient environment with improved treatment adherence and developing clinical insight, social-cognitive deficits are a viable treatment target.

Conclusions

Anosognosia is a common feature of schizophrenia. Many of the symptoms of schizophrenia directly arise from challenges in evaluating the validity and plausibility of certain experiences. Impairments in the accuracy of self-assessment appear to be related to part of the larger picture of cognitive deficits in schizophrenia, while overt biases seem to be a common and central feature of self-assessment in schizophrenia. The combination of IA/IB and possible decision-making that involves an alternative reality, can lead to self-reports that are truly uninformative when attempting to make a judgment regarding functioning.

Research has suggested dysfunctions in several different brain regions being implicated in various forms of IA and IB deficits. General awareness seems related to dysfunctions in the prefrontal cortex and specific brain structures are implicated in success in momentary judgments regarding the accuracy of socially relevant decisions. Better functioning in these regions is associated with better social outcomes, suggesting that the ability to activate critical brain regions "on demand" to make socially relevant self-assessments leads to better social outcomes.

The implications of anosognosia are broad and certain treatments (i.e., antipsychotic medications) that are commonly avoided by people with schizophrenia because of impairments in clinical insight may actually hold the promise for the first inroads into impairments in awareness. Treatment of IB requires targeting a variety of attitudes related to perceptions of abilities and past achievements. The eventual goal of these treatments would be realistic self-assessment, which we have shown to have the immediate potential to improve functioning in several different domains. Clinical stability induced by medication adherence does not seem to have a direct impact on cognitive performance,[75] but recent studies suggest that clinical stability may be a prerequisite for training gains in learning-based therapies.[76] As noted above, sustained psychotic symptoms appear to have the potential to lead to wide-ranging deterioration in brain functioning.

Naturally, value judgments are embedded in considering evaluating refusal of treatments associated with anosognosia. On the one hand, refusing treatment for illness, even if it is potentially terminal, is generally accepted in the United States. On the other hand, anosognosia adds an extra layer of complexity to the decision-making process because individuals are not aware of their illness. Would an individual choose to have the illness treated if they did not have anosognosia? It is further complicated when a refusal to accept treatment leads to risk for others or the patient themselves. Thus, anosognosia presents a complex dilemma. Would your life be better if you accepted treatment or is refusal, despite possessing the previously mentioned "without knowledge of the disease," simply a fundamental right of self-determination? Obviously, as treatments targeting anosognosia are further developed, it is our hope that this discussion is actually not required.

References

1. Gainotti G. History of anosognosia. *Front Neurol Neurosci*. 2019;**44**:75–82. doi: 10.1159/000494954.

2. Sartorius N, Shapiro R, Kimura M, Barrett K. WHO international pilot study of schizophrenia. *Psychol Med*. 1972 Nov;**2**(4):422–425. doi: 10.1017/s0033291700045244.

3. Carpenter WT Jr, Strauss JS, Bartko JJ. Flexible system for the diagnosis of schizophrenia: report from the WHO International Pilot Study of Schizophrenia. *Science*. 1973 Dec 21;**182**(4118):1275–1278. doi: 10.1126/sci- ence.182.4118.1275.

4. Amador XF, Strauss DH, Yale SA, et al. Assessment of insight in psychosis. *Am J Psychiatry*. 1993;**150**(6):873–879. doi:10.1176/ajp.150.6.873

5. Amador XF, Flaum M, Andreasen NC, et al. Awareness of illness in schizophrenia and schizoaffective and mood disorders. *Arch Gen Psychiatry*. 1994;**51**(10):826–836. doi:10.1001/archpsyc.1994.03950100074007

6. Amador XF, Gorman JM. Psychopathologic domains and insight in schizophrenia. *Psychiatr Clin North Am*. 1998;**21**(1):27–42. doi:10.1016/s0193-953x(05)70359-2

7. Ventura J, Subotnik KL, Han S, et al. The relationship between sex and functional outcome in first-episode schizophrenia: the role of premorbid adjustment and insight. *Psychol Med*. 2023;**53**(14):6878–6887. doi:10.1017/S0033291723000442

8. Penney D, Sauvé G, Mendelson D, et al. Immediate and sustained outcomes and moderators associated with metacognitive training for psychosis: a systematic review and meta-analysis. *JAMA Psychiatry*. 2022;**79**(5):417–429. doi:10.1001/jamapsychiatry.2022.0277

9. Beck AT, Baruch E, Balter JM, Steer RA, Warman DM. A new instrument for measuring insight: the Beck Cognitive Insight Scale. *Schizophr Res.* 2004; **68**(2–3):319–329. doi:10.1016/S0920-9964(03)00189-0

10. Medalia A, Thysen J. Insight into neurocognitive dysfunction in schizophrenia. *Schizophr Bull.* 2008;**34** (6):1221–1230. doi:10.1093/schbul/sbm144

11. Parellada M, Boada L, Fraguas D, et al. Trait and state attributes of insight in first episodes of early-onset schizophrenia and other psychoses: a 2-year longitudinal study. *Schizophr Bull.* 2011;37(1):38–51. doi:10.1093/schbul/sbq109

12. Buckley PF, Wirshing DA, Bhushan P, et al. Lack of insight in schizophrenia: impact on treatment adherence. *CNS Drugs.* 2007;**21**(2):129–141. doi:10.2165/00023210-200721020-00004

13. Lehrer DS, Lorenz J. Anosognosia in schizophrenia: hidden in plain sight. *Innov Clin Neurosci.* 2014;**11**(5–6):10–17.

14. Köther U, Veckenstedt R, Vitzthum F, et al. "Don't give me that look" – overconfidence in false mental state perception in schizophrenia. *Psychiatry Res.* 2012;**196**(1):1–8. doi:10.1016/j.psychres.2012.03.004

15. Balzan R, Delfabbro P, Galletly C, Woodward T. Confirmation biases across the psychosis continuum: the contribution of hypersalient evidence-hypothesis matches. *Br J Clin Psychol.* 2013;**52**(1):53–69. doi:10.1111/bjc.12000

16. Damiani S, Donadeo A, Bassetti N, et al. Understanding source monitoring subtypes and their relation to psychosis: a systematic review and meta-analysis. *Psychiatry Clin Neurosci.* 2022;**76** (5):162–171. doi:10.1111/pcn.13338

17. Velligan DI, Sajatovic M, Hatch A, Kramata P, Docherty JP. Why do psychiatric patients stop antipsychotic medication? A systematic review of reasons for nonadherence to medication in patients with serious mental illness. *Patient Prefer Adherence.* 2017;**11**:449–468. doi:10.2147/PPA.S124658

18. O'Connor JA, Ellett L, Ajnakina O, et al. Can cognitive insight predict symptom remission in a first episode psychosis cohort?. *BMC Psychiatry.* 2017;**17**(1):54. doi:10.1186/s12888-017-1210-9

19. Gould F, McGuire LS, Durand D, et al. Self-assessment in schizophrenia: accuracy of evaluation of cognition and everyday functioning. *Neuropsychology.* 2015;**29** (5):675–682. doi:10.1037/neu0000175

20. Benoit A, Harvey PO, Bherer L, Lepage M. Does the Beck Cognitive Insight Scale predict response to cognitive remediation in schizophrenia? *Schizophr Res Treatment.* 2016;**2016**:6371856. doi:10.1155/2016/6371856

21. Alameda L, Golay P, Baumann P, et al. Assertive outreach for "difficult to engage" patients: A useful tool for a subgroup of patients in specialized early psychosis intervention programs. *Psychiatry Res.* 2016;**239**:212–219. doi: 10.1016/j.psychres.2016.03.010

22. Fleming SM, Weil RS, Nagy Z, Dolan RJ, Rees G. Relating introspective accuracy to individual differences in brain structure [published correction appears in *Science.* 2012 May 11;**336**(6082):670]. *Science.* 2010;**329**(5998):1541–1543. doi:10.1126/science.1191883

23. Morgan O, Strassnig MT, Moore RC, et al. Accuracy of immediate self-assessment of neurocognitive test performance: associations with psychiatric diagnosis and longitudinal psychotic symptoms. *J Psychiatr Res.* 2022; **156**:594–601. doi:10.1016/j .jpsychires.2022.10.069

24. Gould F, Sabbag S, Durand D, Patterson TL, Harvey PD. Self-assessment of functional ability in schizophrenia: milestone achievement and its relationship to accuracy of self-evaluation. *Psychiatry Res.* 2013;**207**(1–2):19–24. doi:10.1016/j .psychres.2013.02.035

25. Moritz S, Woodward TS, Jelinek L, Klinge R. Memory and metamemory in schizophrenia: a liberal acceptance account of psychosis. *Psychol Med.* 2008;**38** (6):825–832. doi:10.1017/S0033291707002553

26. Helzer EG, Dunning D. Why and when peer prediction is superior to self-prediction: the weight given to future aspiration versus past achievement. *J Pers Soc Psychol.* 2012;**103**(1):38–53. doi:10.1037/a0028124

27. Holshausen K, Bowie CR, Mausbach BT, Patterson TL, Harvey PD. Neurocognition, functional capacity, and functional outcomes: the cost of inexperience. *Schizophr Res.* 2014;**152**(2–3):430–434. doi:10.1016/j .schres.2013.08.004

28. Strassnig M, Kotov R, Fochtmann L, et al. Associations of independent living and labor force participation with impairment indicators in schizophrenia and bipolar disorder at 20-year follow-up. *Schizophr Res.* 2018;**197**:150–155. doi:10.1016/j.schres.2018.02.009

29. Balzan RP, Woodward TS, Delfabbro P, Moritz S. Overconfidence across the psychosis continuum: a calibration approach. *Cogn Neuropsychiatry.* 2016;**21** (6):510–524. doi:10.1080/13546805.2016.1240072

30. Jones MT, Deckler E, Laurrari C, et al. Confidence, performance, and accuracy of self-assessment of social cognition: A comparison of schizophrenia patients and healthy controls. *Schizophr Res Cogn.* 2019;**19**:002-2. doi:10.1016/j.scog.2019.01.002

31. Ehrlinger J, Johnson K, Banner M, Dunning D, Kruger J. Why the unskilled are unaware: further explorations of (Absent) self-insight among the

incompetent. *Organ Behav Hum Decis Process.* 2008;**105**(1):98–121. doi:10.1016/j.obhdp.2007.05.002

32. Badal VD, Depp CA, Pinkham AE, Harvey PD. Dynamics of task-based confidence in schizophrenia using seasonal decomposition approach. *Schizophr Res Cogn.* 2023; **32**:100278.

33. Perez MM, Tercero BA, Penn DL, Pinkham AE, Harvey PD. Overconfidence in social cognitive decision making: correlations with social cognitive and neurocognitive performance in participants with schizophrenia and healthy individuals. *Schizophr Res.* 2020;**224**:51–57.

34. Engh JA, Sundet K, Simonsen C, et al. Verbal learning contributes to cognitive insight in schizophrenia independently of affective and psychotic symptoms. *Prog Neuropsychopharmacol Biol Psychiatry.* 2011;**35** (4):1059–1063. doi:10.1016/j.pnpbp.2011.02.021

35. Tercero BA, Perez MM, Mohsin N, et al. Using a Meta-cognitive Wisconsin Card Sorting Test to measure introspective accuracy and biases in schizophrenia and bipolar disorder. *J Psychiatr Res.* 2021;**140**:436–442.

36. Gorora ME, Dalkner N, Moore RC, et al. A meta-cognitive Wisconsin Card Sorting Test in people with schizophrenia and bipolar disorder: Self-assessment of sorting performance. *Psychiatry Res.* 2024;**334**:115831. doi:10.1016/j.psychres.2024.115831

37. Moritz S, Stojisavlevic M, Göritz AS, Riehle M, Scheunemann J. Does uncertainty breed conviction? On the possible role of compensatory conviction in jumping to conclusions and overconfidence in psychosis. *Cogn Neuropsychiatry.* 2019;**24**(4):284–299. doi:10.1080/13546805.2019.1642863

38. Buchy L, Woodward TS, Liotti M. A cognitive bias against disconfirmatory evidence (BADE) is associated with schizotypy. *Schizophr Res.* 2007;**90**(1– 3):334–337. doi:10.1016/j.schres.2006.11.012

39. Stone ER, Opel RB. Training to improve calibration and discrimination: the effects of performance and environmental feedback. *Organ Behav Hum Decis Process.* 2000;**83**(2):282–309. doi:10.1006/obhd.2000.2910

40. Nassar MR, Waltz JA, Albrecht MA, Gold JM, Frank MJ. All or nothing belief updating in patients with schizophrenia reduces precision and flexibility of beliefs. *Brain.* 2021;**144**(3):1013–1029. doi:10.1093/brain/awaa453

41. Coltheart M, Davies M. Failure of hypothesis evaluation as a factor in delusional belief. *Cogn Neuropsychiatry.* 2021;**26**(4):213–230.

42. Moritz S, Göritz AS, Gallinat J, et al. Subjective competence breeds overconfidence in errors in psychosis. A hubris account of paranoia. *J Behav Ther Exp Psychiatry.* 2015;**48**:118–124. doi:10.1016/j.jbtep.2015.02.011

43. Harvey PD, Earle-Boyer EA, Weilgus MS, Levinson JC. Encoding, memory, and thought disorder in schizophrenia and mania. *Schizophr Bull.* 1986; **12** (2):252–261. doi:10.1093/schbul/12.2.252

44. Luck SJ, Hahn B, Leonard CJ, Gold JM. The hyperfocusing hypothesis: a new account of cognitive dysfunction in schizophrenia. *Schizophr Bull.* 2019;**45** (5):991–1000. doi:10.1093/schbul/sbz063

45. Flashman LA, McAllister TW, Johnson SC, et al. Specific frontal lobe subregions correlated with unawareness of illness in schizophrenia: a preliminary study. *J Neuropsychiatry Clin Neurosci.* 2001; **13**(2):255–257. doi:10.1176/jnp.13.2.255

46. McEvoy JP, Hartman M, Gottlieb D, et al. Common sense, insight, and neuropsychological test performance in schizophrenia patients. *Schizophr Bull.* 1996;**22**(4):635–641. doi:10.1093/schbul/22.4.635

47. Lysaker PH, Bell MD, Bryson G, Kaplan E. Neurocognitive function and insight in schizophrenia: support for an association with impairments in executive function but not with impairments in global function. *Acta Psychiatr Scand.* 1998;**97**(4):297–301. doi:10.1111/j.1600-0447.1998.tb10003.x

48. Simon V, De Hert M, Wampers M, Peuskens J, van Winkel R. The relation between neurocognitive dysfunction and impaired insight in patients with schizophrenia. *Eur Psychiatry.* 2009;**24**(4):239–243. doi:10.1016/j.eurpsy.2008.10.004

49. Shad MU, Tamminga CA, Cullum M, Haas GL, Keshavan MS. Insight and frontal cortical function in schizophrenia: a review. *Schizophr Res.* 2006; **86**(1– 3):54–70. doi:10.1016/j.schres.2006.06.006

50. Harvey PD. Domains of cognition and their assessment. *Dialogues Clin Neurosci.* 2019;**21** (3):227–237. doi:10.31887/DCNS.2019.21.3/pharvey

51. Palaniyappan L, Mallikarjun P, Joseph V, Liddle PF. Appreciating symptoms and deficits in schizophrenia: right posterior insula and poor insight. *Prog Neuropsychopharmacol Biol Psychiatry.* 2011;**35** (2):523–527. doi:10.1016/j.pnpbp.2010.12.008

52. Fleming SM, Dolan RJ. The neural basis of metacognitive ability. *Philos Trans R Soc Lond B Biol Sci.* 2012;**367**(1594):1338–1349. doi:10.1098/rstb.2011.0417

53. Pinkham AE, Klein HS, Hardaway GB, Kemp KC, Harvey PD. Neural correlates of social cognitive introspective accuracy in schizophrenia. *Schizophr Res.* 2018;**202**:166–172. doi:10.1016/j.schres.2018.07.001

54. Howes OD, Whitehurst T, Shatalina E, et al. The clinical significance of duration of untreated psychosis: an umbrella review and random-effects meta-analysis. *World Psychiatry*. 2021;**20**(1):75–95. doi:10.1002/wps.20822

55. Zoghbi AW, Lieberman JA, Girgis RR. The neurobiology of duration of untreated psychosis: a comprehensive review. *Mol Psychiatry*. 2023;**28**(1):168–190. doi:10.1038/s41380-022-01718-0

56. Davis KL, Buchsbaum MS, Shihabuddin L, et al. Ventricular enlargement in poor-outcome schizophrenia. *Biol Psychiatry*. 1998;**43**(11):783–793.

57. Badal VD, Depp CA, Harvey PD, et al. Confidence, accuracy judgments and feedback in schizophrenia and bipolar disorder: a time series network analysis. *Psychol Med*. 2023;**53**(9):4200–4209. doi:10.1017/S0033291722000939

58. Gohari E, Moore RC, Depp CA, et al. Momentary severity of psychotic symptoms predicts overestimation of competence in domains of everyday activities and work in schizophrenia: an ecological momentary assessment study. *Psychiatry Res*. 2022;**310**:114487. doi:10.1016/j.psychres.2022.114487

59. Mervis JE, Vohs JL, Lysaker PH. An update on clinical insight, cognitive insight, and introspective accuracy in schizophrenia-spectrum disorders: symptoms, cognition, and treatment. *Expert Rev Neurother*. 2022;**22**(3):245–255. doi:10.1080/14737175.2022.2049757

60. Nicolò G, Dimaggio G, Popolo R, et al. Associations of metacognition with symptoms, insight, and neurocognition in clinically stable outpatients with schizophrenia. *J Nerv Ment Dis*. 2012;**200**(7):644–647. doi:10.1097/NMD.0b013e31825bfb10

61. Saravanan B, Jacob KS, Johnson S, et al. Outcome of first-episode schizophrenia in India: longitudinal study of effect of insight and psychopathology. *Br J Psychiatry*. 2010;**196**(6):454–459.

62. Allan S, Mcleod H, Bradstreet S, et al. Understanding implementation of a digital self-monitoring intervention for relapse prevention in psychosis: protocol for a mixed method process evaluation. *JMIR Res Protoc*. 2019; **8**(12):e15634. doi:10.2196/15634

63. Pinkham AE, Harvey PD, Penn DL. Paranoid individuals with schizophrenia show greater social cognitive bias and worse social functioning than non-paranoid individuals with schizophrenia. *Schizophr Res Cogn*. 2016;**3**: 33–38. doi:10.1016/j.scog.2015.11.002

64. Pinkham AE, Harvey PD, Penn DL. Social cognition psychometric evaluation: results of the final validation study. *Schizophr Bull*. 2018;**44**(4):737–748. doi:10.1093/schbul/sbx117

65. Silberstein JM, Pinkham AE, Penn DL, Harvey PD. Self-assessment of social cognitive ability in schizophrenia: association with social cognitive test performance, informant assessments of social cognitive ability, and everyday outcomes. *Schizophr Res*. 2018;**199**:75–82. doi:10.1016/j.schres.2018.04.015

66. Dressing H, Foerster K, Gass P. Are stalkers disordered or criminal? Thoughts on the psychopathology of stalking. *Psychopathology*. 2011; **44**(5):277–282. doi:10.1159/000325060

67. Salvatore G, Lysaker PH, Popolo R, et al. Vulnerable self, poor understanding of others' minds, threat anticipation and cognitive biases as triggers for delusional experience in schizophrenia: a theoretical model. *Clin Psychol Psychother*. 2012;**19**(3):247–259. doi:10.1002/cpp.746

68. Vaskinn A, Rokicki J, Bell C, et al. Violent offending in males with or without schizophrenia: a role for social cognition?. *Schizophr Bull*. 2024; **50**(3):663–672. doi:10.1093/schbul/sbad151

69. Lysaker PH, Erickson M, Ringer J, et al. Metacognition in schizophrenia: the relationship of mastery to coping, insight, self-esteem, social anxiety, and various facets of neurocognition. *Br J Clin Psychol*. 2011;**50**(4):412–424. doi:10.1111/j.2044-8260.2010.02003.x

70. Penn D, Roberts DL, Munt ED, et al. A pilot study of social cognition and interaction training (SCIT) for schizophrenia. *Schizophr Res*. 2005;**80**(2–3):357–359. doi:10.1016/j.schres.2005.07.011

71. Combs DR, Adams SD, Penn DL, et al. Social Cognition and Interaction Training (SCIT) for inpatients with schizophrenia spectrum disorders: preliminary findings. *Schizophr Res*. 2007;**91**(1–3):112–116. doi:10.1016/j.schres.2006.12.010

72. Dark F, Scott JG, Baker A, et al. Randomized controlled trial of social cognition and interaction training compared to befriending group. *Br J Clin Psychol*. 2020;**59**(3):384–402. doi:10.1111/bjc.12252

73. Kurtz MM, Gagen E, Rocha NB, Machado S, Penn DL. Comprehensive treatments for social cognitive deficits in schizophrenia: A critical review and effect-size analysis of controlled studies. *Clin Psychol Rev*. 2016;**43**:80–89. doi:10.1016/j.cpr.2015.09.003

74. Yeo H, Yoon S, Lee J, Kurtz MM, Choi K. A meta-analysis of the effects of social-cognitive training in schizophrenia: The role of treatment characteristics and study quality. *Br J Clin Psychol*. 2022;**61**(1):37–57. doi:10.1111/bjc.12320

75. Buckley PF, Harvey PD, Bowie CR, Loebel A. The relationship between symptomatic remission and neuropsychological improvement in schizophrenia patients switched to treatment with ziprasidone. *Schizophr Res.* 2007;**94**(1–3):99–106. doi:10.1016/j.schres.2006.12.032

76. Nuechterlein KH, Ventura J, Subotnik KL, et al. A randomized controlled trial of cognitive remediation and long-acting injectable risperidone after a first episode of schizophrenia: improving cognition and work/school functioning. *Psychol Med.* 2022;**52**(8):1517–1526. doi:10.1017/S0033291720003335

6

How Antipsychotics Work in Schizophrenia
A Primer on Mechanisms

Jonathan M. Meyer

Introduction

Schizophrenia spectrum disorders are characterized by core central nervous system (CNS) domains: positive symptoms (hallucinations, delusions, disorganized speech/behavior); negative symptoms (apathy/avolition, diminished expression); and cognitive dysfunction (deficits in working memory, processing speed, executive function).[1] Positive symptoms are necessary to establish the diagnosis, but patients vary considerably in both the presentation of those symptoms, and the extent and severity of negative symptoms and cognitive deficits. Other associated features of schizophrenia include high rates of substance use disorders,[2] persistent depressive symptoms,[3] and twofold higher rates of aggression,[4] with the latter being a product of inadequately controlled positive symptoms or of impulsivity not motivated by psychosis.[5] A distinct neurobiological substrate underlies each of these symptom clusters, and multiple neurotransmitters are implicated in the dysfunction of relevant circuits, particularly dopamine, glutamate, acetylcholine (ACh), and serotonin.[6-9]

Given the complex neurobiology of schizophrenia, and the reality that each individual has their own distinct clinical presentation, no antipsychotic effectively remediates the totality of the three primary symptom domains, with cognitive dysfunction and negative symptoms exhibiting limited benefit from most agents.[10,11] This limitation is likely rooted in the common mechanism of action for most antipsychotics approved prior to 2024: dopamine D_2 receptor blockade. This mechanism is responsible for any improvements in positive symptoms, but has limited independent benefit for negative and cognitive symptoms. D_2 receptor blockade is also inadequate to manage positive symptoms in roughly one-third of patients (i.e., those with treatment resistant schizophrenia [TRS]).[12-14] Although D_2 receptor binding has been the model for most antipsychotics, there are two agents whose primary antipsychotic mechanism lies outside

of this domain: clozapine, and the first of a new class of medication that lacks any D_2 receptor affinity (xanomeline) but instead works by stimulating a subset of muscarinic cholinergic receptors.[15,16] Clozapine binds weakly to the D_2 receptor, but it clearly possesses other mechanisms. To date clozapine remains the only medication with proven efficacy in TRS, namely those with inadequate positive symptom response to D_2 binding antipsychotics.[12,17] Moreover, clozapine exhibits other unique clinical properties in patients with schizophrenia, including reduction in suicidal behavior and impulsive aggression, and alleviation of psychogenic polydipsia (i.e., excessive water drinking related to poorly controlled psychosis).[4,17] Clozapine's mechanisms of action remain incompletely understood despite US approval for TRS on September 26, 1989, although one hypothesis is discussed below in the section on TRS.[18] Importantly, despite advances in the neuropharmacology of schizophrenia, there is no compelling evidence that any other antipsychotic, including the new muscarinic receptor activators, are effective substitutes for clozapine in TRS, or for schizophrenia patients with persistent aggression or suicidality not responsive to D_2 receptor modulating agents.[17]

Positive symptoms

Although clozapine's efficacy profile has not been replicated, D_2 receptor binding antipsychotics and muscarinic antipsychotic agents share a core property: reduction in dopamine neurotransmission. How this is achieved varies greatly between the two classes of medication, but that difference is best understood in the context of the dopamine dysfunction inherent to positive symptoms.[13] Human imaging studies demonstrate that the positive symptoms in schizophrenia patients *who are not treatment resistant* are associated with excess presynaptic production of dopamine in the associative striatum (Figure 6.1).[13,18] This understanding was not

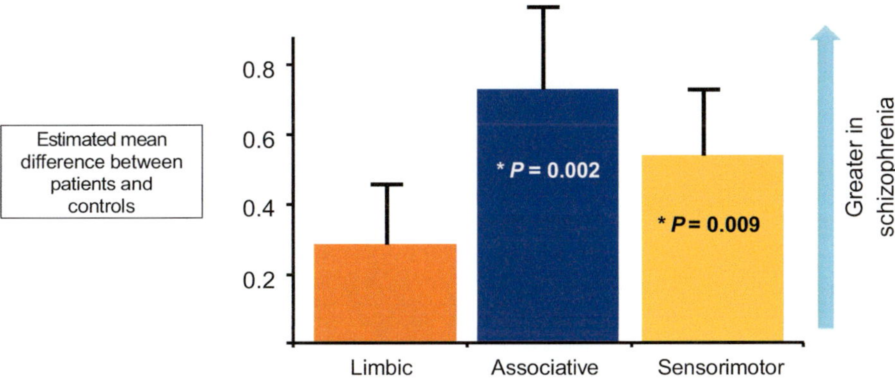

Figure 6.1 Imaging findings note presynaptic dopamine dysfunction (excessive turnover and release) in the associative and adjacent sensorimotor areas of the striatum for patients with schizophrenia when compared to control subjects.[13]

present in the early 1950s when two competing antipsychotic mechanisms became commercially available: depletion of dopamine from presynaptic neurons by reserpine,[19] or blockade of postsynaptic dopamine receptors by chlorpromazine.[20] The first widely imitated antipsychotic, chlorpromazine (Thorazine®), was initially synthesized in 1950 as an improvement on an earlier compound promethazine (Phenergan®). The goal was to develop a more potent medication to induce a nonnarcotic state of "artificial hibernation" and thereby ease anesthetic induction and postsurgery recovery.[20] The connection with dopamine was only later elucidated by Arvid Carlsson, a discovery that garnered Carlsson the Nobel Prize in Physiology or Medicine in 2000.[20] Carlsson's insight was to connect the finding that motor symptoms of Parkinson's disease were related to loss of dopamine producing neurons, and the observation that medications effective for positive psychotic symptoms (e.g., chlorpromazine or reserpine) were associated with a reversible form of drug-induced parkinsonism (DIP). From those facts he deduced in 1963 that antipsychotic medications must be blocking dopamine receptors, or, in the case of reserpine, act by depleting dopamine from presynaptic stores.[21] Carlsson's inductive leap was that the underlying pathophysiology of positive symptoms must somehow relate to excessive dopamine in a specific brain circuit, thereby formulating the dopamine hypothesis of schizophrenia. Animal models characterized the dopamine tracts involved in positive symptoms, and modern human imaging studies confirmed the association of positive symptoms with excessive dopamine turnover in the associative striatum and adjacent portions of the sensorimotor striatum.[13]

Although positive symptoms are a presynaptic problem of dopamine overproduction and release, the presynaptic mechanism inherent to reserpine (blockade of the vesicular monoamine transporter type 2 [VMAT2]) was abandoned as the basis for future antipsychotics by the early 1960s after trials of another VMAT2 inhibitor tetrabenazine.[22] Tetrabenazine shared reserpine's core mechanism and lacked reserpine's effects on blood pressure, but it proved no more effective than reserpine or chlorpromazine, and was often associated with akathisia (restlessness) and DIP at the doses needed to control psychosis.[23,24] With VMAT2 inhibition reaching a dead end, Carlsson's discovery that chlorpromazine's impact on positive psychotic symptoms rested in dopamine receptor blockade facilitated development of compounds that shared its mechanism (D_2 receptor antagonism), but without chlorpromazine's risk for sedation, orthostasis, and anticholinergic adverse effects (e.g., dry mouth, memory impairment, constipation).[25] Subsequent generations of D_2 acting antipsychotics were later developed that possessed lower risk for DIP, tardive dyskinesia (TD), and other movement disorders related to D_2 receptor blockade[14]; however, *when used in equivalent dosages*, all antipsychotics were comparably effective in non-TRS patients (Table 6.1).[26]

Following the demise of presynaptic acting VMAT2 inhibitors, the mechanism of action for every antipsychotic approved through 2023 involved blockade of postsynaptic dopamine D_2 receptors. As illustrated in Figure 6.2, these agents did not address the presynaptic basis of positive symptoms, but managed this problem by interfering with dopamine binding at postsynaptic receptors.[14] These antipsychotics

Table 6.1 Antipsychotics listed alphabetically and by primary mechanism for positive symptom reduction

First generation (D_2 receptor antagonists)	Second generation (D_2 receptor antagonists)	Second generation (D_2 receptor partial agonists)	Muscarinic M_1/M_4 receptor stimulating agents
Chlorpromazine, Fluphenazine, Haloperidol, Perphenazine	Asenapine, Clozapine[a], Iloperidone, Lumateperone, Lurasidone, Olanzapine, Paliperidone, Quetiapine, Risperidone, Ziprasidone	Aripiprazole, Brexpiprazole, Cariprazine	Xanomeline-trospium

[a] Clozapine is the only effective medication for treatment-resistant schizophrenia

were nonselective, and acted at D_2 receptors throughout the CNS and in the periphery yielding several unfortunate consequences. At the level of the dopamine synapse, D_2 antagonists blocked postsynaptic D_2 receptors but also blocked the shorter variant D_{2S} receptors present on presynaptic neurons.[14] As these presynaptic D_{2S} receptors are inhibitory, blocking dopamine's activity further disinhibits presynaptic dopamine release. The level of receptor occupancy required for D_2 antagonists to overcome this effect was not understood when antipsychotics first became available, and efficacy was established for dosage ranges that managed positive symptoms while minimizing as much as possible motor adverse effects.[14] Only in the late 1980s did imaging studies find that at least 65% postsynaptic D_2 receptor occupancy was associated with positive symptom reduction, while >80% receptor occupancy was associated with higher rates of motor adverse effects resulting from D_2 blockade in the dorsal striatum (referred to as extrapyramidal side effects in the older literature): DIP, akathisia, and TD. The proverbial "sweet spot" for D_2 receptor occupancy was thus in the range of 65%–80%, but with significant interindividual heterogeneity noted in the correlation between occupancy, response, and tolerability.[27] First-generation antipsychotics (FGAs) had significantly higher rates of D_2-related motor effects compared to second-generation antipsychotics (SGAs), as the latter possessed an inherent mechanism to mitigate this risk in the form of serotonin 2A ($5HT_{2A}$) receptor antagonism.[28,29] Three dopamine partial agonist antipsychotics (DPAs) were developed (aripiprazole, brexpiprazole, cariprazine) that also have lower risk of motor side effects than FGAs due to their weak intrinsic dopaminergic activity.[14] Because these agents weakly stimulate postsynaptic D_2 receptors, imaging studies noted that DPAs became effective for positive symptoms at 80%–

100% D_2 receptor occupancy. This level of D_2 occupancy would pose significant tolerability problems for antagonist antipsychotics, but the intrinsic dopamine activity of the DPAs results in relatively low rates of DIP and akathisia.[14]

Two other unfortunate consequences of D_2 receptor antagonism are sexual dysfunction from blockade of D_2 receptors in the hypothalamic–pituitary axis (HPA), and glucose dysregulation.[14] As dopamine inhibits prolactin release from the HPA, D_2 receptor blockade can induce hyperprolactinemia of sufficient severity to lower sex hormone levels resulting in menstrual irregularities, gynecomastia or galactorrhea, decreased libido, and bone density loss.[14,30] Blockade of D_2 receptors on insulin secreting pancreatic β-cells and in glucose sensing hypothalamic cells impairs glycemic control, thereby putting patients at risk for metabolic syndrome and diabetes mellitus.[31]

Xanomeline is a muscarinic M_1 and M_4 receptor agonist initially developed to improve cognition in Alzheimer's disease, but was surprisingly found to exert antipsychotic properties in those patients despite being devoid of any D_2 receptor binding.[32] Subsequent animal research discovered that the dopamine neurons associated with positive symptoms receive cholinergic and glutamatergic stimulatory input, and that stimulation of M_1 and M_4 receptors lessen the extent of this input. Cholinergic input to the relevant dopamine tracts originates from a midbrain structure, the laterodorsal tegmental nucleus (LDT).[8,16] LDT neurons possess an abundance of inhibitory M_4 autoreceptors – therefore, any agent which stimulates M_4 receptors will decrease LDT ACh output, with the net result being decreased ACh stimulation of presynaptic dopamine outflow and a reduction in positive symptoms.[16,33] Although there is cholinergic stimulation of dopaminergic neurons in motor areas of the striatum, this cholinergic pathway (the pedunculopontine nucleus) is primarily controlled

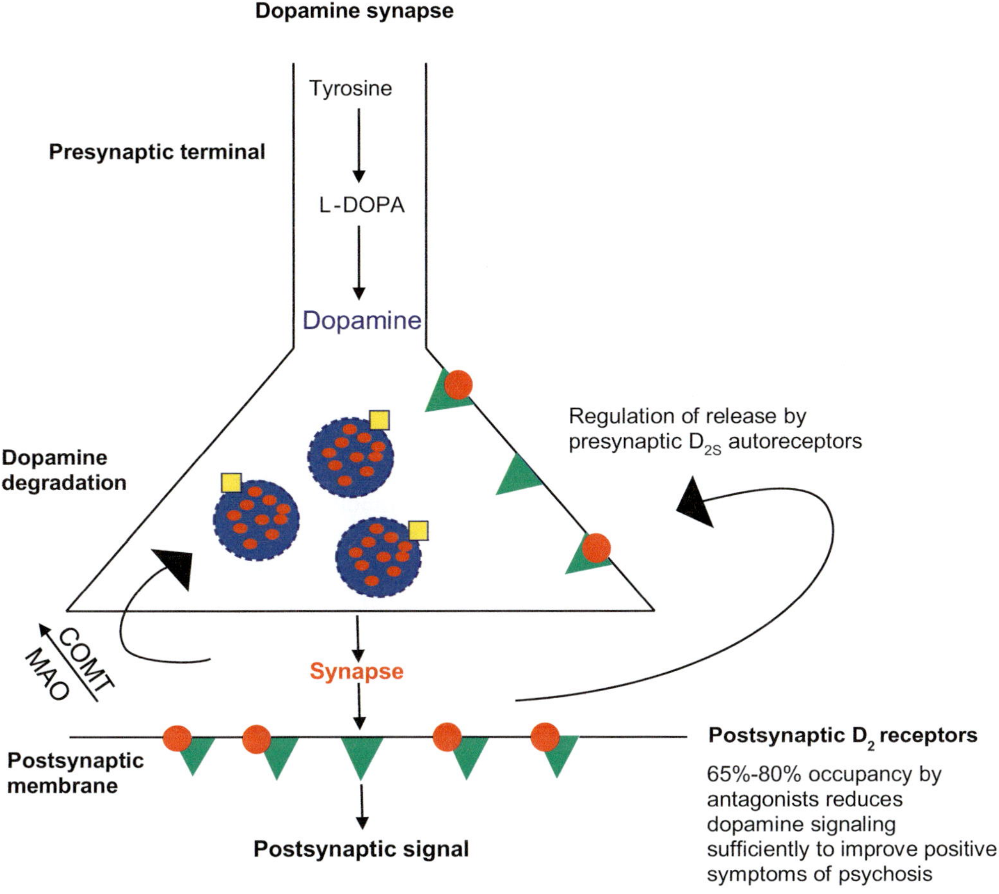

Figure 6.2 How dopamine D_2 receptor binding antipsychotics work at dopamine synapses.[14]
Scheme: Dopamine – red circles; blue dotted circles – presynaptic vesicles containing dopamine; yellow squares – vesicular monoamine transporter type 2 (VMAT2); dopamine D_2 receptors – green triangles.
Abbreviations: MAO: monoamine oxidase; COMT: catechol *O*-methyltransferase.
Legend: Dopamine is produced in the presynaptic neuron by conversion from tyrosine to L-dopa and then to dopamine. Dopamine is inserted into presynaptic vesicles by VMAT2, and is released into the synapse upon neuronal stimulation. Excess synaptic dopamine is broken down via the enzymes COMT or MAO. D_2 antagonist antipsychotics bind to both presynaptic and postsynaptic D_2 receptors. Blocking dopamine on the presynaptic autoreceptor further disinhibits presynaptic dopamine release. To improve positive symptoms, D_2 antagonist antipsychotics must block 65%–80% of postsynaptic receptors. The three dopamine partial agonist antipsychotics require 80%–100% postsynaptic receptor occupancy for effective antipsychotic activity.

by activity at M_2 autoreceptors. Muscarinic M_4 receptor stimulating molecules (agonists or positive allosteric modulators) thus work presynaptically to reduce positive symptoms, yet they do so without D_2 receptor binding, and they act selectively, sparing motor areas from effects on dopamine neurotransmission.[33]

Muscarinic M_1 receptor activation also acts selectively to decrease presynaptic dopamine output, but the antipsychotic effect arises via modulation of the stimulatory glutamate signal that originates in the prefrontal cortex (PFC).[16] Glutamate signaling from the PFC is decreased by stimulating M_1 receptors on inhibitory GABA-ergic interneurons in the PFC. Increased activity of these GABA-ergic interneurons acts as a brake on glutamate outflow, with the net result seen as less glutamate stimulated dopamine release and less positive symptoms.[16] Stimulation of M_1 receptors is associated with gastrointestinal adverse effects, so xanomeline was subsequently combined with trospium, an anticholinergic medication that does not appreciably cross the blood–brain barrier and thus mitigates the procholinergic adverse effects of peripheral M_1 agonism without interfering with xanomeline's CNS mechanism.[15,34,35] Use of anticholinergics with extensive CNS penetration (e.g., benztropine, diphenhydramine) is strongly discouraged when treating patients with schizophrenia due to their deleterious cognitive effects,[36] but there is now another reason to eschew these agents: they will interfere with the action of muscarinic receptor stimulating antipsychotics.[37] On the basis of three positive trials, xanomeline-trospium received FDA approval on September 26, 2024, exactly 35 years after that for clozapine. Unlike the example of clozapine, xanomeline's mechanism is better understood and forms the basis for a new class of muscarinic receptor stimulating agents currently undergoing clinical trials for schizophrenia and other psychotic disorders.[16] The obvious advantage lies in the fact that their selective presynaptic mechanism reduces dopamine overactivity, but without the motor or endocrine adverse effects seen with D_2 receptor binding antipsychotics.[16] Moreover, the presynaptic mechanism provided by muscarinic receptor stimulating antipsychotics can work cooperatively with postsynaptic D_2 receptor blockade to lessen the impact of excessive dopamine signaling.[38] For that reason, clinicians and researchers who work in the field of schizophrenia are eagerly awaiting data from a randomized study of xanomeline-trospium or placebo added adjunctively to D_2 acting antipsychotics. This trial (A Study to Assess Efficacy and Safety of Adjunctive KarXT in Subjects With Inadequately Controlled Symptoms of Schizophrenia; NCT05145413) is due to report data in 2025.

Clozapine for TRS or schizophrenia with persistent aggression

One-third of patients living with schizophrenia are treatment resistant, and thus realize little to no positive symptom reduction from D_2 receptor modulation.[12] Imaging studies indicate that TRS is associated with relatively normal striatal dopamine synthesis, not the excessive presynaptic dopamine turnover and release typically associated with positive symptoms, thus explaining why these patients derive limited benefit from D_2 receptor blockade.[6] At least 40% of those with TRS will respond to clozapine, while response to other antipsychotics, even at high dosages, is typically <5%.[39,40] When imaged with proton magnetic resonance spectroscopy, response to clozapine in TRS patients is associated with reduction of the glutamate signal in the caudate, but the exact mechanism by which clozapine exerts this effect is not sufficiently characterized to the extent it has been replicated by other molecules.[18] Given the

high prevalence of TRS, use of clozapine becomes critical to competency restoration when persistent positive symptom severity impedes adjudication.[41]

Clozapine possesses another unique benefit – an effect on aggression that is independent of its impact on psychosis symptoms.[4] Multiple factors, especially substance misuse, underlie behaviors that bring patients with psychotic disorders into contact with the criminal justice system.[42] Poorly controlled positive symptoms are an important contributor to elevated violence risk in patients living with schizophrenia, so aggression remains a core target of antipsychotic therapy.[43] However, it should be noted that the most common form of interpersonal violence in forensic inpatient populations is not psychotically driven – it is impulsive aggression related to inadequate control over response to provocative stimuli.[5,42] A detailed analysis of 839 assaults among chronically aggressive state hospital patients noted that only 17% were motivated by psychosis (or mania), while 54% were impulsive, and the remaining 29% were planned or predatory in nature.[44] When persistent aggression or violence in schizophrenia patients is due to undertreated psychosis, the usual treatment algorithm is followed to address positive symptoms.[5] When aggressive behaviors in that patient population are impulsive, the most strongly evidence-based pharmacological intervention is clozapine.[4,5] A 2024 review of clozapine's anti-aggression effects found that this property existed for impulsive aggression in patients whose positive symptoms were adequately controlled.[4] One of the most compelling pieces of evidence was the findings from a prospective, double-blind trial of clozapine, olanzapine, and haloperidol in persistently aggressive male state hospital patients with modest levels of psychotic symptoms.[45,46] That study found clozapine superior to the other medications for acts of aggression, with no differences between the three medications on psychosis symptoms; moreover, clozapine's antiaggression effect was particularly evident in patients with greater baseline levels of cognitive dysfunction.[45,46]

Clozapine's treatment-related adverse effects and hematological monitoring requirements are a burden for patients with schizophrenia, and often dissuade clinicians from its use despite the absence of evidence-based options for TRS or persistent impulsive aggression.[17] As decades of research have failed to uncover the mix of receptor activities that result in its unparalleled effectiveness, it is incumbent that clinicians working with forensic populations develop expertise in prescribing clozapine.[47,48] As noted in the literature, the failure to prescribe clozapine to TRS patients or schizophrenia patients with persistent aggression is deemed to be below the standard of care as it deprives incarcerated patients of the fundamental right to effective treatment.[49,50]

Negative symptoms

The differential diagnosis of negative symptoms includes those which are inherent to the diagnosis of schizophrenia (i.e., primary) or those due to other causes such as depression, anxiety, or medication induced adverse effects.[51] It should be noted that antipsychotic trials of acutely exacerbated adult schizophrenia patients find negative symptom improvement, but the extent of this improvement is highly correlated with positive symptom reduction, a phenomenon known as pseudospecificity.[52-54] Stable, modestly symptomatic patients with persistent moderate/severe primary negative symptoms achieve limited negative symptom benefit from most antipsychotics.[51] Although the complex neurobiology of negative symptoms has thwarted attempts at developing approved agents, they remain an important treatment target given the high prevalence and associated disability. It is worth noting that the DPA cariprazine demonstrated comparative benefit on negative symptoms versus the D_2 receptor antagonist SGA risperidone in a 26-week randomized, double-blind, controlled trial (n = 461), with a modest effect size of 0.31.[55] Among the three DPAs, cariprazine possesses the highest affinity for the D_3 receptor, and it is the only one in this antipsychotic class effective as monotherapy for bipolar depression.[56,57] Although patients with moderate or severe depressive symptoms were excluded from that trial, it is unclear if cariprazine's negative symptom impact lies outside of its antidepressant mechanisms, or is an epiphenomenon of these receptor activities.

Cognitive dysfunction

Cognitive impairment associated with schizophrenia (CIAS) is a common and disabling feature of the disorder clinically recognized for over a century. It was the presence of prominent cognitive disturbance that led Emil Kraepelin to arrive at the term dementia praecox (premature dementia) for this psychotic disorder.[14] CIAS has two aspects in common with negative symptoms: (1) there can be secondary causes of cognitive dysfunction that must be addressed (e.g., benzodiazepines, CNS acting anticholinergics, sedatives) and (2) the complex neurobiology of CIAS and the heterogeneity of

symptoms has hindered progress in producing effective agents.[9] Nonetheless, ongoing studies continue to focus on this disabling feature of schizophrenia, with medications in clinical trials that work by stimulating N-methyl-D-aspartate (NMDA) glutamate receptors.[58,59] The underlying hypothesis driving development of these agents is that hypofunction of NMDA receptors residing on PFC GABA-ergic interneurons contributes to CIAS.[60] The NMDA receptor possesses a binding site for glutamate, and a co-agonist site that binds either glycine or D-serine.[61] The leading candidates stimulate the co-agonist site by one of two strategies: inhibiting glycine reuptake to increase synaptic levels of glycine (iclepertin), or inhibiting the metabolism of D-serine thereby increasing its synaptic levels (luvadaxistat).[58,59] Sadly, luvadaxistat failed to meet its primary endpoints in a second phase 2 study and further research was abandoned by the manufacturer.[62]

The discovery of xanomeline's antipsychotic properties not only opened new avenues for positive symptom control, it also refocused attention on one aspect of schizophrenia neurobiology that relates to CIAS, and which may be improved by xanomeline's M_1 receptor agonism: low muscarinic M_1 receptor expression.[63,64] Although initially noted in postmortem specimens,[64] subsequent imaging studies found modestly decreased M_1 receptor density in unmedicated antipsychotic naïve schizophrenia patients compared to age-matched peers without schizophrenia.[65] Further research noted that 25% of schizophrenia patients have ≥75% decreased M_1 receptor density, a subgroup referred to as having the muscarinic receptor deficit subgroup (MRDS).[64] Schizophrenia patients with MRDS show widespread decreases in cortical M_1 receptors, altered patterns of M_1 receptor gene promoter methylation, and lower levels of muscarinic M_1 receptor mRNA compared to controls.[65] Notably, non-MRDS patients with schizophrenia do not differ in these measures from control individuals. Not surprisingly, lower levels of muscarinic M_1 receptor expression are associated with poorer performance in verbal learning and memory and more severe negative symptoms in medication free psychotic patients.[65]

Since any pool of schizophrenia patients possessing severe cognitive deficits would be enriched with those having MRDS, the hypothesis that xanomeline's M_1 receptor stimulation might improve CIAS was explored as a secondary outcome measure in clinical trials.[66] Neuroimaging for low M_1 expression was not possible, but analysis of the double-blind phase 2b

Table 6.2 Xanomeline-trospium treatment effect on cognitive performance by baseline impairment in a double-blind, placebo-controlled phase 2b trial[a] [66]

		LS mean change from baseline at day 35		
	Treatment arm	Estimate (SE)	*p* Value	Cohen's *d*
Minimally impaired	KarXT (n = 34)	−0.18 (0.13)	0.19	0.22
	Placebo (n = 65)	−0.22 (0.15)	0.15	0.28
	KarXT vs. placebo	0.04 (0.16)	0.79	0.05
Impaired	KarXT (n = 23)	0.57 (0.19)	**0.01**	**0.61**
	Placebo (n = 37)	0.07 (0.13)	0.59	0.09
	KarXT vs. placebo	0.50 (0.22)	**0.03**	**0.50**

Least squares (LS) means and *p* values are derived from post hoc analysis of covariance (ANCOVA) models, with covariates of site, gender, age, and baseline performance.

[a] For this exploratory analysis, individuals with a high degree of test subdomain intraindividual variability were removed as this is typically reflective of noncompliance with test procedures or otherwise invalid data.

study found differential cognitive benefits from xanomeline stratified by level of impairment.[66] As seen in Table 6.2, the cognitive impact of xanomeline devolved only to the subgroup with clinically significant cognitive impairment (defined as a baseline composite cognitive battery score more than one standard deviation below the normative mean).[66] This finding of cognitive benefit in cognitively impaired patients, presumably from xanomeline's M_1 activity, aligns with the concept that more severe forms of CIAS are associated with MRDS, while schizophrenia patients with limited cognitive dysfunction likely have CNS M_1 expression and activity closer to the norm. Importantly, the association of xanomeline treatment with improved cognitive function in impaired patients was replicated in exploratory analyses from the two phase three studies.[67] These positive results represent the first breakthrough in CIAS treatment, findings that should be particularly noteworthy to the field of forensic psychiatry. For schizophrenia patients who are not treatment resistant but whose level of cognitive dysfunction remains an impediment to competency restoration, xanomeline may offer potential hope to address CIAS symptoms that interfere with mastery of court material and effective interaction with attorneys and other court personnel.

positive symptom reduction. Yet 2024 saw a revolution in positive symptom treatment, providing clinicians two means to manage the consequences of presynaptic dopamine overactivity: blocking dopamine from binding to postsynaptic dopamine D_2 receptors, or reducing presynaptic dopamine release by stimulation of muscarinic M_1 and M_4 receptors. Importantly, muscarinic receptor stimulation not only avoids the motor and endocrine adverse effects of nonselective D_2 blockade, clinical trials of xanomeline-trospium noted cognitive benefits among patients with significant levels of cognitive dysfunction. The promise of cognitive improvement had not been realized previously and hopefully diminishes the level of clinical nihilism when confronted with this important problem. Despite these advances, clozapine remains the only effective medication for resistant schizophrenia or schizophrenia patients with persistent impulsive aggression, and its complex interplay of pharmacological activities has defied replication in molecules with improved tolerability. Given the absence of other effective options for TRS or persistent impulsive aggression, all clinicians who treat patients with schizophrenia must be adept at using clozapine – it is the standard of care.

Conclusion

Despite the disability resulting from negative symptoms and cognitive dysfunction, the clinical effect of antipsychotics was historically dependent on D_2 receptor blockade and the benefit largely confined to

References

1. Marder SR, Cannon TD. Schizophrenia. *N Engl J Med.* 2019;**381**(18): 1753–1761. doi:10.1056/NEJMra1808803

2. Siddiqui S, Mehta D, Coles A, et al. Psychosocial interventions for individuals with comorbid psychosis and substance use disorders: systematic review and meta-analysis of randomized studies. *Schizophr Bull.* 2024;doi:10.1093/schbul/sbae101

3. Ceskova E. Pharmacological strategies for the management of comorbid depression and schizophrenia. *Expert Opin Pharmacother.* 2020;**21**(4): 459–465. doi:10.1080/ 14656566.2020.1717466

4. Faden J, Citrome L. A systematic review of clozapine for aggression and violence in patients with schizophrenia or schizoaffective disorder. *Schizophr Res.* 2024;**268**:265–281. doi:10.1016/ j.schres.2023.11.008

5. Meyer JM, Cummings MA, Proctor G, Stahl SM. Psychopharmacology of persistent violence and aggression. *Psychiatr Clin North Am.* 2016;**39**(4): 541–556.

6. Egerton A, Murphy A, Donocik J, et al. Dopamine and glutamate in antipsychotic-responsive compared with antipsychotic-nonresponsive psychosis: a multicenter positron emission tomography and magnetic resonance spectroscopy study (STRATA). *Schizophr Bull.* 2021;**47**(2): 505–516. doi:10.1093/schbul/sbaa128

7. Iasevoli F, Avagliano C, D'Ambrosio L, et al. Dopamine dynamics and neurobiology of non-response to antipsychotics, relevance for treatment resistant schizophrenia: a systematic review and critical appraisal. *Biomedicines.* 2023;**11**(3): 895. doi:10.3390/biomedicines11030895

8. McCutcheon RA, Weber LAE, Nour MM, Cragg SJ, McGuire PM. Psychosis as a disorder of muscarinic signalling: psychopathology and pharmacology. *Lancet Psychiatry.* 2024;**11**(7):554–565. doi:10.1016/S2215-0366(24)00100-7

9. Howes OD, Bukala BR, Beck K. Schizophrenia: from neurochemistry to circuits, symptoms and treatments. *Nat Rev Neurol.* 2024;**20**(1):22–35. doi:10.1038/ s41582-023-00904-0

10. Kantrowitz JT, Correll CU, Jain R, Cutler AJ. New developments in the treatment of schizophrenia: an expert roundtable. *Int J Neuropsychopharmacol.* 2023;**26**(5): 322–330. doi:10.1093/ijnp/pyad011

11. Howes OD, Dawkins E, Lobo MC, Kaar SJ, Beck K. New drug treatments for schizophrenia: a review of approaches to target circuit dysfunction. *Biol Psychiatry.* 2024;**96**(8):638–650. doi:10.1016/j .biopsych.2024.05.014

12. Howes OD, McCutcheon R, Agid O, et al. Treatment-resistant schizophrenia: Treatment Response and Resistance in Psychosis (TRRIP) working group consensus guidelines on diagnosis and terminology.

Am J Psychiatry. 2017;**174**(3):216–229. doi:10.1176/ appi.ajp.2016.16050503

13. McCutcheon RA, Abi-Dargham A, Howes OD. Schizophrenia, dopamine and the striatum: from biology to symptoms. *Trends Neurosci.* 2019;**42**(3): 205–220. doi:10.1016/j.tins.2018.12.004

14. Meyer JM. Pharmacotherapy of psychosis and mania. In: Brunton LL, ed. *Goodman & Gilman's The Pharmacological Basis of Therapeutics*, 14th ed. McGraw-Hill; 2022:357–384.

15. Kaul I, Sawchak S, Walling DP, et al. Efficacy and safety of xanomelinetrospium chloride in schizophrenia: a randomized clinical trial. *JAMA Psychiatry.* 2024;**81** (8):749–756. doi:10.1001/jamapsychiatry.2024.0785

16. Paul SM, Yohn SE, Brannan SK, Neugebauer NM, Breier A. Muscarinic receptor activators as novel treatments for schizophrenia. *Biol Psychiatry.* 2024;**96** (8):627–637. doi:10.1016/j.biopsych.2024.03.014

17. Meyer JM, Stahl SM. *The Clozapine Handbook—Stahl's Handbooks.* Cambridge University Press; 2019:317.

18. McQueen G, Sendt KV, Gillespie A, et al. Changes in brain glutamate on switching to clozapine in treatment-resistant schizophrenia. *Schizophr Bull.* 2021;**47**(3):662–671. doi:10.1093/schbul/sbaa156

19. Bleuler M, Stoll WA. Clinical use of reserpine in psychiatry: comparison with chlorpromazine. *Ann N Y Acad Sci.* 1955;**61**(1):167–173. doi:10.1111/ j.1749-6632.1955.tb42463.x

20. Lopez-Munoz F, Alamo C, Cuenca E, et al. History of the discovery and clinical introduction of chlorpromazine. *Ann Clin Psychiatry* 2005;**17** (3):113–135. doi:10.1080/10401230591002002

21. Carlsson A, Lindqvist M. Effect of chlorpromazine or haloperidol on formation of 3-methoxytyramine and normetanephrine in mouse brain. *Acta Pharmacol Toxicol (Copenh).* 1963;**20**:140–144. doi:10.1111/ j.16000773.1963.tb01730.x

22. Quinn GP, Shore PA, Brodie BB. Biochemical and pharmacological studies of RO 1-9569 (tetrabenazine), a nonindole tranquilizing agent with reserpine-like effects. *J Pharmacol Exp Ther.* 1959;**127**(1):103–109.

23. Smith ME. Clinical comparison of tetrabenazine (Ro 1-9569), reserpine and placebo in chronic schizophrenics. *Dis Nerv Syst.* 1960;**21**(3 Suppl):120–123.

24. Ashcroft GW, Macdougall EJ, Barker PA. A comparison of tetrabenazine and chlorpromazine in chronic schizophrenia. *J Ment Sci.* 1961;**107**: 287–93. doi:10.1192/bjp.107.447.287

25. Janssen PA. The evolution of the butyrophenones, haloperidol and trifluperidol, from meperidine-like 4-phenylpiperidines. *Int Rev Neurobiol.* 1965;**8**:221–263. doi:10.1016/s0074-7742(08)60759-x

26. Huhn M, Nikolakopoulou A, Schneider-Thoma J, et al. Comparative efficacy and tolerability of 32 oral antipsychotics for the acute treatment of adults with multi-episode schizophrenia: a systematic review and network meta-analysis. *The Lancet.* 2019;**394** (10202):939–951. doi:10.1016/ s0140-6736(19)31135-3

27. Kapur S, Zipursky R, Jones C, Remington G, Houle S. Relationship between dopamine D(2) occupancy, clinical response, and side effects: a double-blind PET study of first-episode schizophrenia. *Am J Psychiatry.* 2000;**157**(4):514–520.

28. Bubser M, Backstrom JR, Sanders-Bush E, Roth BL, Deutch AY. Distribution of serotonin 5-HT(2A) receptors in afferents of the rat striatum. *Synapse.* 2001;**39**(4):297–304. doi:10.1002/1098-2396(20010315)39:4<29 7::Aid-syn1012>3.0.Co;2-q

29. Navailles S, De Deurwaerdère P. Presynaptic control of serotonin on striatal dopamine function. *Psychopharmacology (Berl).* 2011;**213**(2–3):213–242. doi:10.1007/s00213-010-2029-y

30. Dibonaventura M, Gabriel S, Dupclay L, Gupta S, Kim E. A patient perspective of the impact of medication side effects on adherence: results of a cross-sectional nationwide survey of patients with schizophrenia. *BMC Psychiatry.* 2012;**12**:20. doi:10.1186/1471-244x-12-20

31. Castellani LN, Pereira S, Kowalchuk C, et al. Antipsychotics impair regulation of glucose metabolism by central glucose. *Mol Psychiatry.* 2022;**27** (11):4741–4753. doi:10.1038/s41380-022-01798-y

32. Bodick NC, Offen WW, Levey AI, et al. Effects of xanomeline, a selective muscarinic receptor agonist, on cognitive function and behavioral symptoms in Alzheimer disease. *Arch Neurol.* 1997;**54**(4):465–473. doi:10.1001/ archneur.1997.00550160091022

33. Yohn SE, Weiden PW, Felder CC, Stahl SM. Muscarinic acetylcholine receptors for psychotic disorders: bench-side to clinic. *Trends Pharmacol Sci.* 2022;**43**(12):1098–1112. doi:10.1016/j.tips.2022.09.006

34. Brannan SK, Sawchak S, Miller AC, et al. Muscarinic cholinergic receptor agonist and peripheral antagonist for schizophrenia. *N Engl J Med.* 2021;**384**(8):717–726. doi:10.1056/NEJMoa2017015

35. Kaul I, Sawchak S, Correll CU, et al. Efficacy and safety of the muscarinic receptor agonist KarXT (xanomeline-trospium) in schizophrenia (EMERGENT-2) in the USA: results from a randomised, double-blind, placebo-controlled, flexible-dose phase 3 trial. *Lancet.* 2024;**403** (10422):160–170. doi:10.1016/s0140-6736(23)02190-6

36. Joshi YB, Thomas ML, Braff DL, et al. Anticholinergic medication burden-associated cognitive impairment in schizophrenia. *Am J Psychiatry.* 2021;**178** (9):838–847. doi:10.1176/appi.ajp.2020.20081212

37. Barak S, Weiner I. The M$_1$/M$_4$ preferring agonist xanomeline reverses amphetamine-, MK801- and scopolamine-induced abnormalities of latent inhibition: putative efficacy against positive, negative and cognitive symptoms in schizophrenia. *Int J Neuropsychopharmacol.* 2011;**14**(9):1233–1246. doi:10.1017/s1461145710001549

38. Kinon BJ, Leucht S, Tamminga C, et al. Rationale for adjunctive treatment targeting multiple mechanisms in schizophrenia. *J Clin Psychiatry.* 2024;**85**(3):23nr15240. doi:10.4088/JCP .23nr15240

39. Kane J, Honigfeld G, Singer J, Meltzer H. Clozapine for the treatment-resistant schizophrenic. A double-blind comparison with chlorpromazine. *Arch Gen Psychiatry.* 1988;**45**(9):789–796.

40. Siskind D, Siskind V, Kisely S. Clozapine response rates among people with treatment-resistant schizophrenia: data from a systematic review and metaanalysis. *Can J Psychiatry.* 2017;**62**(11): 772–777. doi:10.1177/07067437 177 18167

41. Singh A, Delgado D, Ventura MI, et al. Clozapine use and forensic outcomes in psychiatric inpatients deemed incompetent to stand trial. *J Am Acad Psychiatry Law.* 2022;**50**(3):427–433. doi:10.29158/ jaapl.210123-21

42. Lambe S, Cooper K, Fazel S, Freeman D. Psychological framework to understand interpersonal violence by forensic patients with psychosis. *Br J Psychiatry.* 2024;**224**(2):47–54. doi:10.1192/bjp.2023.132

43. Whiting D, Gulati G, Geddes JR, Dean K, Fazel S. Violence in schizophrenia: triangulating the evidence on perpetration risk. *World Psychiatry.* 2024; **23** (1):158–160. doi:10.1002/wps.21171

44. Quanbeck CD, McDermott BE, Lam J, et al. Categorization of aggressive acts committed by chronically assaultive state hospital patients. *Psychiatr Serv.* 2007;**58**(4):521–528. doi:10.1176/appi. ps.58.4.521

45. Krakowski MI, Czobor P, Citrome L, Bark N, Cooper TB. Atypical antipsychotic agents in the treatment of violent patients with schizophrenia and schizoaffective disorder. *Arch Gen Psychiatry.* 2006;**63** (6):622–629.

46. Krakowski MI, Czobor P. Executive function predicts response to antiaggression treatment in schizophrenia: a randomized controlled trial. *J Clin Psychiatry.* 2012;**73**(1):74–80. doi:10.4088/JCP.11m07238

47. Tibrewal P, Nair PC, Gregory KJ, et al. Does clozapine treat antipsychotic-induced behavioural supersensitivity through glutamate modulation within the striatum? *Mol Psychiatry.* 2023; **28**(5):1839–1842. doi:10.1038/s41380-023-02026-x

48. Naguy A, Alhazeem H. Clozapine prescripers – dogmatic or pragmatic? *Psychopharmacol Bull*. 2024;**54** (2):46–50.

49. Zarzar TR, Williams JB, Pruette ME, Sheitman BB. A legal right to clozapine therapy for incarcerated individuals with treatment-resistant schizophrenia. *Psychiatr Serv*. 2021;**72**(4):482–484. doi:10.1176/appi .ps.202000845

50. Zarzar TR. Clozapine proficiency as a milestone in psychiatric training. *JAMA Psychiatry*. 2024;**81** (7):639–640. doi:10.1001/jamapsychiatry.2024.0702

51. Correll CU, Schooler NR. Negative symptoms in schizophrenia: a review and clinical guide for recognition, assessment, and treatment. *Neuropsychiatr Dis Treat*. 2020;**16**:519–534. doi:10.2147/NDT.S225643

52. Hopkins SC, Ogirala A, Loebel A, Koblan KS. Understanding antipsychotic drug treatment effects: a novel method to reduce pseudospecificity of the positive and negative syndrome scale (PANSS) factors. *Innov Clin Neurosci*. 2017;**14**(11–12):54–58.

53. Hopkins SC, Ogirala A, Loebel A, Koblan KS. Transformed PANSS factors intended to reduce pseudospecificity among symptom domains and enhance understanding of symptom change in antipsychotic-treated patients with schizophrenia. *Schizophr Bull*. 2018;**44**(3):593–602. doi:10.1093/schbul/ sbx101

54. Hopkins SC, Ogirala A, Loebel A, Koblan KS. Characterization of specific and distinct patient types in clinical trials of acute schizophrenia using an uncorrelated PANSS score matrix transform (UPSM). *Psychiatry Res*. 2020;**294**:113569. doi:10.1016/j .psychres.2020.113569

55. Nemeth G, Laszlovszky I, Czobor P, et al. Cariprazine versus risperidone monotherapy for treatment of predominant negative symptoms in patients with schizophrenia: a randomised, double-blind, controlled trial. *Lancet*. 2017;**389**(10074):1103–1113. doi:10.1016/ S0140-6736(17)30060-0

56. Girgis RR, Slifstein M, D'Souza D, et al. Preferential binding to dopamine D_3 over D_2 receptors by cariprazine in patients with schizophrenia using PET with the D_3/D_2 receptor ligand $[^{11}C]$-(+)-PHNO. *Psychopharmacology (Berl)*. 2016;**233**(19– 20):3503–3512. doi:10.1007/s00213-016-4382-y

57. Stahl SM. Mechanism of action of cariprazine. *CNS Spectr*. 2016;**21**(2):123–127. doi:10.1017/ s1092852916000043

58. Rosenbrock H, Desch M, Wunderlich G. Development of the novel GlyT1 inhibitor, iclepertin (BI 425809), for the treatment of cognitive impairment associated with schizophrenia. *Eur Arch Psychiatry Clin Neurosci*. 2023;**273**(7):1557–1566. doi:10.1007/s00406 -023-01576-z

59. Murthy V, Hanson E, DeMartinis N, et al. INTERACT: a randomized phase 2 study of the DAAO inhibitor luvadaxistat in adults with schizophrenia. *Schizophr Res*. 2024;**270**:249–257. doi:10.1016/j .schres.2024.06.017

60. Tamminga CA. The neurobiology of cognition in schizophrenia. *J Clin Psychiatry*. 2006;**67**(Suppl 9):9–13; discussion 36–42.

61. Peng A, Chai J, Wu H, et al. New therapeutic targets and drugs for schizophrenia beyond dopamine D_2 receptor antagonists. *Neuropsychiatr Dis Treat*. 2024;**20**:607–620. doi:10.2147/ndt.S455279

62. Neurocrine Biosciences Inc. Neurocrine Biosciences provides update on ERUDITE™ phase 2 data for luvadaxistat in adults with cognitive impairment associated with schizophrenia. www.neurocrine.com/ our-company/news-and-media/news/neurocrine-bio sciences-provides-update-on-erudite-phase-2-data-fo r-luvadaxistat-in-adults-with-cognitive-impairment-a ssociated-with-schizophrenia/. Accessed September 12, 2024.

63. Gibbons AS, Scarr E, Boer S, et al. Widespread decreases in cortical muscarinic receptors in a subset of people with schizophrenia. *Int J Neuropsychopharmacol*. 2013;**16**(1):37–46. doi:10.1017/s1461145712000028

64. Dean B, Haroutunian V, Scarr E. Lower levels of cortical [3H]pirenzepine binding to postmortem tissue defines a sub-group of older people with schizophrenia with less severe cognitive deficits. *Schizophr Res*. 2023;**255**:274–282. doi:10.1016/j.schres.2023.03.035

65. Dean B, Scarr E. Muscarinic M_1 and M_4 receptors: hypothesis driven drug development for schizophrenia. *Psychiatry Res*. 2020;**288**:112989. doi:10.1016/j.psychres.2020.112989

66. Sauder C, Allen LA, Baker E, et al. Effectiveness of KarXT (xanomeline-trospium) for cognitive impairment in schizophrenia: post hoc analyses from a randomised, double-blind, placebo-controlled phase 2 study. *Transl Psychiatry*. 2022;**12**(1):491. doi:10.1038/s41398-022- 02254-9

67. Horan W, Sauder C, Harvey PD, et al. The impact of KarXT on cognitive impairment in acute schizophrenia: replication in pooled data from phase 3 trials. *Poster 88 presented at the 2024 Annual Congress of the Schizophrenia International Research Society, 3– 7 April 2024, Florence, Italy*; 2024.

Do Antipsychotics Work in People with Schizophrenia?

A Review of Outcomes and Effect Sizes

Christoph U. Correll

Introduction

Schizophrenia is a severe and still very often chronic mental disorder that can profoundly affect a person's thoughts, feelings, and behaviors.[1] Schizophrenia impacts approximately 20 million people worldwide[2] and often begins in late adolescence or early adulthood.[3] Schizophrenia is characterized by a constellation of positive symptoms (hallucinations, delusions, disorganized thinking or behaviors), negative symptoms (anhedonia, avolition, amotivation, affective flattening, alogia) cognitive dysfunction (attention, memory, speed of processing, executive functioning, social cognition), and often also mood symptoms.[1] Without effective treatment, schizophrenia leads to substantial disability, repeated hospitalizations, social isolation, homelessness, and a 5–10% lifetime suicide risk.[1,4]

While the causes of schizophrenia are multifactorial and still only insufficiently understood, spanning genetic, neurodevelopmental, and environmental factors,[5,6] the effective management of schizophrenia depends critically on early, sustained, and evidence-based pharmacological, psychoeducational, psychological, and psychosocial interventions.[7–10] Among these, antipsychotics remain the cornerstone for people diagnosed with schizophrenia.[4] It is important, though, not to confuse the outcomes and treatment needs of people living with schizophrenia with those of people diagnosed with other types of psychotic disorders, including the very heterogeneous group of "first-episode psychosis," which is a mixture of disorders with varying outcomes both with and without antipsychotic treatment.[4,11]

However, antipsychotic medications are frequently the subject of public criticism and activist skepticism. Critics often cite modest trial results in moderately ill patients, high nonresponse rates, and substantial side effects to argue that antipsychotics "don't work."

This chapter provides a different view from this negative narrative, with a comprehensive, accessible, and data-driven synthesis of the evidence. Drawing on relevant meta-analyses, the concept of effect sizes, and real-world outcome data – including competency restoration, suicide reduction, and relapse prevention – and by comparing outcomes of antipsychotics with those of commonly used medications to treat chronic medical disorders, this chapter highlights that antipsychotics are among the most effective interventions in medicine for chronic illnesses.

On the other hand, gaps in antipsychotic efficacy clearly remain.[12] These gaps include limited efficacy of current antipsychotics for negative symptoms and cognitive dysfunction, as well as residual and resistant positive symptoms despite adherence to currently available antipsychotics, as well as reward dysfunction and comorbid substance use disorders. Furthermore, although more recently approved antipsychotics have been shown to be safer and better tolerated, antipsychotics do have varying degrees of adverse effects,[13] which can limit functionality and decrease quality of life.[14] Moreover, treatment resistance rates are about 20% in patients with first-episode schizophrenia and 40% in patients with multiepisode schizophrenia.[15] Finally, recovery rates remain small, being about 22% in patients with first-episode schizophrenia[16] and 11% in patients with multiepisode schizophrenia,[17] and, by themselves, antipsychotics cannot help people find friends, romantic partners, or jobs, as there are "no skills in pills." However, through treatment-related symptomatic stability, antipsychotics can enable people living with schizophrenia to take fuller advantage of psychological, psychosocial, and supported education and employment interventions to help them achieve their life goals.[18]

Taken together, this chapter rebuts held opinions that antipsychotics "don't work" through an evaluation of meta-analyses, clinical trial data, and real-world effectiveness studies, showing that antipsychotics not only work comparably to – or better than – many standard treatments used in general medicine, but also are essential to improving both symptoms and long-term outcomes in people living with schizophrenia.

Mechanism of action and balancing benefits and risks

Antipsychotic medications primarily act by modulating dopaminergic transmission, particularly through antagonism or partial agonism of postsynaptic D_2 dopamine receptors in the associative striatum pathway, and this is thought to underlie the positive symptoms of schizophrenia.[19,20] However, the pharmacology of these drugs is far more nuanced. While first-generation antipsychotics (FGAs) predominantly block postsynaptic dopamine receptors, many second-generation antipsychotics (SGAs) also interact with serotonin (5-HT$_{2A}$), histamine (H$_1$), adrenergic (α1) and cholinergic receptors.[19] Clozapine, in particular, exhibits a unique receptor profile[21] and remains the gold standard for treatment-resistant schizophrenia.[22]

FGAs can effectively reduce positive symptoms but are often associated with neuromotor side effects. SGAs have broader receptor activity with improved tolerability, but some have relevant cardiometabolic risks, including weight gain and glucose and lipid abnormalities.[23] Long-acting injectable antipsychotics (LAIs) have emerged as a valuable strategy to address the challenge of nonadherence – a major contributor to relapse – by providing sustained drug release and improving treatment continuity.[24,25] Meta-analyses across different study designs, including randomized controlled trials, cohort studies, and pre–post or mirror-image studies, have demonstrated 8–56% reductions in relapse/hospitalization rates with LAIs compared to oral formulations,[26] with particular superiority in real-world studies and those using patients as their own controls.[26,27] Despite these benefits, underutilization of LAIs persists due to clinician hesitancy and perceived patient resistance.[25,28]

Nevertheless, both acute and long-term adverse effects are a real concern.[13] FGAs, especially high-potency FGAs, such as haloperidol, are associated with considerable rates of neuromotor side effects, such as acute dystonia, parkinsonism, akathisia, and tardive dyskinesia.[29–32] SGAs tend to have more favorable neuromotor profiles but pose cardiometabolic risks, including weight gain, insulin resistance, and dyslipidemia, as well as metabolic syndrome,[33,34] each of which being a risk factor for cardiovascular illness, the most common cause of mortality in people with schizophrenia.[35] Both some FGAs and some SGAs are associated with prolactin elevation and related sexual dysfunction,[36] as well as a possible increased risk for breast cancer.[37,38]

Strategies to mitigate these risks include selecting or switching to agents with lower cardiometabolic (e.g., aripiprazole, brexpiprazole, cariprazine, lumateperone, lurasidone, ziprasidone)[39,40] or other side-effect burdens, using the lowest effective dose,[41,42] monitoring cardiometabolic parameters regularly, using treatments targeting metabolic syndrome parameters,[43–45] and incorporating lifestyle interventions.[39] LAIs can also help maintain therapeutic levels while reducing the peak–trough fluctuations that contribute to side effects.[46]

Efficacy and effect sizes: How well do antipsychotics work?

Importantly, however, the benefits of antipsychotic treatment overall outweigh the risks considerably when viewed generally from an individual and population health perspective.[4] Moreover, premature discontinuation of treatment – often driven by challenges with illness insight and/or insufficiently managed adverse effect burdens – is a major driver of relapse, hospitalization, and suicide risk.[47]

Benefits and harms of treatments in medicine are most meaningfully quantified using statistical measures called "effect sizes." These metrics provide a standardized way to compare the magnitude of a treatment's efficacy or effectiveness or adverse effect risk across different medications, studies, and even conditions.[48] The most widely used effect size in psychiatry for continuous outcomes, such as changes in symptoms or blood test measures, is the standardized mean difference (SMD).[49] The SMD is typically reported as Cohen's d effect size, whereby the number above or below 0 (i.e., no difference) indicates the magnitude of either the increase or decrease in the value, respectively, compared to a control condition or to baseline when comparing outcomes within a treatment group. By convention, an effect size of 0.2 is considered small, of 0.5 is considered medium, and of 0.8 and above is considered large.[49] The advantage of SMDs over weighted mean differences (WMDs), which can only be calculated for studies using the exact same rating scale, is that effects can be pooled across different rating instruments, as the difference between the groups is expressed as the amount of standard deviation units, which can be added and for which mean values can be calculated.

For the continuous outcome of time to event (e.g., time until relapse), hazard ratios (HRs) are typically used, whereby the decimal value above or below 1 (i.e., no difference) indicates the percentage risk that is increased or decreased, respectively, compared to a control condition. For categorical outcomes, such as response, remission, recovery, or relapse, the absolute experimental event rate (EER) is compared with the control event rate (CER), resulting in relative effect size measures, such as odds ratios (ORs) or risk ratios (RRs).[48] The advantage of RRs is that they can be converted into a risk difference (RD) and then to either the number needed to treat (NNT) for benefits or the number needed to harm (NNH) for negative effects, whereby the resultant full number represents the number of people one needs to expose to the experimental agents to get one additional good (i.e., NNT) or one additional bad (i.e., NNH) outcome compared to the control condition.

When examining the question of whether or not antipsychotics work, these metrics provide a powerful and interpretable comparative evidence base, which can demonstrate that antipsychotics not only work, but are even among the most effective pharmacologic treatments in medicine. Clearly, not everyone improves when taking such drugs, and antipsychotics are also associated with adverse effects that can be bothersome or even dangerous, but this is also a reality for common medications used in somatic medicine.

In a review of meta-analytic results of anti-psychotic efficacy, Leucht et al. compared these results using 13 different effect size measures.[48] The authors examined mean difference (MD), SMD, NNT derived from SMD, OR, RR, and RD derived from SMD, as well as drug response and placebo response in percentages. Applying these indices to meta-analyses comparing antipsychotic drugs with placebo for acute schizophrenia, the authors reported a difference of all antipsychotics pooled versus placebo (105 trials, n = 22,741 participants) of MD 9.4 (95% confidence interval (CI) = 8.4–10.2) Positive and Negative Syndrome Scale (PANSS) total points, SMD: 0.47 (95% CI = 0.42–0.51), NNT: 5

(95% CI = 5–6), OR: 2.34 (95% CI = 2.14–2.52), RR: 1.67 (95% CI = 1.59–1.73), RD: 20% (95% CI = 18–22), and proportion of patients improved on drug: 50% (95% CI = 48–52) compared to proportion of patients improved on placebo: 30%. Taken together, these indices, plus others that are less often used in publications, indicated a substantial but not a large superiority of anti-psychotics versus placebo. The authors noted that the chronicity of the patients in most of the trials should be considered, as people with first-episode and early-phase illness may experience better anti-psychotic response.[50,51]

These effect sizes become more powerful when contextualized across medical disciplines and their drug classes. In a review of results from 94 meta-analyses, including 48 drugs used in 20 medical diseases and 16 drugs used in 8 psychiatric disorders, Leucht et al.[52] observed that while some general medical drugs clearly had greater effect sizes than psychotropic medications, the psychiatric drugs were not generally less efficacious than the general medical drugs. This finding was subsequently confirmed.[53] Looking specifically at antipsychotics for people with schizophrenia, the effect size for the improvement of total psychopathology in patients with an acute exacerbation of schizophrenia was SMD = 0.43 versus placebo, which was similar to the median effect size across all medical drugs examined.[52] However, while acute symptom reduction is critical, the long-term effectiveness of anti-psychotics is even more compelling. One of the most replicated findings in psychiatric research is that sustained antipsychotic treatment substantially reduces the risk of relapse in patients with schizophrenia. Thus, when patients responding to anti-psychotics were continued on the same antipsychotic or discontinued, the effect size more than doubled from SMD = 0.43 to a RR-derived SMD = 0.92 for relapse prevention (Figure 7.1).[52] This difference in relapse rates, which was not related to the speed of antipsychotic discontinuation,[54] trans-lated into a NNT of 3, with NNTs < 10 being gener-ally clinically relevant and ≤ 5 being strongly clinically relevant.[55]

When comparing the meta-analytic efficacy of medical drugs for the prevention of a negative medical outcome with the NNT of 3 for the prevention of relapse with antipsychotics, it becomes evident that the effect size for antipsychotics in schizophrenia is

Table 7.1 Efficacy of antipsychotics and common medical medications in preventing a negative outcome

Treatment	Studies	Patients	Outcome	PBO	Drug	ARD	NNT[a]	SMD[b]
Antipsychotics[c]	62	6,392	Schizophrenia relapse	57.0%	22.0%	38.0%	3	0.92
Statins[d]	14	90,056	Major CVD event	18.0%	14.0%	4.0%	25	0.15
ACE inhibitors[d]	5	18,229	CVD events	18.0%	14.0%	4.0%	25	0.16
Metformin[d]	11	12,840	Type 2 diabetes mellitus mortality	6.0%	2.7%	2.3%	31	0.03
Aspirin[d]	16	17,000	Secondary prevention of severe CVD events	8.2%	6.7%	1.5%	67	0.12

[a] Smaller number indicates greater medication efficacy.

[b] Larger number indicates greater medication efficacy.

[c] Based on Leucht et al. (2012).[52]

[d] Based on Leucht et al. (2015).[53]

ACE = angiotensin-converting enzyme; ARD = absolute risk difference; CVD = cardiovascular disease; NNT = number needed to treat; SMD = standardized mean difference.

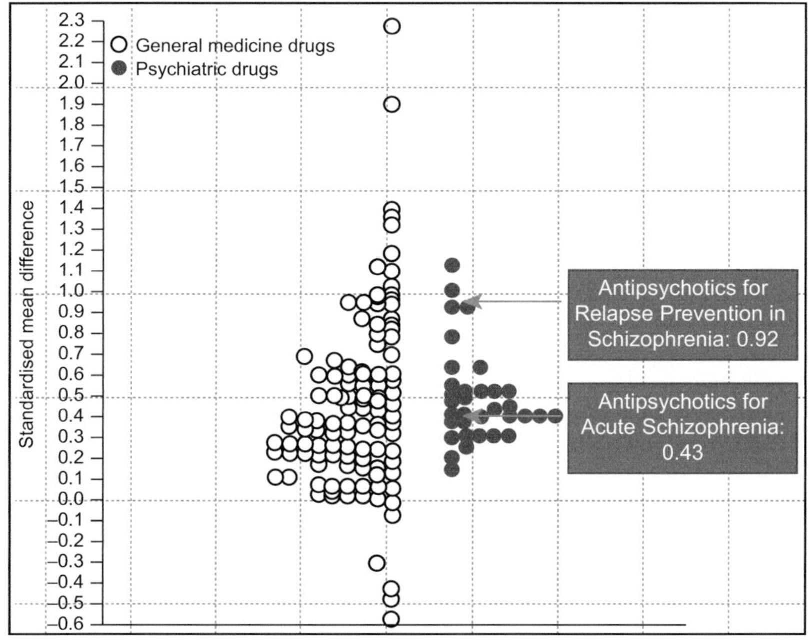

Figure 7.1 Standardized effect sizes for the efficacy of psychiatric and general medical drug treatments versus placebo

Adapted from Leucht et al. (2012).[52]

10–20-fold greater (with smaller NNTs indicating greater efficacy; Table 7.1).[52] Specifically, the NNT for prevention of a major cardiovascular disease event with statins and angiotensin-converting enzyme (ACE) inhibitors was 25, and the NNT for the same effect was 67 for aspirin. Similarly, the preventive effect for mortality in type 2 diabetes with metformin was NNT = 31. In addition to antipsychotics having a stronger preventive effect relative to placebo, in absolute numbers more patients with such conditions have relapse as the targeted negative outcome prevented with antipsychotics. This advantage in absolute numbers is due to the fact that negative cardiovascular and mortality events were relatively less frequent (6–18% on placebo versus 2.7–14% on the drug) than schizophrenia relapses (57% on placebo versus 22% on antipsychotics; Table 7.1).

Beyond symptoms, treatment persistence, and relapse prevention

However, the benefits of antipsychotics extend beyond acute symptom improvement, maintenance of the effect, and prevention of relapses or hospitalizations. While acute symptom reduction is a basic need and the long-term effectiveness of antipsychotics is critical, functional outcomes and beneficial effects on longevity are even more compelling.

In a nationwide Swedish database study using a within-subject design, the risk of sickness absence or of receiving disability pension during antipsychotic use was compared with antipsychotic non-use during a maximum of 11 years of follow-up.[56] Among the cohort of patients with first-episode non-affective psychosis (n = 21,551; age range: 16–45 years), 45.9% had work disability during the median length of follow-up of 4.8 years. Altogether, the risk of work disability was significantly lower during use compared with nonuse of any antipsychotic (adjusted HR [aHR] = 0.65, 95% CI = 0.59–0.72), with the greatest benefit observed for LAIs (aHR = 0.46, 95% CI = 0.34–0.62). aHRs were similar during the periods of <2 years, 2–5 years, and >5 years since diagnosis, indicating that ongoing antipsychotic treatment was associated with approximately 30–50% lower risk of work disability versus nonuse of antipsychotics in the same individuals, which held true even beyond 5 years after first diagnosis, being highly important for the promotion of functional recovery.

Additional real-world evidence supports improvements in functioning and legal outcomes. A recent study of 3,166 adults (mean age: 38.6 ± 12.6 years), 76.5% with schizophrenia spectrum disorders in California's forensic state hospital system who were deemed Incompetent to Stand Trial, showed that as many as 86.5% of them were successfully restored to competency, with 98.8% discharged on antipsychotic medications.[57] Patients treated with antipsychotic monotherapy demonstrated higher restoration rates compared to those requiring additional mood stabilizers, indicating that more complex or severely ill patients require additional interventions. These findings underscore the beneficial role that antipsychotics can play beyond reducing psychotic symptoms, aiding the restoration of humanistically relevant functional capacity for participation in legal proceedings. These functional improvements can then extend beyond the courtroom, facilitating reintegration for individuals with severe mental illness into the community.

In a related study, postdischarge outcomes among 4,056 adult Florida Medicaid enrollees with schizophrenia (69%) or bipolar disorder (31%) were examined.[58] While altogether 1,263 participants (31%) were arrested at least once during follow-up, those adhering to outpatient treatment had a significantly lower risk of any arrests (misdemeanor or felony) and of misdemeanor arrests. Among patients with schizophrenia spectrum disorders, engagement in outpatient services – including medication adherence – significantly reduced criminal justice involvement.

Finally, the gold-standard outcome in medicine is the reduction of mortality risk. This outcome is particularly relevant for people with schizophrenia, who experience as many as 15.37 years of potential life lost (95% CI = 14.18–16.55), being third only to commonly comorbid substance-use disorders (20.38 years [95% CI = 18.65–22.11]) and eating disorders (16.64 years [95% CI = 7.45–25.82]).[59] In this context, recent studies are highly relevant, not only confirming an increased mortality risk for people with schizophrenia compared to the general population and other mental disorders, but also demonstrating that antipsychotic treatment was able to significantly reduce this increased risk.

For example, in a meta-analysis of 135 studies, including 4,536,447 people with schizophrenia, 1,115,600,059 general population controls and 3,827,955 other psychiatric illness controls, all-cause mortality was significantly increased in people with schizophrenia versus any nonschizophrenia control group (RR = 2.52, 95% CI = 2.38–2.68; Figure 7.2).[60] The increased mortality risk was most pronounced in people with first-episode (RR = 7.43, 95% CI = 4.02–13.75, n = 2) and incident (i.e., earlier-phase) schizophrenia (RR = 3.52, 95% CI = 3.09–4.00, n = 7) compared to the general population. The specific-cause mortality was highest for suicide/injury–poisoning/undetermined non-natural cause (RR = 9.76–8.42). Compared to individuals with schizophrenia aged ≥40 years, those aged <40 years had significantly increased all-cause and suicide-related mortality, and comorbid substance-use disorder significantly increased all-cause mortality (RR = 1.62, 95% CI = 1.47–1.80). However,

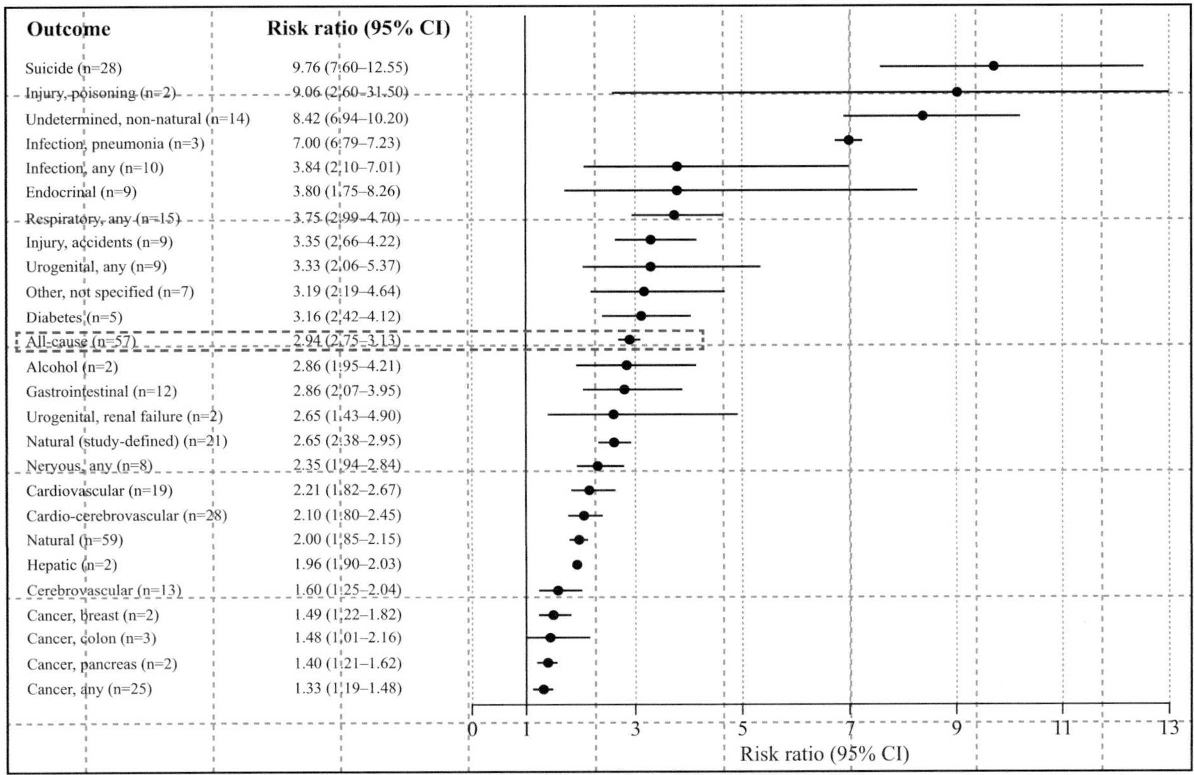

Figure 7.2 All-cause and specific-cause mortality estimates in people with schizophrenia compared to the general population
CI = confidence interval.
Based on Correll et al. (2022).[60]

importantly, antipsychotics were protective against all-cause mortality compared to no antipsychotic use (RR = 0.71, 95% CI = 0.59–0.84, n = 11), with the largest effects observed for SGA-LAIs (RR = 0.39, 95% CI = 0.27–0.56), clozapine (RR = 0.43, 95% CI = 0.34–0.55), any LAI (RR = 0.47, 95% CI = 0.39–0.58), and any SGA (RR = 0.53, 95% CI = 0.44–0.63; Figure 7.3).[60]

Similarly, a nationwide Finnish register-based study sought to determine the factors associated with mortality and to demonstrate their impact on expected life-years in patients with schizophrenia.[61] In these analyses, factors that significantly increased all-cause mortality were cardiovascular disease (HR = 2.41, 95% CI = 2.34–2.49), liver disease (HR = 1.98, 95% CI = 1.78–2.21), renal disease (HR = 1.63, 95% CI = 1.56–1.70), longer duration of previous hospitalizations (HR = 1.96, 95% CI = 1.90–2.02), diabetes (HR = 1.40, 95% CI = 1.35–1.45), history of switching antipsychotics, likely indicating instability (HR = 1.39, 95% CI = 1.35–1.44), history of substance abuse (HR = 1.38, 95% CI = 1.30–1.46), and past or present use of benzodiazepines (HR = 1.12, 95% CI = 1.09–1.16). Conversely, and importantly, factors that significantly reduced all-cause mortality were use of antipsychotics (HR = 0.46, 95% CI = 0.45–0.47), past or present use of lipid-modifying agents (HR = 0.71, 95% CI = 0.68–0.73), antidepressant use (HR = 0.87, 95% CI = 0.85–0.90), and lithium use (HR = 0.90, 95% CI = 0.86–0.95).[61]

These expected and general population-consistent findings of cardiovascular disease and diabetes being associated with increased mortality risk in people with schizophrenia, combined with the significant protective effects of antipsychotics, have led to what has been called the "mortality paradox."[62] This seeming paradox stems from the fact that antipsychotics can have adverse cardiovascular and diabetes effects – especially clozapine, which was one of the most mortality-reducing agents. This seeming paradox has been resolved, however, by a Finnish database study using a within-subject design.[63] In this study, adults aged <65 years diagnosed with schizophrenia were subdivided into four cohorts based on

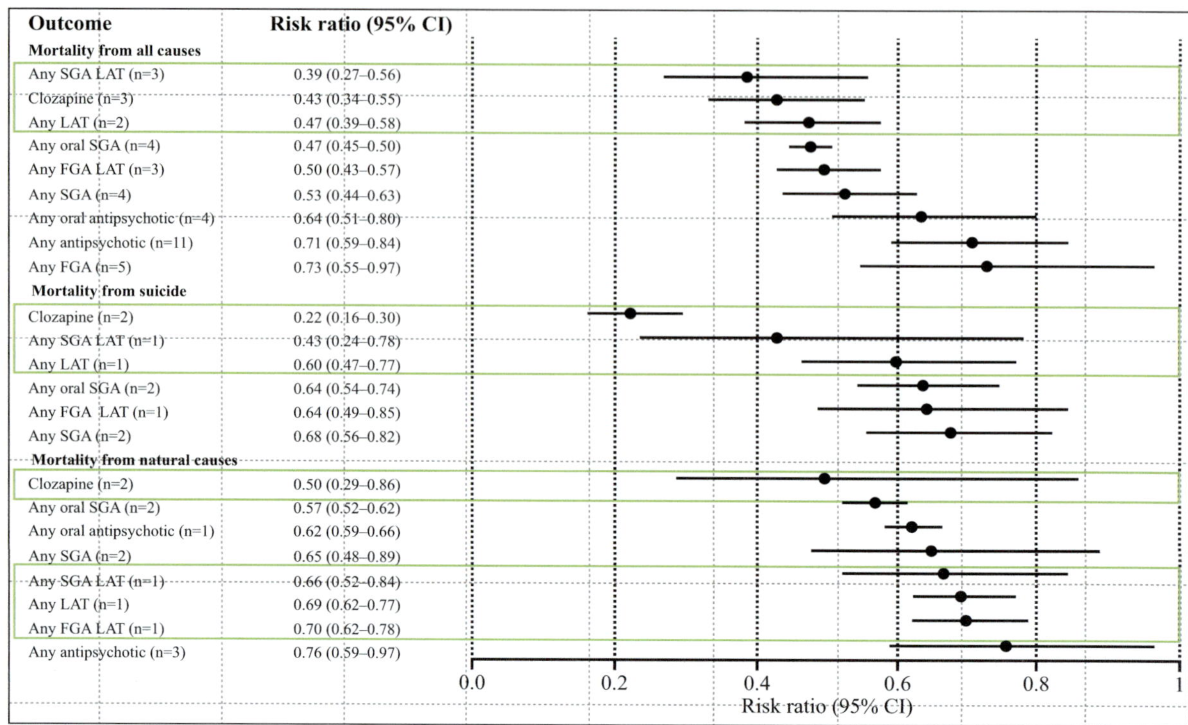

Figure 7.3 Reduction in all-cause and specific-cause mortality in people with schizophrenia dependent on antipsychotic versus no antipsychotic treatment

CI = confidence interval; FGA = first-generation antipsychotic ; LAT = long-acting therapy; SGA = second-generation antipsychotic. Based on Correll et al. (2022).[60]

cardiometabolic drug use during the follow-up period, namely statin (n = 14,047), antidiabetic (n = 13,070), antihypertensive (n = 17,227), and beta-blocker (n = 21,464) users. The results suggested an indirect, mediating protective effect of antipsychotics use via not only reduced illness severity, psychosis-related stress, and potentially improved healthy lifestyle behaviors, but also increased persistence of secondary preventive medical drugs, offsetting the potential increased cardiovascular risk of some antipsychotics, including of clozapine and LAIs, each of which being the most protective against premature mortality,[60,61] and each also being associated with greater adherence to cardiometabolic drugs. Specifically, clozapine (aHR = 0.34–0.55) followed by olanzapine (aHR = 0.43–0.71) were associated the most with reducing discontinuation of all cardiometabolic drug categories.[63]

Taken together, the summarized consistency across metrics and outcomes confirms that antipsychotics provide a measurable benefit, not merely conferring sedation or behavior control, as is sometimes claimed by critics. This antipsychotic efficacy includes acute reduction of symptoms and prevention of relapse, but it also extends across symptom domains, including functional areas, reflecting true antipsychotic efficacy and effectiveness, thereby not just representing non-specific trial participation or placebo effects and not being due to sedative properties or "chemical restraint" effects, as has sometimes been claimed.

Integrating antipsychotic use with psychosocial care and global guidelines

While antipsychotic medications are foundational in the treatment of schizophrenia, they are most effective when embedded within a broader biopsychosocial framework. Comprehensive care includes not only pharmacologic treatment but also individual and family psychoeducation, cognitive behavioral therapy, supported employment, social skills training, and case management services.[10]

International and national guidelines consistently advocate for multimodal interventions, also emphasizing person-centered care, early intervention, and the integration of pharmacological and psychosocial therapies.[64,65] These models combine the backbone of antipsychotic treatment with psychotherapy, supported education/employment, and assertive outreach to optimize functional outcomes. Evidence suggests that early integrated interventions – also called "coordinated specialty care" – for people with first-episode and early-phase illness improves engagement, reduces relapses, and increases the likelihood of recovery compared to usual community care.[66]

Moreover, recent clinical care models increasingly emphasize digital health tools, measurement-based care, and shared decision-making as core components of modern schizophrenia management.[67–69] Digital adherence tools (e.g., smart pill bottles, digital blister packs), symptom-tracking apps, and telepsychiatry offer scalable ways to enhance the monitoring and personalization of care. Thus, ultimately, antipsychotics are most impactful when used as part of a comprehensive treatment strategy that respects patient autonomy, addresses environmental and social factors, and targets recovery, not merely symptom suppression.

Conclusions

While no single treatment is universally effective, the evidence unequivocally supports the use of antipsychotics as essential components of care for people with schizophrenia. Based on the data reviewed in this chapter, the evidence is clear and consistent: Antipsychotics work in people with schizophrenia. Their efficacy, demonstrated through dozens of meta-analyses, randomized trials, and real-world cohort studies, and measured using multiple effect size indices and long-term outcomes, is robust and comparable to – or even exceeds – that of many accepted treatments in internal medicine. Importantly, antipsychotics do more than reduce symptoms. They restore stability, prevent relapse, enable functional recovery, reduce the likelihood of incarceration, help patients regain competency in legal contexts, and reduce the increased risk of premature mortality due to any cause, suicide, and common medical conditions.

However, these advantages are obviously – as for other medical conditions and treatments – based on group mean values and proportions. Hence, not all patients with schizophrenia can and will benefit sufficiently across all desired domains, or they might not benefit at all from antipsychotic treatment. Moreover, some acute or long-term side effects will limit the use and benefits of antipsychotics for relevant subgroups of patients. This situation means that better overall treatments or better specific treatments for individuals and subgroups of patients with schizophrenia still need to be sought, and that individualized care is in dire need. Moreover, the best outcomes can be obtained when pharmacological treatment is embedded in a framework of psychosocial support and individualized care.

Based on this evidence, mental health professionals, policymakers, and advocates should feel confident in asserting: Yes, antipsychotics work for people with schizophrenia. Their continued use – combined with strategies to enhance adherence, reduce side effects, and promote recovery – is not a matter of debate, but one of responsibility. Dismissing the value of antipsychotics on the basis of side effects or ideological positions undermines the lived experience of millions who benefit from them. Such a position also misleads policymakers, families, and even patients, who may forego potentially lifesaving treatment due to such misinformation. Antipsychotics, especially when paired with psychosocial and psychological interventions, are foundational to current schizophrenia care.

The path forward is not to question whether antipsychotics work, but to determine how best to deploy them safely, equitably, and in alignment with patient goals. A truly recovery-oriented system must integrate pharmacological and psychosocial care, address stigma, and empower individuals to reclaim meaningful lives. We must shift the public discourse from polarized skepticism to informed understanding. The lives of patients – and the integrity of psychiatric practice – depend on it.

References

1. Kahn RS, Sommer IE, Murray RM, et al. Schizophrenia. *Nat Rev Dis Primers.* 2015;1:15067. doi: 10.1038/nrdp.2015.67.

2. Solmi M, Seitidis G, Mavridis D, et al. Incidence, prevalence, and global burden of schizophrenia – Data, with critical appraisal, from the Global Burden of Disease (GBD) 2019. *Mol Psychiatry.* 2023;**28**(12):5319–5327. doi: 10.1038/s41380-023-02138-4.

3. Solmi M, Radua J, Olivola M, et al. Age at onset of mental disorders worldwide: Large-scale meta-analysis of 192 epidemiological studies. *Mol Psychiatry.* 2022;**27**(1):281–295. doi: 10.1038/s41380-021-01161-7.

4. Correll CU, Rubio JM, Kane JM. What is the risk–benefit ratio of long-term antipsychotic treatment in people with schizophrenia? *World Psychiatry.* 2018;**17**(2):149–160. doi: 10.1002/wps.20516.

5. McCutcheon RA, Krystal JH, Howes OD. Dopamine and glutamate in schizophrenia: Biology, symptoms and treatment. *World Psychiatry.* 2020;**19**(1):15–33. doi: 10.1002/wps.20693.

6. Pillinger T, D'Ambrosio E, McCutcheon R, Howes OD. Is psychosis a multisystem disorder? A meta-review of central nervous system, immune, cardiometabolic, and endocrine alterations in first-episode psychosis and perspective on potential models. *Mol Psychiatry.* 2019;**24**(6):776–794. doi: 10.1038/s41380-018-0058-9.

7. Huhn M, Nikolakopoulou A, Schneider-Thoma J, et al. Comparative efficacy and tolerability of 32 oral antipsychotics for the acute treatment of adults with multi-episode schizophrenia: a systematic review and network meta-analysis. *Lancet.* 2019;**394**(10202):939–951. doi: 10.1016/S0140-6736(19)31135-3

8. Solmi M, Cortese S, Vita G, et al. An umbrella review of candidate predictors of response, remission, recovery, and relapse across mental disorders. *Mol Psychiatry.* 2023;**28**(9):3671–3687. doi: 10.1038/s41380-023-02298-3.

9. Ostuzzi G, Bertolini F, Tedeschi F, et al. Oral and long-acting antipsychotics for relapse prevention in schizophrenia-spectrum disorders: A network meta-analysis of 92 randomized trials including 22,645 participants. *World Psychiatry.* 2022;**21**(2):295–307. doi: 10.1002/wps.20972.

10. Solmi M, Croatto G, Piva G, et al. Efficacy and acceptability of psychosocial interventions in schizophrenia: Systematic overview and quality appraisal of the meta-analytic evidence. *Mol Psychiatry.* 2023;**28**(1):354–368. doi: 10.1038/s41380-022-01727-z.

11. Wunderink L, Nieboer RM, Wiersma D, Sytema S, Nienhuis FJ. Recovery in remitted first-episode psychosis at 7 years of follow-up of an early dose reduction/discontinuation or maintenance treatment strategy: Long-term follow-up of a 2-year randomized clinical trial. *JAMA Psychiatry.* 2013;**70**(9):913–920. doi: 10.1001/jamapsychiatry.2013.19.

12. Correll CU. What are we looking for in new antipsychotics? *J Clin Psychiatry.* 2011;**72**(Suppl 1):9–13. doi: 10.4088/JCP.10075su1.02.

13. Solmi M, Murru A, Pacchiarotti I, et al. Safety, tolerability, and risks associated with first- and second-generation antipsychotics: A state-of-the-art clinical review. *Ther Clin Risk Manag.* 2017;**13**:757–777. doi: 10.2147/TCRM.S117321.

14. Tandon R, Lenderking WR, Weiss C, et al. The impact on functioning of second-generation antipsychotic medication side effects for patients with schizophrenia: a worldwide, cross-sectional, web-based survey. *Ann Gen Psychiatry.* 2020;**19**:42. doi: 10.1186/s12991-020-00292-5.

15. Diniz E, Fonseca L, Rocha D, et al. Treatment resistance in schizophrenia: a meta-analysis of prevalence and correlates. *Braz J Psychiatry.* 2023;**45**(5):448–458. doi: 10.47626/1516-4446-2023-3126.

16. Hansen HG, Speyer H, Starzer M, et al. Clinical recovery among individuals with a first-episode schizophrenia an updated systematic review and meta-analysis. *Schizophr Bull.* 2023;**49**(2):297–308. doi: 10.1093/schbul/sbac.

17. Jääskeläinen E, Juola P, Hirvonen N, et al. A systematic review and meta-analysis of recovery in schizophrenia. *Schizophr Bull.* 2013;**39**(6):1296–1306. doi: 10.1093/schbul/sbs130.

18. Correll CU, Ismail Z, McIntyre RS, Rafeyan R, Thase ME. Patient functioning, life engagement, and treatment goals in schizophrenia. *J Clin Psychiatry.* 2022;**83**(5):LU21112AH2. doi: 10.4088/JCP.LU21112AH2.

19. Meyer JM. How antipsychotics work in schizophrenia: A primer on mechanisms. *CNS Spectr.* 2024;**30**(1):e6. doi: 10.1017/S1092852924002244.

20. Correll CU, Abi-Dargham A, Howes O. Emerging treatments in schizophrenia. *J Clin Psychiatry.* 2022;**83**(1):SU21024IP1. doi: 10.4088/JCP.SU21024IP1.

21. de Bartolomeis A, Vellucci L, Barone A, et al. Clozapine's multiple cellular mechanisms: What do we know after more than fifty years? A systematic review and critical assessment of translational mechanisms relevant for innovative strategies in treatment-resistant schizophrenia. *Pharmacol Ther.* 2022;**236**:108236. doi: 10.1016/j.pharmthera.2022.108236.

22. Howes OD, McCutcheon R, Agid O, et al. Treatment-resistant schizophrenia: Treatment Response and Resistance in Psychosis (TRRIP)

Working Group Consensus Guidelines on Diagnosis and Terminology. *Am J Psychiatry.* 2017;**174**(3):216–229. doi: 10.1176/appi .ajp.2016.16050503.

23. Kane JM, Correll CU. Past and present progress in the pharmacologic treatment of schizophrenia. *J Clin Psychiatry.* 2010;**71**(9):1115–1124. doi: 10.4088/ JCP.10r06264yel.

24. Correll CU, Citrome L, Haddad PM, et al. The use of long-acting injectable antipsychotics in schizophrenia: Evaluating the evidence. *J Clin Psychiatry.* 2016;**77** (Suppl 3):1–24. doi: 10.4088/JCP.15032su1.

25. Haddad PM, Correll CU. Long-acting antipsychotics in the treatment of schizophrenia: Opportunities and challenges. *Expert Opin Pharmacother.* 2023;**24**(4):473–493. doi: 10.1080/ 14656566.2023.2181073.

26. Kishimoto T, Hagi K, Kurokawa S, Kane JM, Correll CU. Long-acting injectable versus oral antipsychotics for the maintenance treatment of schizophrenia: A systematic review and comparative meta-analysis of randomised, cohort, and pre–post studies. *Lancet Psychiatry.* 2021;**8**(5):387–404. doi: 10.1016/S2215-0366(21)00039-0.

27. Efthimiou O, Taipale H, Radua J, et al. Efficacy and effectiveness of antipsychotics in schizophrenia: Network meta-analyses combining evidence from randomised controlled trials and real-world data. *Lancet Psychiatry.* 2024;**11**(2):102–111. doi: 10.1016/ S2215-0366(23)00366-8.

28. Kane JM, McEvoy JP, Correll CU, Llorca PM. Controversies surrounding the use of long-acting injectable antipsychotic medications for the treatment of patients with schizophrenia. *CNS Drugs.* 2021;**35**(11):1189–1205. doi: 10.1007/s40263-021-00861-6.

29. Wu H, Siafis S, Wang D, et al. Antipsychotic-induced akathisia in adults with acute schizophrenia: A systematic review and dose-response meta-analysis. *Eur Neuropsychopharmacol.* 2023;**72**:40–49. doi: 10.1016/j.euroneuro.2023.03.015.

30. Siafis S, Wu H, Wang D, et al. Antipsychotic dose, dopamine D2 receptor occupancy and extrapyramidal side-effects: A systematic review and dose-response meta-analysis. *Mol Psychiatry.* 2023;**28**(8):3267–3277. doi: 10.1038/s41380-023-02203-y.

31. Carbon M, Kane JM, Leucht S, Correll CU. Tardive dyskinesia risk with first- and second-generation antipsychotics in comparative randomized controlled trials: A meta-analysis. *World Psychiatry.* 2018;**17**(3):330–340. doi: 10.1002/wps.20579.

32. Carbon M, Hsieh CH, Kane JM, Correll CU. Tardive dyskinesia prevalence in the period of second-generation antipsychotic use: A meta-analysis.

J Clin Psychiatry. 2017;**78**(3):e264–e278. doi: 10.4088/ JCP.16r10832.

33. Pillinger T, McCutcheon RA, Vano L, et al. Comparative effects of 18 antipsychotics on metabolic function in patients with schizophrenia, predictors of metabolic dysregulation, and association with psychopathology: A systematic review and network meta-analysis. *Lancet Psychiatry.* 2020;**7**(1):64–77. doi: 10.1016/S2215-0366(19)30416-X.

34. Burschinski A, Schneider-Thoma J, Chiocchia V, et al. Metabolic side effects in persons with schizophrenia during mid- to long-term treatment with antipsychotics: A network meta-analysis of randomized controlled trials. *World Psychiatry.* 2023;**22**(1):116–128. doi: 10.1002/wps.21036.

35. Correll CU, Solmi M, Veronese N, et al. Prevalence, incidence and mortality from cardiovascular disease in patients with pooled and specific severe mental illness: A large-scale meta-analysis of 3,211,768 patients and 113,383,368 controls. *World Psychiatry.* 2017;**16**(2):163–180. doi: 10.1002/wps.20420.

36. Zhu Y, Zhang C, Siafis S, et al. Prolactin levels influenced by antipsychotic drugs in schizophrenia: A systematic review and network meta-analysis. *Schizophr Res.* 2021;**237**:20–25. doi: 10.1016/j .schres.2021.08.013.

37. Solmi M, Lähteenvuo M, Tanskanen A, et al. Antipsychotic use and risk of breast cancer in women with severe mental illness: Replication of a nationwide nested case–control database study. *Schizophr Bull.* 2024;**50**(6):1471–1481. doi: 10.1093/schbul/sbae058.

38. Taipale H, Solmi M, Lähteenvuo M, et al. Antipsychotic use and risk of breast cancer in women with schizophrenia: A nationwide nested case–control study in Finland. *Lancet Psychiatry.* 2021;**8**(10):883–891. doi: 10.1016/S2215-0366(21) 00241-8.

39. Firth J, Siddiqi N, Koyanagi A, et al. The Lancet Psychiatry Commission: A blueprint for protecting physical health in people with mental illness. *Lancet Psychiatry.* 2019;**6**(8):675–712. doi: 10.1016/S2215-0366(19)30132-4.

40. Siskind D, Gallagher E, Winckel K, et al. Does switching antipsychotics ameliorate weight gain in patients with severe mental illness? A systematic review and meta-analysis. *Schizophr Bull.* 2021;**47**(4):948–958. doi: 10.1093/schbul/sbaa191.

41. Højlund M, Kemp AF, Haddad PM, Neill JC, Correll CU. Standard versus reduced dose of antipsychotics for relapse prevention in multi-episode schizophrenia: A systematic review and meta-analysis of randomised controlled trials. *Lancet Psychiatry.* 2021;**8**(6):471–486. doi: 10.1016/S2215-0366(21) 00078-X.

42. Ostuzzi G, Vita G, Bertolini F, et al. Continuing, reducing, switching, or stopping antipsychotics in individuals with schizophrenia-spectrum disorders who are clinically stable: A systematic review and network meta-analysis. *Lancet Psychiatry*. 2022;**9**(8):614–624. doi: 10.1016/S2215-0366(22)00158-4.

43. Vancampfort D, Firth J, Correll CU, et al. The impact of pharmacological and non-pharmacological interventions to improve physical health outcomes in people with schizophrenia: A meta-review of meta-analyses of randomized controlled trials. *World Psychiatry*. 2019;**18**(1):53–66. doi: 10.1002/wps.20614.

44. Buzea CA, Manu P, Dima L, Correll CU. Drug–drug interactions involving combinations of antipsychotic agents with antidiabetic, lipid-lowering, and weight loss drugs. *Expert Opin Drug Metab Toxicol*. 2022;**18**(11):729–744. doi: 10.1080/17425255.2022.2147425.

45. Buzea CA, Dima L, Correll CU, Manu P. Drug–drug interactions involving antipsychotics and antihypertensives. *Expert Opin Drug Metab Toxicol*. 2022;**18**(4):285–298. doi: 10.1080/17425255.2022.2086121.

46. Correll CU, Kim E, Sliwa JK, et al. Pharmacokinetic characteristics of long-acting injectable antipsychotics for schizophrenia: An overview. *CNS Drugs*. 2021;**35**(1):39–59. doi: 10.1007/s40263-020-00779-5.

47. Kane JM, Kishimoto T, Correll CU. Non-adherence to medication in patients with psychotic disorders: Epidemiology, contributing factors and management strategies. *World Psychiatry*. 2013;**12**(3):216–26. doi: 10.1002/wps.20060.

48. Leucht S, Siafis S, Engel RR, et al. How efficacious are antipsychotic drugs for schizophrenia? An interpretation based on 13 effect size indices. *Schizophr Bull*. 2022;**48**(1):27–36. doi: 10.1093/schbul/sbab094.

49. Andrade C. Mean difference, standardized mean difference (SMD), and their use in meta-analysis: As simple as it gets. *J Clin Psychiatry*. 2020;**81**(5):20f13681. doi: 10.4088/JCP.20f13681.

50. Zhu Y, Li C, Huhn M, et al. How well do patients with a first episode of schizophrenia respond to antipsychotics: A systematic review and meta-analysis. *Eur Neuropsychopharmacol*. 2017;**27**(9):835–844. doi: 10.1016/j.euroneuro.2017.06.011.

51. Correll CU, Tocco M, Hsu J, Goldman R, Pikalov A. Short-term efficacy and safety of lurasidone versus placebo in antipsychotic-naïve vs. previously treated adolescents with an acute exacerbation of schizophrenia. *Eur Psychiatry*. 2022;**65**(1):1–35. doi: 10.1192/j.eurpsy.2022.11.

52. Leucht S, Hierl S, Kissling W, Dold M, Davis JM. Putting the efficacy of psychiatric and general medicine medication into perspective: Review of meta-analyses. *Br J Psychiatry*. 2012;**200**(2):97–106. doi: 10.1192/bjp.bp.111.096594.

53. Leucht S, Helfer B, Gartlehner G, Davis JM. How effective are common medications: A perspective based on meta-analyses of major drugs. *BMC Med*. 2015;**13**:253. doi: 10.1186/s12916-015-0494-1.

54. Leucht S, Tardy M, Komossa K, et al. Antipsychotic drugs versus placebo for relapse prevention in schizophrenia: A systematic review and meta-analysis. *Lancet*. 2012;**379**(9831):2063–2071. doi: 10.1016/S0140-6736(12)60239-6.

55. Citrome L. Compelling or irrelevant? Using number needed to treat can help decide. *Acta Psychiatr Scand*. 2008;**117**(6):412–419. doi: 10.1111/j.1600-0447.2008.01194.x

56. Solmi M, Taipale H, Holm M, et al. Effectiveness of antipsychotic use for reducing risk of work disability: Results from a within-subject analysis of a Swedish national cohort of 21,551 patients with first-episode nonaffective psychosis. *Am J Psychiatry*. 2022;**179**(12):938–946. doi: 10.1176/appi.ajp.21121189

57. Faizi A, McDermott B, Warburton K. Do antipsychotic medications work: An exploration using competency to stand trial as the functional outcome. *CNS Spectr*. 2025;**30**(1):e29.

58. Van Dorn RA, Desmarais SL, Petrila J, Haynes D, Singh JP. Effects of outpatient treatment on risk of arrest of adults with serious mental illness and associated costs. *Psychiatr Serv*. 2013;**64**(9):856–862. doi: 10.1176/appi.ps.201200406.

59. Chan JKN, Correll CU, Wong CSM, et al. Life expectancy and years of potential life lost in people with mental disorders: A systematic review and meta-analysis. EClinicalMedicine. 2023;**65**:102294. doi: 10.1016/j.eclinm.2023.102294.

60. Correll CU, Solmi M, Croatto G, et al. Mortality in people with schizophrenia: A systematic review and meta-analysis of relative risk and aggravating or attenuating factors. *World Psychiatry*. 2022;**21**(2):248–271. doi: 10.1002/wps.20994.

61. Correll CU, Bitter I, Hoti F, et al. Factors and their weight in reducing life expectancy in schizophrenia. *Schizophr Res*. 2022;**250**:67–75. doi: 10.1016/j.schres.2022.10.019.

62. Solmi M, Correll CU. The antipsychotic paradox: Lessons regarding determinants of premature mortality. *Eur Neuropsychopharmacol*. 2022;**62**:1–3. doi: 10.1016/j.euroneuro.2022.05.014.

63. Solmi M, Tiihonen J, Lähteenvuo M, et al. Antipsychotics use is associated with greater adherence to cardiometabolic medications in patients with schizophrenia: Results from a nationwide, within-subject design study.

Schizophr Bull. 2022;**48**(1):166–175. doi: 10.1093/schbul/sbab087.

64. McCutcheon RA, Pillinger T, Varvari I, et al. INTEGRATE: International guidelines for the algorithmic treatment of schizophrenia. *Lancet Psychiatry.* 2025;**12**(5):384–394. doi: 10.1016/S2215-0366(25)00031-8.

65. Correll CU, Martin A, Patel C, et al. Systematic literature review of schizophrenia clinical practice guidelines on acute and maintenance management with antipsychotics. *Schizophrenia (Heidelb).* 2022;**8**(1):5. doi: 10.1038/s41537-021-00192-x.

66. Correll CU, Galling B, Pawar A, et al. Comparison of early intervention services vs treatment as usual for early-phase psychosis: A systematic review, meta-analysis, and meta-regression. *JAMA Psychiatry.* 2018;**75**(6):555–565. doi: 10.1001/jamapsychiatry.2018.0623.

67. Hau C, Xia W, Ryan S, et al. Smartphone monitoring and digital phenotyping apps for schizophrenia: A review of the academic literature. *Schizophr Res.* 2025;**281**:237–248. doi: 10.1016/j.schres.2025.05.019.

68. Byun AJS, Lane E, Langholm C, et al. Towards clinical subtypes in schizophrenia: Integrating cognitive, functional, and digital phenotyping assessments. *Mol Psychiatry.* 2025;**30**:4641–4650. doi: 10.1038/s41380-025-03054-5.

69. Torous J, Linardon J, Goldberg SB, et al. The evolving field of digital mental health: Current evidence and implementation issues for smartphone apps, generative artificial intelligence, and virtual reality. *World Psychiatry.* 2025;**24**(2):156–174. doi: 10.1002/wps.21299.

Do Antipsychotic Medications Work?
An Exploration Using Competency to Stand Trial as the Functional Outcome

Ambarin Faizi, Barbara E. McDermott, and Katherine Warburton

The advancement of antipsychotic medications represents a significant leap in our ability to treat severe mental illness, thus ensuring that individuals can be treated effectively and humanely within the legal system.
—*Justice Sandra Day O'Connor,* Riggins v. Nevada *(1992)*

Introduction

The evolution of treatments in psychiatry has significantly transformed over the past century, moving from rudimentary and often inhumane practices to sophisticated pharmacological interventions. The serendipitous discovery of chlorpromazine as a sedative by Henri Laborit, a French surgeon, led to its trial in psychiatric patients due to its observed calming effect. Chlorpromazine demonstrated remarkable efficacy in reducing psychotic symptoms in psychiatric patients, leading to its widespread adoption in psychiatric hospitals.[1] The discovery of chlorpromazine marked a turning point, as it was the first antipsychotic medication that effectively managed symptoms of psychosis and laid the groundwork for the development of numerous other antipsychotic medications.[1]

The literature contains robust evidence establishing the use of antipsychotic medication in the treatment of schizophrenia and other psychotic disorders primarily via a reduction in the positive symptoms of psychosis (delusions, hallucinations).[2-5] The landmark, Clinical Antipsychotic Trials of Intervention Effectiveness (CATIE)[6] study, for instance, compared multiple antipsychotic medications, including both first-generation (typical) and second-generation (atypical) antipsychotics. This large-scale, multiphase study found that while all tested medications were effective in managing psychotic symptoms, differences in side effect profiles significantly influenced patient adherence and outcomes. Multiple studies have demonstrated similar results (CUtLASS, SOHO).[7,8] Along these lines, a meta-analysis conducted by Leucht and colleagues[9] provided evidence that long-acting injectable antipsychotics (LAIs) were more effective in preventing relapse compared to their oral counterparts. This study reviewed data from multiple randomized trials and concluded that injectable formulations provided more consistent drug levels, which helped maintain symptom control and reduce relapse rates, thereby offering a valuable option for patients with adherence issues. Several studies support the advantages of long-acting injectables in relapse prevention and reducing hospitalization.[10-12]

The development of these above-described medications with demonstrated efficacy in treating the positive psychotic symptoms of major mental disorders spurred the deinstitutionalization movement of the 1960s and 70s, which sought to reduce the population of mental health patients in institutional settings by shifting the treatment to community-based environments. Unfortunately, this deinstitutionalization movement also led to unintended consequences, such as transinstitutionalization and criminalization of mental illness.[13] Incarceration rates are notably high among individuals with mental illness, particularly those with psychotic disorders such as schizophrenia.[14] Approximately 24% of local jail inmates in the United States have reported symptoms of a psychotic disorder, such as delusions or hallucinations, according to the Bureau of Justice Statistics report from 2006.[15] Although this statistic has remained stable over time, recent reports continue to highlight a significant presence of psychotic disorders among the incarcerated population. The overrepresentation of people with psychotic illness in the legal system is underscored by the ballooning referrals for competency to stand trial (CST) evaluations over the past decade. Estimates of the annual number of competence evaluations have previously ranged from 19,000 to 60,000, but more recent estimates suggest that approximately 94,000 evaluations are conducted annually in the United States.[16]

CST is a fundamental concept in forensic psychiatry and legal proceedings, ensuring that defendants possess the mental capacity to understand the nature and consequences of the legal process and participate adequately in their defense. The landmark case *Dusky* v. *United States* (1960) established the standard for competency, requiring that defendants have a rational and factual understanding of the proceedings against them and be able to consult with their attorney with a reasonable degree of rational understanding.[17] Meta-analyses by Nicholson and Kugler[18] and Pirelli et al.[19] revealed several indicators related to the finding of incompetence to stand trial, notably that individuals diagnosed with a psychotic disorder were eight times more likely to be deemed incompetent than individuals without a psychotic disorder. Active psychosis, including delusions and hallucinations, can distort an individual's perception of reality, making it challenging for them to engage meaningfully in the legal process.[20]

Antipsychotic medications play a vital role in effectively treating symptoms of psychosis but what impact do they have on improving functional abilities to enable individuals to understand the legal process and participate in their defense? While the efficacy of antipsychotic medications in symptom reduction is well established, their success in restoring the functional competencies necessary for CST is less recognized. Wall and Lee[21] emphasize that competency encompasses more than just an absence of psychotic symptoms; it involves a complex interplay of cognitive, emotional, and behavioral capacities. Mossman[22] conducted a comprehensive study that identified antipsychotic medications as essential in restoring competency in defendants diagnosed with schizophrenia and other psychotic disorders. His research demonstrated that with appropriate pharmacological treatment, a significant proportion of incompetent defendants could be restored to competency. His findings were further supported by Cochrane and colleagues[23] who reviewed the impact of psychotropic medications on trial competency, emphasizing the role of antipsychotics in alleviating symptoms that impede legal competence. Their review highlighted that effective treatment of psychotic symptoms was

crucial for restoring cognitive and functional abilities necessary for trial competency. They describe the consistently high response rate to antipsychotic medication treatment as "remarkable."

Our study's focus on functional outcomes is predicated on the understanding that competency restoration involves a comprehensive recovery of abilities. This includes the capacity to comprehend the charges against oneself, the roles of various courtroom personnel, and the potential consequences of legal decisions. The *Dusky* v. *United States* (1960) ruling emphasizes the necessity for defendants to have both a rational and factual understanding of legal proceedings, which inherently involves higher-level cognitive and functional capabilities. By focusing on these outcomes, our study substantiates the effectiveness of antipsychotic medications in not only reducing symptoms but also improving the functional abilities required for legal competency.

The main purpose of our research was to examine the effectiveness of antipsychotic medication on the real-world functional outcomes of competency restoration. Traditional measures of antipsychotic efficacy primarily focus on the reduction of positive psychotic symptoms such as hallucinations and delusions. While these are crucial for acute symptom management, they do not necessarily translate into the practical abilities required for a defendant to be deemed competent to stand trial. CST requires more than symptom reduction; it necessitates higher-level cognitive and functional abilities to understand court proceedings, communicate effectively with legal counsel, and participate meaningfully in one's defense.[19,21] This study examines over 3,000 individuals in California's state hospital system who were deemed incompetent to stand trial (IST) to determine if antipsychotic medications are not just effective in symptom relief but also have utility in restoring complex functional capabilities.

Methods

This research was approved by the State of California Committee for the Protection of Human Subjects and the University of California, Davis School of Medicine Institutional Review Board (IRB). The IRB granted a waiver of informed consent.

The study was conducted at the Department of State Hospital (DSH) hospitals using data collected from the records of individuals found IST and committed to DSH for restoration. Of the five existing hospitals in the DSH system, only four provide competency restoration treatment. In these four DSH hospitals, over 85% of the beds are dedicated to patients under forensic commitments, comprised primarily of patients found incompetent to stand trial (IST), Not Guilty by Reason of Insanity (NGRI), and Offenders with Mental Disorders (OMD; a California statute that civilly commits offenders as dangerous after a determinate sentence), with a small number of other commitment types. Although DSH also funds numerous jail-based competence restoration programs in CA, only hospital admissions were examined in this study.

The records of patients found IST and admitted for restoration to competence between the dates of February 1, 2018 through January 31, 2019 were included in the study. At the time of data collection, California statute required that, with few exceptions, defendants found IST for a felony be committed to a locked facility for restoration to competence. Only offenders found IST for misdemeanors and a limited number of non-violent felonies were by statute eligible for community restoration. The maximum length of commitment for restoration of offenders with felony charges was 3 years at the time the majority of this study was conducted. On January 1, 2019, the maximum length of commitment was reduced to 2 years.

Procedure

All patients were admitted directly from referring county jails. When committed to DSH, courts are required to submit documentation for each individual, which includes documentation of the committing offense and the arrest report associated with the committing offense, the report(s) written by the forensic evaluator(s), the criminal arrest history, any jail medical records available at the time of commitment, and various court documents associated with the commitment (primarily minute orders). A document capturing all relevant information was developed and coders were trained in extracting necessary information for the records. All coders were required to evidence consistency in coding data during this training.

For discharge data, the electronic data systems maintained by DSH were accessed to obtain discharge date, discharge commitment type (primarily restored to competence vs no substantial likelihood of restoration [NSL]), and discharge diagnoses. When restoration status seemed implausible based on the length of hospitalization, the associated court report for that admission was accessed to confirm the evaluator's opinion. All four hospitals provided access to court reports to confirm discharge recommendations; all reports were examined when the length of hospitalization was one year or longer. When inconsistencies were found, the electronic system indicated restoration whereas the report recommended that the individual be returned to court as NSL. In no case did the electronic data system indicate NSL and the report recommended restoration. Note that the outcome measure in this study was the restoration opinion contained in the report. The judicial decision regarding this opinion was not obtained.

For diagnosis, we accessed the electronic data management system that tracks treatment team diagnosis. For this study, we opted to use discharge diagnosis, as admission diagnosis is often unreliable due to the treatment team's unfamiliarity with patients on admission. Moreover, because the electronic data management system tracks treatment team diagnosis, which may not align with the diagnosis contained in the court report, we opted to only access the electronic system.

To determine the types of medications used for restoration, we accessed the electronic data system documenting medications. This system maintains records of all medications prescribed during the individual's hospitalization. Because of the complexity of prescribing practices in long-term care facilities and the types of individuals found not competent to stand trial (typically diagnosed with either a psychotic disorder or a cognitive disorder), we examined the data to document the use of two classes of medications: antipsychotics (either typical or atypical) and mood stabilizers. Dosage was not recorded for these analyses. Each individual was reported as either prescribed an antipsychotic (yes/no) or a mood stabilizer (yes/no). Each patient was categorized as discharged on neither an antipsychotic nor a mood stabilizer, only an antipsychotic, only a mood stabilizer, or on both an antipsychotic and a mood stabilizer.

Participants

There were a total of 3,166 unduplicated IST admissions during the specified time period. Twenty-two individuals were recommitted during the year this study was conducted, only one of whom was committed as IST for a new offense. The remainder were recommitted for the same offense after their initial restoration. For these 22 individuals, only their first admission was retained in the dataset.

As can be seen in Table 8.1, women comprised 17.6% of the admissions (n = 556), with the remainder (n = 2,610, 82.4%) described as male. Approximately one-third of the admissions were White (n = 1,046, 33.1%), with slightly less than one-third Hispanic (n = 994, 31.4%). The remainder were either Black (n = 896, 28.3%) or of another ethnic background, including American Indian and Asian (n = 226, 7.1%). The age of the patients on admission ranged from 18 to 92, with an average age of 38.6 (std = 12.6). The majority of patients had documentation of at least one prior inpatient psychiatric admission as an adult (n = 1,756, 56.5%), although many records did not indicate any

Table 8.1 Demographic and clinical characteristics of the sample

–	n (%)
Gender	
Female	556 (17.6)
Male	2610 (82.4)
Race	
African-American	896 (28.3)
Caucasian	1046 (33.1)
Hispanic	994 (31.4)
Other Non-white	226 (7.1)
Prior psychiatric treatment	
Inpatient (as an adult)	1756 (56.5)
None	802 (25.8)
Only juvenile/outpatient/ nonpsychiatric provider	551 (17.7)
Commitment offense	
Assault/battery	1157 (37.1)
Theft	404 (12.9)
Robbery	254 (8.1)
Criminal threats	253 (8.1)
Miscellaneous	172 (5.5)
Obstruction of justice	171 (5.5)
Homicide offenses	164 (5.3)
Arson	147 (4.7)
Failure to register (sex offense)	52 (1.7)
Other	75 (2.4)

prior psychiatric history, either inpatient or outpatient (n = 802, 25.8%). The remainder had documentation that reflected a history of mental health treatment only as a juvenile, as an outpatient, or receiving psychiatric medications from a non-mental health provider (n = 551, 17.7%). Most admissions were English speaking (n = 2,956, 94.7%), although 127 were documented as speaking Spanish as their primary language (4.1%). A very small percentage had records that reflected speaking another language (n = 36, 1.2%). Only the most serious felony offense for which the person was found IST was recorded as the commitment offense. The most common commitment offense was assault/battery (n = 1,157, 37.1%), followed by theft (n = 404, 12.9%), robbery (n = 254, 8.1%), criminal threats (n = 253, 8.1%), miscellaneous charges (typically vandalism, n = 172, 5.5%), obstruction of justice (171, 5.5%), homicide offenses (164, 5.3%), arson (n = 147, 4.7%), failure to register as a sex offender (n = 52, 1.7%), and other (kidnapping, white collar crimes, major driving offenses, escape, (n = 75, 2.4%)).

Data analysis

Data were analyzed using SPSS version 29. Statistical analyses included frequency distributions and descriptive statistics to provide information regarding basic demographics. Chi-square and mean differences analyses were conducted to assess differences in categorical and continuous variables respectively.

Results

Of the 3166 individuals admitted during the specified time period, 2,733 (86.5%) were discharged as restored to competence and 392 (12.5%) were discharged as NSL. The remaining 41 were not discharged and were either returned to court as competent but remained in the hospital to maintain competence (n = 18, 0.6%) or remained in the hospital under a different commitment (for example, found NGRI and hospitalization continued under that commitment, n = 23, 0.7%).

Our primary hypothesis was that antipsychotic medication was critical and effective in restoring patients found not competent to stand trial. As can be seen from Table 8.2, fully 98.8% of individuals admitted as IST were discharged on an antipsychotic, with the majority discharged on an antipsychotic alone (70.9%) and an additional 27.9% on both an antipsychotic and a mood stabilizer. This

Table 8.2 Restoration status by discharge medication

–	Neither antipsychotic nor mood stabilizer N (%)	Only antipsychotic N (%)	Antipsychotic plus mood stabilizer N (%)	Only mood stabilizer
Restored	34 (94.4)	1984 (89.6)	711 (81.6)	4 (100)
Returned as no substantial likelihood	2[a] (5.6)	230 (10.4)	160 (18.4)	0 (0)
Total	36 (1.1)	2214 (70.9)	871 (27.9)	4 (0.1)

[a] DC diagnosis of a neurocognitive disorder

Table 8.3 Restoration to competence by discharge diagnoses

Discharge diagnosis	Total sample with discharge diagnosis, outcome, and medication N (%)	Percent discharged as restored to competence N (%)	Percent discharged as no substantial likelihood N (%)
Schizophrenia	1169 (38.0)	987 (84.4)	182 (15.6)
Schizoaffective disorder	483 (15.7)	420 (87.0)	63 (13.0)
Bipolar disorder	261 (8.5)	252 (96.6)	9 (3.4)
Unspecified schizophrenia spectrum and other psychotic disorders	703 (22.8)	655 (93.2)	48 (6.8)
Neurocognitive disorders	73 (2.4)	29 (39.7)	44 (60.3)
Delusional disorder	32 (1.0)	30 (93.8)	2 (6.3)
Other mental health disorders	132 (4.3)	120 (90.9)	12 (9.1)
No major mental health disorder	226 (7.3)	220 (97.3)	6 (2.7)
Total	3079	2713 (88.1)	366 (11.9)

table also demonstrates that almost 90% of individuals discharged on only an antipsychotic were believed to be restored to competence, in comparison to patients discharged on a combination of an antipsychotic and a mood stabilizer, where only slightly more than 80% of these individuals were believed restored. When patients were discharged on neither an antipsychotic nor a mood stabilizer, close to 95% were restored to competence. The two patients returned to court as NSL and on neither of the targeted medications had a primary diagnosis of a neurocognitive disorder. All patients discharged on only a mood stabilizer were restored to competence (X^2 (3) = 38.5, p < .001). This table clearly shows that individuals for whom an antipsychotic was not sufficient were less likely to be restored than any other group.

Since psychiatric medications may not be the treatment of choice for certain disorders (for example neurocognitive disorders are unlikely to respond to antipsychotic medications), we examined the discharge diagnoses associated with medications and restoration status. Tables 8.3–8.5 clarify the relationship between diagnosis, medications, and discharge status. As can be seen from Table 8.3, the plurality of patients received a diagnosis of schizophrenia; the second largest diagnostic category was unspecified schizophrenia spectrum and other psychotic disorders, followed by schizoaffective disorder. Combined with delusional disorder, these four diagnostic categories, whose

Table 8.4 Restoration to competence by discharge diagnosis – discharged only on an antipsychotic

Discharge diagnosis	Percent of sample discharged on antipsychotic alone N (% of total sample)	Percent discharged as restored to competence N (%)	Percent discharged as no substantial likelihood N (%)
Schizophrenia	880 (75.5)	766 (87.0)	114 (13.0)
Schizoaffective disorder	239 (49.8)	218 (91.2)	21 (8.8)
Bipolar disorder	158 (60.8)	153 (96.8)	5 (3.2)
Unspecified schizophrenia spectrum and other psychotic disorders	563 (80.7)	530 (94.1)	33 (5.9)
Neurocognitive disorders	52 (76.5)	20 (38.5)	32 (61.5)
Delusional disorder	26 (83.9)	25 (96.2)	1 (3.8)
Other mental health disorders	93 (75.0)	85 (91.4)	8 (8.6)
No major mental health disorder	180 (84.9)	176 (97.8)	4 (2.2)
Total	2191 (72.1)	1973 (90.1)	218 (9.9)

Table 8.5 Restoration to competence by discharge diagnosis – discharged on antipsychotic and mood stabilizer

Discharge diagnosis	Percent of sample discharged on both antipsychotic and mood stabilizer N (% of total sample)	Percent discharged as restored to competence N (%)	Percent discharged as no substantial likelihood N (%)
Schizophrenia	286 (24.5)	218 (76.2)	68 (23.8)
Schizoaffective disorder	241 (50.2)	199 (82.6)	42 (17.4)
Bipolar disorder	102 (39.2)	98 (96.1)	4 (3.9)
Unspecified schizophrenia spectrum and other psychotic disorders	135 (19.3)	120 (88.9)	15 (11.1)
Neurocognitive disorders	16 (23.5)	6 (37.5)	10 (62.5)
Delusional disorder	5 (16.1)	4 (80.0)	1 (20.0)
Other mental health disorders	31 (25.0)	27 (87.1)	4 (12.9)
No major mental health disorder	32 (15.1)	30 (93.8)	2 (6.2)
Total	848 (27.9)	702 (82.8)	146 (17.2)

primary symptoms are psychotic in nature, comprised over 75% of the total sample. Notably, three diagnoses evidenced restoration rates of less than 90%: schizophrenia, schizoaffective disorder, and neurocognitive disorders. Not surprisingly, neurocognitive disorders had substantially lower restoration rates than any other diagnosis (less than 40% were restored to competence) although they comprised a very small percentage of the total sample.

Table 8.4 provides restoration rates and the percentage of the total sample who were returned to court prescribed only an antipsychotic. Not surprisingly, two diagnostic categories evidenced a lower percentage of patients returned to court – as either restored or NSL – on only an antipsychotic. Less than 50% of individuals with a diagnosis of schizoaffective disorder were returned to court only prescribed an antipsychotic; slightly more than 60% of individuals with a diagnosis of bipolar disorder were discharged prescribed only an antipsychotic.

Table 8.5 documents the diagnostic comparisons for restoration rates in individuals who required the addition of a mood stabilizer to their medication regimen. As can be seen in this table, substantially more people who required adjunctive medication were unlikely to be restored for most diagnoses with two notable exceptions: bipolar disorder and neurocognitive disorders.

Table 8.6 Days in hospital by diagnosis – discharged restored

Discharge diagnosis	Days in hospital Mean (Std)
Schizophrenia[b]	145.0 (121.0)
Schizoaffective disorder[c]	130.5 (103.7)
Bipolar disorder[d]	107.0 (86.1)
Unspecified schizophrenia spectrum and other psychotic disorder[d]	107.5 (94.2)
Neurocognitive disorders[a]	179.7 (109.4)
Delusional disorder[d]	97.4 (67.1)
Other mental health disorders[d]	78.4 (62.0)
No major mental health disorder	77.4 (74.9)

[a] Neurocognitive disorders longer than all others

[b] Schizophrenia different than all others

[c] Schizoaffective different than all others

[d] All statistically same

Individuals with these diagnoses evidenced a similar restoration rate with or without the addition of a mood stabilizer (96.8 and 96.1 for bipolar disorder and 38.5 and 37.5 for neurocognitive disorders).

Table 8.6 provides the length of stay by discharge diagnosis for patients who were returned to court as restored to competence. Not surprisingly, individuals diagnosed with neurocognitive disorders required the longest hospitalization (average of almost 6 months), followed by individuals diagnosed with schizophrenia (slightly less than 5 months). Patients diagnosed with schizoaffective disorder also differed from all other diagnostic categories with a discharge length of stay of slightly more than 4 months. All other diagnostic categories evidenced lengths of stay of approximately 3.5 months or less. The shortest lengths of stay were found in individuals with either no major mental health disorder (i.e., personality disorders and substance use disorders) or nonpsychotic mental health disorders (e.g., anxiety disorders). Interestingly, individuals with a diagnosis of a delusional disorder evidenced a relatively brief length of stay of approximately 3 months.

Figure 8.1 depicts the restoration discharge length of stay by diagnosis for individuals restored on an antipsychotic alone compared to those requiring the addition of a mood stabilizer. As can be seen from this graphic, individuals requiring the addition of a mood stabilizer evidenced longer discharge lengths of stay in general (F(7,2659) = 2.012, p = .05). However, for three diagnostic categories (unspecified

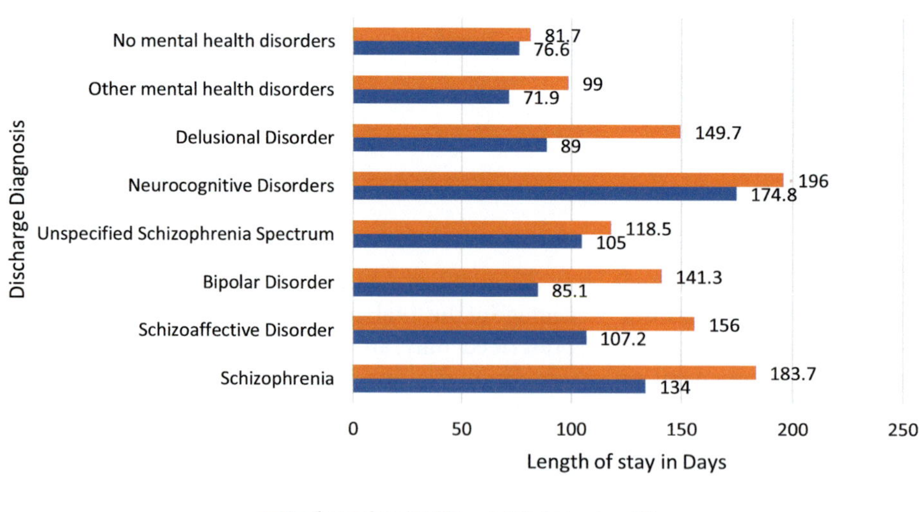

Figure 8.1 Days in hospital by diagnosis and medication – discharge restored.

schizophrenia spectrum and other psychotic disorders, neurocognitive disorders, and no major mental health disorders) the differences were not statistically significant.

Discussion

Our data provide compelling evidence that antipsychotic medications are critical in restoring competency to proceed with criminal charges. Our primary question was, "Do antipsychotic medications work?," with an operational definition of "work" entirely different than most research on these medications. We were not attempting to understand if antipsychotic medication reduced psychotic symptoms. As noted previously, there is ample evidence that in the majority of individuals diagnosed with a psychotic disorder, both first-generation (typical) and second-generation (atypical) antipsychotic medications reduce the positive symptoms of psychosis.[2–8] Moreover, there is some research that suggests that certain atypical medications reduce cognitive or negative symptoms observed in some psychotic disorders.[4–5] But is that definition of "work" enough? A recent New York Times opinion essay[24] argued that merely decreasing or eliminating symptoms was an inadequate definition of work. The author noted that while approximately 60% of individuals with a psychotic disorder experience symptom remission or reduction, some studies describe worsening outcomes with long-term maintenance of these medications, noting "profound side effects" associated with these medications. The author argued that because of these negative outcomes, antipsychotic medications should not be a mandatory component of treatment and that alternative interventions should be explored. Admittedly, despite their efficacy in managing the positive symptoms of schizophrenia, medications such as chlorpromazine (known as first-generation or typical antipsychotics) are associated with adverse events such as extrapyramidal symptoms (EPS) like tardive dyskinesia.[25] The introduction of clozapine in the 1970s marked the beginning of the second-generation antipsychotics, also known as atypical antipsychotics. These medications aimed to balance efficacy and adverse reactions, although they introduced other challenges such as metabolic side effects, including weight gain and diabetes.[26] Recent advancements in antipsychotic therapy have focused on optimizing efficacy, minimizing side effects, and improving patient adherence. LAIs have been developed to enhance treatment adherence by providing sustained drug release, reducing the need for daily medication.[27] These formulations have demonstrated efficacy in preventing relapse and improving outcomes in schizophrenia.[28] Even more recently, in September 2024 the FDA approved an antipsychotic medication that employs a novel mechanism of action for reducing psychotic symptoms, which may further reduce negative side effects.[29] This reduction in side effects may increase adherence and improve long-term outcomes.

Our study's findings underscore the pivotal role of antipsychotic medications in restoring functional capacity via the restoration of CST among individuals diagnosed with severe mental illness, particularly psychotic disorders. The efficacy of antipsychotics in reducing symptoms of psychosis is well-established, yet our research highlights their critical role in restoring the functional capabilities necessary for CST. Among the 3,166 individuals admitted as IST, 86.5% were successfully restored to competency, with 98.8% of these individuals discharged on an antipsychotic regimen, highlighting the crucial role these medications play in not only symptom reduction but also in functional restoration.

One of the key findings of our study is the differential outcomes observed among individuals prescribed a combination of antipsychotics and mood stabilizers versus those on antipsychotic monotherapy. Patients requiring the addition of mood stabilizers demonstrated longer lengths of stay and higher rates of being deemed as having no substantial likelihood of restoration to competency, indicating a more complex and treatment-resistant illness. This finding is consistent with an international study[30] in 2020 which demonstrates that patients with schizophrenia who received adjunctive treatment with mood stabilizers are more severely ill and less responsive to monotherapy treatments. In our study specifically, while 89.6% of individuals discharged on antipsychotic monotherapy were restored to competency, this rate decreased to 81.6% for those on both an antipsychotic and a mood stabilizer. These findings suggest that the presence of mood instability or comorbid conditions, such as schizoaffective or bipolar disorder, contributes to the complexity of psychotic illness, necessitating more intensive and prolonged treatment efforts.

Our study also sheds light on the treatability of delusional disorder with antipsychotic medications, a disorder traditionally viewed as more resistant to treatment than other psychotic disorders. Notably, our data indicate that individuals diagnosed with the delusional disorder who were treated with antipsychotics had a restoration rate of 93.8% and a relatively brief length of stay of approximately 3 months, compared to an average of 5 months for patients with schizophrenia. A critical aspect of this more rapid response to medication may lie in the symptom profile of these two diagnostic categories. The literature documents a wide range of symptoms associated with a schizophrenic process, which can include the previously described positive symptoms as well as negative symptoms, including various deficits in cognitive functioning. In contrast, most literature describing symptoms associated with delusional disorder documents that cognitive function remains intact regardless of medication intervention.[31–33] This diagnostic difference in symptom profiles may lead to a more rapid restoration rate. Regardless, our data supports emerging literature[34–36] that suggests delusional disorder can indeed be effectively managed with antipsychotic medication, leading to significant functional improvement and restoration of competency.

A key strength of our study is its large sample size of 3,166 individuals, which enhances the generalizability of our findings across diverse treatment settings. Additionally, our focus on functional outcomes provides a more comprehensive understanding of the effectiveness of antipsychotic medications beyond mere symptom reduction.

However, our study is not without limitations. The reliance on discharge diagnoses may introduce variability in diagnostic accuracy, and the absence of dosage data limits our ability to assess the impact of specific medication regimens. Future research should explore the role of dosage and the potential benefits of combining pharmacological and non-pharmacological interventions to optimize functional outcomes.

Conclusions

The use of antipsychotic medication has been validated by extensive clinical research demonstrating its efficacy in managing symptoms of several mental disorders such as schizophrenia and bipolar disorder. Antipsychotics reduce delusions, hallucinations, and other psychotic features, allowing patients to function more effectively in daily life. While critics may argue that compulsory mental health care overemphasizes medication, it is crucial to note that antipsychotics, when appropriately administered and managed, can significantly improve patients' quality of life, prevent relapse, and support long-term recovery and stability.

In conclusion, our study affirms the vital role of antipsychotic medications in restoring competency among individuals with severe mental illness, particularly those with psychotic disorders. The effectiveness of antipsychotic medications, including in the treatment of delusional disorder and comorbid mood symptoms, provides a hopeful outlook for restoring functionality and increasing independence in a vulnerable patient population. While the introduction of antipsychotic medication catalyzed the deinstitutionalization movement and was heralded as a shift toward greater societal integration for individuals with mental illness, the current state of individuals with severe mental illness and criminal legal system involvement reflects a significant divergence from that vision. Rather than being fully realized as an evidence-based treatment mechanism for facilitating meaningful community reintegration, medications are often used primarily to stabilize individuals for participation in the criminal legal system. This highlights an unfortunate systemic shortfall in achieving the intended promise of community-based care.

References

1. Delay J, Deniker P, Harl JM. Therapeutic use in psychiatry of phenothiazine of central elective action. *Ann Med Psychol (Paris)*. 1952 Jun;**110**(21):112–117. PMID: 12986408.

2. Leucht S, Tardy M, Komossa K, et al. Antipsychotic drugs versus placebo for relapse prevention in schizophrenia: a systematic review and meta-analysis. *Lancet*. 2012 Jun 2;**379**(9831):2063–2071. doi: 10.1016/ S0140-6736(12)60239-6.

3. Howner K, Andiné P, Engberg G, Ekström EH, et al. Pharmacological treatment in forensic psychiatry-a systematic review. *Front Psychiatry*. 2020 Jan 16;**10**:963. doi: 10.3389/ fpsyt.2019.00963.

4. Singh A, Delgado D, Ventura MI, et al. Clozapine use and forensic outcomes in psychiatric inpatients deemed incompetent to stand trial. *J Am Acad Psychiatry Law*. 2022 Sep;**50**(3):427–433. doi: 10.29158/JAAPL.210123-21.

5. Geddes J, Freemantle N, Harrison P, Bebbington P. Atypical antipsychotics in the treatment of schizophrenia: systematic overview and

meta-regression analysis. *BMJ*. 2000 Dec 2;**321** (7273):1371–1376. doi: 10.1136/bmj.321.7273.1371.

6. Lieberman, JA, Stroup, TS, McEvoy, JP, et al. Effectiveness of antipsychotic drugs in patients with chronic schizophrenia. *N Engl J Med*. 2005 Sep 22; **353** (12):1209–1223. doi: 10.1056/NEJMoa051688.

7. Jones PB, Barnes TR, Davies L, et al. Randomized controlled trial of the effect on Quality of Life of second- vs first-generation antipsychotic drugs in schizophrenia: Cost Utility of the Latest Antipsychotic Drugs in Schizophrenia Study (CUtLASS 1). *Arch Gen Psychiatry*. 2006 Oct;**63**(10):1079–1087. doi: 10.1001/archpsyc.63.10.1079.

8. Haro JM, Edgell ET, Novick D, et al. Effectiveness of antipsychotic treatment for schizophrenia: 6-month results of the Pan-European Schizophrenia Outpatient Health Outcomes (SOHO) study. *Acta Psychiatr Scand*. 2005 Mar;**111**(3):220–231. doi: 10.1111/j.1600-0447.2004.00450.x.

9. Leucht C, Heres S, Kane JM, et al. Oral versus depot antipsychotic drugs for schizophrenia – A critical systematic review and meta-analysis of randomized long-term trials. *Schizophr Res*. 2011 Apr; **127**(1–3):83–92. doi: 10.1016/j.schres.2010.11.020.

10. Tiihonen J, Wahlbeck K, Lönnqvist J, et al. Effectiveness of antipsychotic treatments in a nationwide cohort of patients in community care after first hospitalisation due to schizophrenia and schizoaffective disorder: observational follow-up study. *BMJ*. 2006 Jul 29;**333**(7561):224. doi: 10.1136/bmj.38881.382755.2F.

11. Tiihonen J, Haukka J, Taylor M, et al. A nationwide cohort study of oral and depot antipsychotics after first hospitalization for schizophrenia. *Am J Psychiatry*. 2011 Jun;**168**(6):603–609. doi: 10.1176/appi.ajp.2011.10081224.

12. Lambert T, Olivares JM, Peuskens J, et al. Effectiveness of injectable risperidone long-acting therapy for schizophrenia: data from the US, Spain, Australia, and Belgium. *Ann Gen Psychiatry*. 2011 Apr 4;**10**:10. doi: 10.1186/1744-859X-10-10.

13. Hoge SK. Providing transition and outpatient services to the mentally ill released from correctional institutions. In: Greifinger RB, ed. *Public Health Behind Bars*. New York: Springer; 2022:445–460.

14. Ramsay CE, Goulding SM, Broussard B, et al. Prevalence and psychosocial correlates of prior incarcerations in an urban, predominantly African-American sample of hospitalized patients with first-episode psychosis. *J Am Acad Psychiatry Law*. 2011; **39**(1):57–64.

15. James DJ, Glaze LE. Mental health problems of prison and jail inmates. Bureau of Justice Statistics Special Report, NCJ 213600. September 2006.

16. Owen EA, Perry A, Scher DP. Trauma in competency to stand trial evaluations. In: Javier RA, Owen EA, Maddux JA, eds. *Assessing Trauma in Forensic Contexts*. Switzerland AG: Springer Nature; 2020:65–84.

17. *Dusky* v. *United States*, 362 U.S. 402. 1960.

18. Nicholson RA, Kugler KE. Competent and incompetent criminal defendants: a quantitative review of comparative research. *Psychol Bull*. 1991 May;**109**(3):355–370. doi: 10.1037/0033-2909.109.3.355.

19. Pirelli G, Gottdiener WH, Zapf PA. A meta-analytic review of competency to stand trial research. *Psychol Pub Pol'y Law*. 2011;**17**(1):1–53. doi: 10.1037/a0021713.

20. Rosenfeld B, Wall BW. Psychopathology and competence to stand trial. *Crim Justice Behav*. 1998;**25** (4):443–462. doi: 10.1037/a0021713

21. Wall B, Lee R. Assessing competency to stand trial. *Psychiatr Times*. 2020;37(10).

22. Mossman D. Predicting restorability of incompetent criminal defendants. *J Am Acad Psychiatry Law*. 2007;35(1):34–43.

23. Cochrane RE, Herbel BL, Reardon ML, Lloyd KP. The Sell effect: Involuntary medication treatment is a "clear and convincing" success. *Law Hum Behav*. 2013;37(2): 107–116. doi: 10.1037/lhb0000003.

24. Bergner D. A major problem with compulsory mental health care is the medication. *The New York Times*. 2023.

25. Casey DE. Pathophysiology of antipsychotic drug-induced movement disorders. *J Clin Psychiatry*. 2004;**65**(Suppl 9):25–28.

26. Newcomer JW. Second-generation (atypical) antipsychotics and metabolic effects: a comprehensive literature review. *CNS Drugs*. 2005;**19**(Suppl 1):1–93. doi: 10.2165/00023210-200519001-00001.

27. Fleischhacker WW, Meise U, Günther V, Kurz M. Compliance with antipsychotic drug treatment: influence of side effects. *Acta Psychiatr Scand Suppl*. 1994;**382**:11–15.

28. Kishimoto T, Hagi K, Kurokawa S, Kane JM, Correll CU. Long-acting injectable versus oral antipsychotics for the maintenance treatment of schizophrenia: a systematic review and comparative meta-analysis of randomised, cohort, and pre-post studies. *Lancet Psychiatry*. 2021 May;**8** (5):387–404. doi: 10.1016/S2215-0366 (21)00039-0.

29. Meyers JM. How antipsychotics work in schizophrenia: A primer on mechanisms. *CNS Spectrums*, 2024 Dec 2;**30**(1):e6.

30. Lim WK, Chew QH, He YL, et al. Coprescription of mood stabilizers in schizophrenia, dosing, and clinical correlates: An international study. *Hum Psychopharmacol*. 2020;**35**:1–7. doi: 10.1002/hup.2752.

31. Lähteenvuo M, Taipale H, Tanskanen A, Mittendorfer-Rutz E, Tiihonen J. Effectiveness of pharmacotherapies for delusional disorder in a Swedish national cohort of 9076 patients. *Schizophr Res*. 2021 Feb;**228**:367–372. doi: 10.1016/j.schres.2021.01.015.

32. González-Rodríguez A, Seeman MV. Differences between delusional disorder and schizophrenia: a mini narrative review. *World J Psychiatry*. 2022 May 19;**12** (5):683–692. doi: 10.5498/wjp.v12.i5.683.

33. Muñoz-Negro JE, Ibáñez-Casas I, de Portugal E, et al. A psychopathological comparison between delusional disorder and schizophrenia. *Can J Psychiatry*. 2018 Jan;**63**(1):12–19. doi: 10.1177/0706743717706347.

34. Manschreck TC, Khan NL. Recent advances in the treatment of delusional disorder. *Can J Psychiatry*. 2006 Feb;**51**(2):114–119. doi: 10.1177/070674370 605100207.

35. Miola A, Salvati B, Sambataro F, Toffanin T. Aripiprazole for the treatment of delusional disorders: a systematic review. *Gen Hosp Psychiatry*. 2020 Sep Oct;**66**:34–43. doi: 10.1016/ j.genhosppsych.2020.06.012.

36. Gunduz-Bruce H, McMeniman M, et al. Duration of untreated psychosis and time to treatment response for delusions and hallucinations. *Am J Psychiatry*. 2005 Oct;**162**(10):1966–1969. doi: 10.1176/appi.ajp.162.10.1966.

When Do Psychiatric Interventions Work?

An Argument for Using Functional Outcomes When Evaluating the Effectiveness of Treating Schizophrenia

Sean E. Evans

Introduction

Schizophrenia is considered one of the most disabling psychiatric illnesses in the world.[1,2] Schizophrenia is incredibly complex and impacts not only the individual suffering from this illness, but also the families and communities who often struggle with finding ways to support and care for them.[3] Schizophrenia is most often associated with the presentation of its positive symptoms (e.g., hallucinations, delusions, thought disorganization, and paranoia) and negative symptoms (e.g., alogia, blunted and flat affect, stereotyped behaviors and thinking, and social withdrawal) that are used to diagnose the psychiatric illness. Thus, many outcome studies focus on the reduction of these symptoms as measured by such instruments as the Positive and Negative Syndrome Scale (PANSS)[4] or the Brief Psychiatric Rating Scale (BPRS)[5] for measuring the presence and severity of symptoms associated with psychiatric disorders such as schizophrenia. While these instruments have strong psychometric properties and measure an important aspect of the illness, the impact of schizophrenia on functional outcomes goes beyond just the symptomatology of the illness. For instance, individuals with schizophrenia have higher mortality rates and experience more health issues, cognitive deficits, and functional capacity limitations. These individuals have greater involvement in the criminal justice system, increased risk of being both the victims and perpetrators of violence, and increased rates of homelessness, and they often struggle with everyday functioning. Moreover, they report lower levels of quality of life (QoL).

While these topics have been researched by others, to this author's awareness, there has not been a publication that synthesizes the mortality, cognitive, criminal justice, violence, and quality of life-related functional outcomes of schizophrenia, as this chapter attempts to do. Moreover, this chapter will discuss the impacts that pharmacology and outpatient services can have on improving these broader functional outcomes. The author posits that to promote a more holistic, integrated, and meaningful life, clinicians, researchers, and policymakers need to have a broader conceptualization of "real-world" functional outcomes in individuals diagnosed with schizophrenia that extends beyond just management of psychosis symptomatology.

Mortality rates and health status

The diagnosis of schizophrenia is associated with one of the highest mortality risks of all psychiatric disorders.[6] Studies have suggested that individuals diagnosed with severe mental illness (including schizophrenia) die 15–20 years prematurely compared to the general population.[7] While the reduced lifespan of individuals diagnosed with schizophrenia is well-documented, the underlying causes are less well understood. In a systematic review and meta-analysis of 135 cohort studies comparing 4.5 million individuals with schizophrenia to 1.11 billion individuals in the general population, Correll and colleagues examined the risk and attenuating factors associated with mortality in people with schizophrenia.[8] Their findings revealed that the all-cause mortality rate in individuals diagnosed with schizophrenia was 2.9 times higher when compared with the general population.[8] A lower but still statistically significant 1.6-fold increase in all-cause mortality was observed when compared with diseased-matched general population controls.[8]

Suicide was identified as the highest relative risk factor for individuals diagnosed with schizophrenia. Specifically, Correll and colleagues identified a 9.7-fold increase in relative risk, as well as a 7.4-fold increase in relative risk for all-cause mortality for first-episode schizophrenia when compared with the general population.[8] The suicide-related mortality risks were higher for those individuals who were under the age of

40 years.[8] While not examined specifically in this study, others have highlighted that suicide attempts increase with severity of psychotic and depressive symptoms at first psychotic episode.[9]

Other specific causes of mortality, including poisoning (8–9-fold increase) and pneumonia (7-fold increase), were also higher when compared to the general population.[8] The mortality risk remained higher in individuals diagnosed with schizophrenia for infectious, respiratory, and endocrine diseases (3.7–3.8-fold increase), as well as injuries or accidents (3.3-fold increase), when compared to the general population.[8] Unlike suicide-related mortality, natural-cause mortality was not observed as being higher in those under the age of 40 years. Comorbid substance-use disorder (SUD) increases all-cause mortality as well, which is most likely related to the adverse physical impacts of these substances, as well as the adverse impacts related to injury and suicide-related behaviors.[8] Substance use in general, but particularly cannabis use, was associated with poorer antipsychotic medication adherence.[8]

Overall, these findings support the significant impact that schizophrenia has on outcomes related to all-cause mortality compared to the general population. Early and accurate diagnosis, suicide and SUD screening, and treatment in individuals with schizophrenia are critical to reducing these relative risks.[8] Moreover, these findings highlight that earlier detection and treatment are vital for better health and mortality outcomes for individuals diagnosed with schizophrenia.

Functional capacity in everyday functioning

Aside from mortality rates and lifespan, arguably one of the most disabling impacts of schizophrenia is on an individual's ability to manage everyday life. While seemingly straightforward, operationalizing everyday functioning can be quite challenging, as there are many abilities and factors that go into these daily activities, including stable employment, social connections, and independent living. To navigate the demands of daily living, a person must have the ability to perform the necessary life skills, the motivation to perform these skills, and the situational recognition to know when these skills are likely to be successful.[1] Undergirding the ability, motivation, and situational recognition of everyday functioning is a complex interconnection of cognitive performance, functional capacity, social cognition, clinical symptoms, fitness and health status, and environmental factors.[1] While all of these factors are important, this section will focus on the impact of schizophrenia on cognitive performance and functional capacity in daily life tasks.

Cognitive functioning, as measured by neuropsychological assessment, is composed of specific domains, including attention, language, memory and learning, processing speed, and executive functioning. Deficits in these areas can impact a person's ability to efficiently and effectively perform the daily tasks of life. As summarized in Harvey and Strassnig,[1] several studies have shown small to moderate correlations between individual cognitive domains (e.g., attention) with global indices of everyday functioning.[10] Composite scores (i.e., multiple cognitive domains), on the other hand, show moderate to large correlations with everyday functioning.[10,11] Cognitive function is strongly associated with independent residential living,[12] which is a critical aspect of everyday functioning. While cognitive performance is clearly associated with everyday outcomes (e.g., independent living), there is a growing body of literature on the concept of functional capacity as a more direct correlate of day-to-day functioning.

Functional capacity is defined as "an individual's capability, under controlled conditions, to perform tasks and activities that are necessary or desirable in their lives."[13] Given these elements, assessing functional capacity must take into consideration the specific task or ability, the context it is being performed in, and the nature of the disorder or disability that is impacting an individual's functioning.[13] Studies have found that measures of functional capacity are similarly correlated with performance-based neuropsychological measures of real-world functional outcomes.[1,12] While it is still unclear as to how exactly cognitive performance and functional capacity interact, there is growing evidence that functional capacity may have a more direct impact on everyday abilities.[1] Understanding the impacts of cognitive and functional capacity deficits is critical, as there are specific cognitive rehabilitation interventions that can target these areas of challenge. Clinicians, researchers, and policymakers would be remiss if they did not consider cognitive and functional capacity dimensions when conceptualizing real-world functioning.

Criminalization, violence, and homelessness

It is well documented that individuals with serious mental illness (SMI; e.g., schizophrenia, bipolar disorder, schizoaffective disorder) are at increased risk of arrest and incarceration.[14,15] Reports have indicated that approximately 14% of state prisoners, 8% of federal prisoners, and 26% of jail inmates have reported symptoms that are commensurate with "serious psychological distress."[16,17] Moreover, about 43% of state prisoners and 23% of federal prisoners have a history of mental health problems.[16] Individuals with schizophrenia who are incarcerated often experience disruptions in their treatment and can experience significant increases in symptomatology while languishing in jails and prisons. Much has been written on the topic of the criminalization of the mentally ill, and readers are encouraged to review those resources.[18]

While most individuals with schizophrenia are not violent, the presence of psychosis is a well-established risk factor associated with violence.[19] Specifically, individuals with schizophrenia had a 6-month prevalence of 19% violent behavior, with approximately 3.6% of those constituting "serious violent behavior."[20] Serious violent behavior was associated with positive psychotic symptoms (e.g., persecutory ideation), depressive symptoms, childhood conduct problems, and victimization.[20] A similar prevalence of violence in 2–13% of outpatient individuals within a 6-month to 3-year time frame has been observed by others.[21] While the public tends to be more concerned that individuals with schizophrenia are highly likely to commit acts of violence, the research indicates that individuals with SMI are more likely to be the victims of violence. Compared with 2–13% of individuals with SMI perpetrating violence, 20–34% had been violently victimized within the same time frame.[21] Studies that combined both inpatient and outpatient samples reported that 12–22% had perpetrated violence in the past 6–18 months as compared to 35% who were the victims of violence during that same period.[21]

Many factors contribute to homelessness, including victimization of violence (such as domestic violence), poverty, disability, unemployment, adverse childhood experiences, substance abuse, and the presence of SMI.[3] Individuals who are homeless have a higher prevalence of psychiatric disorders, including schizophrenia.[3] A meta-analysis of 31 studies involving 51,925 individuals worldwide showed higher prevalences of psychosis (21.2%) and schizophrenia (10.3%) among homeless people.[3] Homelessness among those with schizophrenia was higher in developing countries (22.2%) as compared to developed countries (8.9%).[3] Overall, this meta-analysis highlights that schizophrenia has a significant impact on incarceration rates, being both the perpetrator and victim of violence, and homelessness.

Quality of life

Most of the research reviewed for this chapter examined "objective" functional measures associated with a diagnosis of schizophrenia. However, an important, often-overlooked perspective associated with schizophrenia is the subjective experience of the one diagnosed with this disabling psychiatric condition. The literature on QoL for those diagnosed with schizophrenia is complex and often contradictory due to a host of factors, including differing operational definitions, measurement methodologies (e.g., subjective QoL versus "objective" measures of QoL), domains measured (e.g., physical, psychological, social, and health-related), and the impacts of symptom severity and the level of insight.[22,23] Early research raised doubts as to the "accuracy" of subjective QoL judgments due to the cognitive impairments and lack of insight related to schizophrenia[24] and findings of poor agreement in self-ratings as compared to clinicians and family members.[25] However, studies have shown that individuals with schizophrenia are able to accurately report on their social deficits and living situations,[26] and comparable convergent validity ratings in perceptions of QoL between individuals and clinicians have been observed.[27] While there are many ways to define the QoL concept, arguably the most recognized definition of QoL is "an individual's perception of their position in life in the context of the culture and value systems in which they live and in relation to their goals, expectations, standards, and concerns."[28] Relevant to the current chapter, recent meta-analyses elucidate the relevance of QoL in the conceptualization of functional outcomes associated with schizophrenia.[29,30]

There is considerable variability in the findings of published studies regarding QoL among individuals diagnosed with schizophrenia. Several recent studies, including two meta-analyses, examining individuals diagnosed with schizophrenia consistently report lower levels of QoL in domains of physical and psychological health, environmental domains (e.g., accessing resources), and in social relationships when compared to the general population and healthy controls.[23,29,30] Longer durations of illness, symptom severity, poverty, and earlier onset of illness were associated with lower subjective reports of QoL.[23,31] While subjective ratings of QoL can vary significantly over a person's lifetime, one study found that the most significant predictor of subjective QoL was age at time of illness onset, with later onset being associated with higher levels of QoL.[31] In this study, earlier age at onset of illness was associated with more relapses, hospitalizations, and poorer outcomes associated with social, occupational, and general functioning.[31]

Overall, these studies underscore the value of considering QoL when conceptualizing overall functional outcomes. As several studies observed, QoL ratings can fluctuate over the course of one's life, and that, despite all of the challenges associated with schizophrenia, some groups reported their subjective QoL to be good.[31] In the next section we will examine the impacts of pharmacological treatment and outpatient services on the functional outcomes reviewed in this chapter.

The impacts of medications and outpatient services on functional outcomes

As noted previously, individuals diagnosed with schizophrenia have higher mortality rates and rates of health issues, significant cognitive deficits and functional capacity limitations, greater involvement in the criminal justice system, increased risk of being both the victims and perpetrators of violence, are overly represented among the homeless, and report lower levels of QoL. While there is no simple solution to these problems, there are some consistent interventions that have been shown to improve the functional outcomes reviewed in this chapter.

Correll and colleagues showed that prescribing antipsychotic medications can protect against all-cause mortality in individuals diagnosed with schizophrenia.[8] Moreover, the second-generation antipsychotics (SGAs), long-acting injectables (LAIs), clozapine, and SGA-LAIs offered the most significant reductions in mortality rates.[8] LAIs and clozapine have been shown to improve rates of continuation of treatment with cardiometabolic medications, such as statins, antidiabetics, and hypertension medications.[32] Moreover, LAIs have been shown to improve medication adherence, relapse prevention, and psychotic symptoms control, as well as improving cognitive functioning in first-episode schizophrenia patients.[33]

Even the simple possession of consistent medication prescriptions, especially during the first 90 days postdischarge, and routine outpatient services represent some of the most significant protections against reincarceration for adults with schizophrenia.[14] High medication possession, which was defined as having medication to cover 80% or more of the days of a 30-day period, was associated with a reduction in arrest.[14] Interestingly, the reduction in arrests with medication possession was not observed for individuals who had medication possession for less than 90 days postdischarge, indicating that consistent medication possession is critical for the observed reductions in arrests.[14] Also, monthly routine outpatient services were associated with reductions in misdemeanor arrests.[14] Those who were arrested utilized systems (e.g., psychiatric hospitalizations and emergency services) associated with higher acute care costs as compared to those who were not arrested; those who were not arrested had higher outpatient and pharmacological costs, which were still considerably lower than the more expensive acute care costs.[14] The economic modeling of Van Dorn and colleagues[14] highlights the potential fiscal impact to state governments with a hypothetical 20% increase of antipsychotic medication upon release from incarceration, which could lead to direct cost savings of USD 1.7 million over a 3-year period.[34] Thus, consistent medication possession among this population could result in direct cost savings for local and state governments by improving efficiency and reducing unnecessary expenditures.

Van Dorn and colleagues have demonstrated that violence perpetration was a positive indicator of both itself and victimization, drug use, and affective symptoms, while cognitive disorganization was associated with a decrease in violence perpetration.[35] Violent victimization was positively indicated by itself and violence perpetration, as well as affective symptoms and alcohol.[35] Their study also showed that violent victimization, alcohol or drug use, and inpatient hospitalization were associated with an increased likelihood of homelessness. The findings of this study support the use of outpatient services (e.g., trauma-informed therapy and cognitive behavioral therapy) and pharmacological interventions that target the affective symptoms associated with schizophrenia, which can reduce events of violence.[35] Similarly, combined pharmacological and psychotherapeutic treatment, well-managed medication side effects, and integration into community programs (as opposed to being institutionalized) have been associated with higher subjective reports of QoL.[23]

Conclusion

While symptom identification and monitoring are critical for diagnostic clarification and treatment, the findings of this brief literature review highlight the critical need to incorporate functional outcomes associated with schizophrenia that extend beyond just symptom management and reduction. The key point of these studies is that *consistent matched treatment that includes both pharmacological and outpatient services* has been shown to improve all functional outcomes. Consistent matched treatment and outpatient services that prioritize improved medication adherence with SGAs, clozapine, and LAIs can significantly improve mortality rates (most notably related to suicide and injury), everyday functioning, and QoL in individuals disabled by schizophrenia. Clinicians are strongly encouraged to incorporate brief health measure screenings to identify illness risk and reduce mortality. Furthermore, consistent matched treatment and outpatient services that incorporate substance abuse screenings and treatment, trauma-informed therapy, cognitive behavioral therapy, and pharmacological treatment that targets both psychosis and affective symptoms have been shown to reduce arrests, violence (both perpetration and victimization) rates, and homelessness. And finally, consistent matched treatment and outpatient services that include neurocognitive and social cognitive training have been shown to improve cognitive and functional capacity dimensions, which are essential for managing everyday life. Better community integration, managed symptoms, improved health, and purposeful living have been shown to improve QoL. Clinicians, researchers, and policymakers need to broaden their conceptualizations of "outcomes" to go beyond the management of psychosis symptomatology. This chapter presents a conceptual framework for advancing more holistic, real-world functional outcomes that promote enhanced community integration and safety, as well as meaningful life experiences for individuals diagnosed with schizophrenia.

References

1. Harvey PD, Strassnig M. Predicting the severity of everyday functional disability in people with schizophrenia: Cognitive deficits, functional capacity, symptoms, and health status. *World Psychiatry*. 2012;**11**(2):73–79.

2. Murray CJ, Lopez AD. Global mortality, disability, and the contribution of risk factors: Global Burden of Disease Study. *Lancet Lond Engl*. 1997;**349**(9063):1436–1442. doi:10.1016/S0140-6736(96)07495-8

3. Ayano G, Tesfaw G, Shumet S. The prevalence of schizophrenia and other psychotic disorders among homeless people: a systematic review and meta-analysis. *BMC Psychiatry*. 2019;**19**(1):370. doi:10.1186/s12888-019-2361-7

4. Kay SR, Fiszbein A, Opler LA. The Positive and Negative Syndrome Scale (PANSS) for schizophrenia. *Schizophr Bull*. 1987;**13**(2):261–276. doi:10.1093/schbul/13.2.261

5. Overall JE, Gorham DR. The Brief Psychiatric Rating Scale. *Psychol Rep*. 1962;**10**:799–812. doi:10.2466/pr0.1962.10.3.799

6. Vermeulen J, van Rooijen G, Doedens P, et al. Antipsychotic medication and long-term mortality risk in patients with schizophrenia; a systematic review and meta-analysis. *Psychol Med*. 2017;**47**(13):2217–2228. doi:10.1017/S0033291717000873

7. Vancampfort D, Rosenbaum S, Schuch F, et al. Cardiorespiratory fitness in severe mental illness: A systematic review and meta-analysis. *Sports Med Auckl NZ*. 2017;**47**(2):343–352. doi:10.1007/s40279-016-0574-1

8. Correll CU, Solmi M, Croatto G, et al. Mortality in people with schizophrenia: A systematic review and meta-analysis of relative risk and aggravating or attenuating factors. *World Psychiatry*. 2022;**21**(2):248–271. doi:10.1002/wps.20994

9. Díaz-Caneja CM, Pina-Camacho L, Rodríguez-Quiroga A, et al. Predictors of outcome in early-onset psychosis: A systematic review. *NPJ Schizophr*. 2015;**1**:14005. doi:10.1038/npjschz.2014.5

10. McClure MM, Bowie CR, Patterson TL, et al. Correlations of functional capacity and neuropsychological performance in older patients with schizophrenia: Evidence for specificity of relationships? *Schizophr Res*. 2007;**89**(1):330–338. doi:10.1016/j.schres.2006.07.024

11. Green MF, Kern RS, Braff DL, Mintz J. Neurocognitive deficits and functional outcome in schizophrenia: Are we measuring the "right stuff"? *Schizophr Bull*. 2000;**26**(1):119–136. doi:10.1093/oxfordjournals.schbul.a033430

12. Bowie CR, Leung WW, Reichenberg A, et al. Predicting schizophrenia patients' real world behavior with specific

neuropsychological and functional capacity measures. *Biol Psychiatry*. 2008;**63**(5):505–511. doi:10.1016/j.biopsych.2007.05.022

13. Patterson TL, Mausbach BT. Measurement of functional capacity: A new approach to understanding functional differences and real-world behavioral adaptation in those with mental illness. *Annu Rev Clin Psychol*. 2010;**6**:139–154. doi:10.1146/annurev.clinpsy.121208.131339

14. Van Dorn RA, Desmarais SL, Petrila J, Haynes D, Singh JP. Effects of outpatient treatment on risk of arrest of adults with serious mental illness and associated costs. *Psychiatr Serv Wash DC*. 2013;**64**(9):856–862. doi:10.1176/appi.ps.201200406

15. Munetz MR, Grande TP, Chambers MR. The incarceration of individuals with severe mental disorders. *Community Ment Health J*. 2001;**37**(4):361–372. doi:10.1023/a:1017508826264

16. Maruschak LM, Bronson J, Alper M. *Indicators of Mental Health Problems Reported by Prisoners: Survey of Prison Inmates, 2016*. Bureau of Justice Statistics; 2021.

17. Bronson J, Berzofsky M. *Indicators of Mental Health Problems Reported by Prisoners and Jail Inmates, 2011–12*. Bureau of Justice Statistics; 2017.

18. Warburton K, Stahl SM, eds. *Decriminalizing Mental Illness*. Cambridge University Press; 2021.

19. Douglas KS, Guy LS, Hart SD. Psychosis as a risk factor for violence to others: A meta-analysis. *Psychol Bull*. 2009;**135**(5):679–706. doi:10.1037/a0016311

20. Swanson J, Van Dorn R, Monahan J, Swartz M. Violence and leveraged community treatment for persons with mental disorders. *Am J Psychiatry*. 2006;**163**(8):1404–1411.

21. Choe JY, Teplin LA, Abram KM. Perpetration of violence, violent victimization, and severe mental illness: Balancing public health concerns. *Psychiatr Serv*. 2008;**59**(2):153–164. doi:10.1176/ps.2008.59.2.153

22. Eack SM, Newhill CE. Psychiatric symptoms and quality of life in schizophrenia: A meta-analysis. *Schizophr Bull*. 2007;**33**(5):1225–1237. doi:10.1093/schbul/sbl071

23. Bobes J, Garcia-Portilla MP, Bascaran MT, Saiz PA, Bouzoño M. Quality of life in schizophrenic patients. *Dialogues Clin Neurosci*. 2007;**9**(2):215–226. doi:10.31887/DCNS.2007.9.2/jbobes

24. Bobes J, García-Portilla P, Sáiz PA, Bascarán T, Bousoño M. Quality of life measures in schizophrenia. *Eur Psychiatry J Assoc Eur Psychiatr*. 2005;**20**(Suppl 3):S313–S317. doi:10.1016/s0924-9338(05)80182-8

25. Sainfort F, Becker M, Diamond R. Judgments of quality of life of individuals with severe mental disorders: Patient self-report versus provider perspectives. *Am J Psychiatry*. 1996;**153**(4):497–502. doi:10.1176/ajp.153.4.497

26. Skantze K, Malm U, Dencker SJ, May PR, Corrigan P. Comparison of quality of life with standard of living in schizophrenic out-patients. *Br J Psychiatry J Ment Sci*. 1992;**161**:797–801. doi:10.1192/bjp.161.6.797

27. Lehman AF, Postrado LT, Rachuba LT. Convergent validation of quality of life assessments for persons with severe mental illnesses. *Qual Life Res Int J Qual Life Asp Treat Care Rehabil*. 1993;**2**(5):327–333. doi:10.1007/BF00449427

28. The World Health Organization Quality of Life Assessment (WHOQOL): Development and general psychometric properties. *Soc Sci Med 1982*. 1998;**46**(12):1569–1585. doi:10.1016/s0277-9536(98)00009-4

29. Dong M, Lu L, Zhang L, et al. Quality of life in schizophrenia: A meta-analysis of comparative studies. *Psychiatr Q*. 2019;**90**(3):519–532. doi:10.1007/s11126-019-09633-4

30. Attepe Özden S, Tekindal M, Tekindal MA. Quality of life of people with schizophrenia: A meta-analysis. *Int J Soc Psychiatry*. 2023;**69**(6):1444–1452. doi:10.1177/00207640231164019

31. Migliorini C, Harvey C, Hou C, et al. Subjective quality of life and schizophrenia: Results from a large cohort study based in Chinese primary care. *BMC Psychiatry*. 2024;**24**(1):86. doi:10.1186/s12888-024-05558-w

32. Solmi M, Tiihonen J, Lähteenvuo M, et al. Antipsychotics use is associated with greater adherence to cardiometabolic medications in patients with schizophrenia: Results from a nationwide, within-subject design study. *Schizophr Bull*. 2022;**48**(1):166–175. doi:10.1093/schbul/sbab087

33. Subotnik KL, Casaus LR, Ventura J, et al. Long-acting injectable risperidone for relapse prevention and control of breakthrough symptoms after a recent first episode of schizophrenia. A randomized clinical trial. *JAMA Psychiatry*. 2015;**72**(8):822–829. doi:10.1001/jamapsychiatry.2015.0270

34. Lin I, Muser E, Munsell M, Benson C, Menzin J. Economic impact of psychiatric relapse and recidivism among adults with schizophrenia recently released from incarceration: A Markov model analysis. *J Med Econ*. 2015;**18**(3):219–229. doi:10.3111/13696998.2014.971161

35. Van Dorn RA, Grimm K, Desmarais SL, et al. Leading indicators of community-based violent events among adults with mental illness. *Psychol Med*. 2017;**47**(7):1179–1191. doi:10.1017/S0033291716003160

Chapter 10

Medications for Psychosis in People with Schizophrenia
What Happens If You Take Them and What Happens If You Don't?

Ambarin Faizi and Stephen M. Stahl

Introduction

Schizophrenia is a severe, chronic psychiatric illness that disrupts perception, cognition, emotion, and function. Despite its low prevalence (approximately 1% globally), it remains one of the leading causes of disability worldwide.[1] While historically viewed as a progressively debilitating mental illness, the disorder has undergone a paradigm shift in understanding. Once associated with treatment nihilism, contemporary research underscores that, with timely and appropriate interventions, individuals diagnosed with schizophrenia can achieve significant symptoms remission and functional recovery.[2–5]

Antipsychotic medications – the cornerstone of schizophrenia treatment for over 70 years – have demonstrable efficacy in reducing psychotic symptoms, preventing relapse, and improving functional outcomes. Yet, the role of long-term pharmacotherapy remains controversial. A vocal minority of critics argue that antipsychotics impair brain function, blunt emotions, and are overprescribed, pointing to naturalistic studies suggesting better outcomes in unmedicated patients. This controversy has led to an urgent clinical and ethical question: Do antipsychotic medications improve long-term outcomes in schizophrenia – or can they worsen them? This question becomes even more pressing when patients intermittently refuse treatment, a common occurrence in clinical practice largely due to anosognosia (poor insight), an unfortunate and prominent symptom of schizophrenia, compounded by experienced or potential medication side effects. As clinicians, we must weigh the potential neurobiological effects of both antipsychotic treatment and untreated psychosis. The stakes are high: Untreated schizophrenia is associated with persistent symptoms, cognitive decline, impaired functioning, poor quality of life, and even premature death.

Our aim is to evaluate the efficacy and necessity of antipsychotic medications in the treatment of schizophrenia, particularly in light of the adverse outcomes observed in patients who intermittently refuse or discontinue treatment. First, we review short-term randomized controlled trials (RCTs), long-term naturalistic studies, real-world forensic outcomes, and emerging neuroimaging evidence to determine whether sustained antipsychotic treatment offers a net benefit in reducing relapse, preserving function, and improving clinical outcomes. We then discuss what we know about the consequences of not taking medications for psychosis in people with schizophrenia, including putative neurotoxic and functional consequences of untreated psychosis.

What happens if people with schizophrenia take antipsychotic medications for psychosis?

Short-term trials

Short-term RCTs form the evidentiary backbone of antipsychotic medication approval. These studies typically last 4–6 weeks and assess symptom reduction using validated scales like the Positive and Negative Syndrome Scale (PANSS) or Brief Psychiatric Rating Scale (BPRS). These trials consistently show that a 20% reduction in symptom severity can be observed within the first 2–4 weeks of treatment. For example, in studies[6] evaluating antipsychotic medications such as risperidone and olanzapine, clinically meaningful improvements typically occur within this initial treatment window. This has led to the understanding that the first few weeks of treatment are critical for assessing early response and predicting longer-term outcomes. Short-term RCTs remain the gold standard for demonstrating the initial efficacy of antipsychotic medications. They consistently show that antipsychotics significantly reduce positive symptoms of schizophrenia, such as delusions and hallucinations. Despite their brevity, their findings are consistent and robust: Antipsychotic medications are significantly more effective than placebo in reducing psychotic symptoms and preventing relapse.[5,7–12]

In one of the most comprehensive meta-analyses of antipsychotic efficacy, Leucht et al.[10] reviewed 167 double-blind RCTs, spanning 60 years of antipsychotic drug trials in acute schizophrenia, with over 28,000 chronically ill participants, and they clarified what constitutes a clinically meaningful treatment response. While regulatory trials often define "response" as a 20% reduction in symptom severity on rating scales such as the PANSS or BPRS, this minimal threshold reflects modest clinical improvement. A 20% reduction may signify early symptom shift, but it does not reliably correlate with improved functioning or reduced suffering. Notably, Leucht and colleagues differentiated this from "good response," defined as a 50% or greater reduction in symptoms scores: a benchmark more strongly associated with robust clinical change, patient-perceived benefit, and readiness for social recovery. Their meta-analysis found that patients treated with antipsychotic medications were more likely to achieve this level of improvement compared to those receiving placebo. These findings strengthen the argument that antipsychotics do more than merely nudge symptoms – they enable substantial and clinically visible improvement in a population in which early and effective treatment can alter long-term trajectories. The findings further reinforce the importance of distinguishing between minimal and meaningful response when evaluating the utility of antipsychotic medications in short-term trials.

In summary, short-term trials robustly support the initial efficacy of treatment with antipsychotic medications.

Long-term trials

Despite the proven efficacy of antipsychotics in short-term trials in people with schizophrenia, a critical question remains: Do these benefits persist in the long term? While short-term RCTs provide critical initial evidence for the efficacy of antipsychotic medication, particularly in reducing acute psychotic symptoms, these trials are inherently limited by their brief duration. In the context of a chronic and relapsing condition like schizophrenia, longer-term outcomes such as sustained remission, functional recovery, and prevention of relapse are more clinically meaningful. However, conducting long-term RCTs in this population presents ethical and practical challenges. Randomizing individuals to prolonged placebo conditions or medication discontinuation is widely considered to be unethical due to the known risk of relapse and potential for serious harm to the individual and others. Furthermore, the chronic nature of schizophrenia, often accompanied by fluctuating insight, impaired adherence, and social instability, makes participant retention in blinded long-term trials difficult. These limitations underscore the importance of real-world data, observational studies, and large registry-based analyses to examine the long-term effectiveness and safety of antipsychotic treatment in naturalistic settings.

The large-scale Schizophrenia Outpatient Health Outcomes (SOHO) study[13] provides support for the long-term effectiveness of antipsychotic medications in real-world settings. Encompassing over 10,000 patients across 10 European countries, SOHO is one of the largest longitudinal studies ever conducted on the outpatient treatment of schizophrenia. The authors observed patients over a 3-year period to assess symptom severity, functional outcomes, and treatment adherence under naturalistic clinical conditions. Importantly, the study reflected the diversity of schizophrenia treatment outside of controlled research environments, offering insights that are directly applicable to everyday psychiatric practice. The findings were unequivocal in supporting the sustained use of antipsychotics. Patients who remained adherent to treatment, particularly with olanzapine and clozapine, demonstrated greater improvements in clinical outcomes, including reductions in positive and negative symptoms, and improvements in quality of life and social functioning, reinforcing the idea that long-term pharmacologic engagement translates to tangible benefits in patient quality of life. Like the Clinical Antipsychotic Trials of Intervention Effectiveness (CATIE) trial,[12] the researchers found olanzapine to be more effective than other antipsychotic medications in the same class. The 6-month results indicating better clinical outcomes, including quality of life and symptom improvement measured with the Clinical Global Impressions (CGI) scale, were also sustained in the 12-month analysis for participants treated with olanzapine and clozapine. The results also confirmed the greater effectiveness of clozapine and supported using combinations of antipsychotics.

Another compelling real-world study[14] offers validation of antipsychotic efficacy beyond short-term RCTs. This study examined outcomes among individuals with serious mental illness, including schizophrenia, who were deemed Incompetent to Stand Trial (IST) and required psychiatric stabilization and competency restoration in a forensic setting. The authors found that among 3,166 individuals found IST, 86.5% were successfully restored to competency within 1 year of antipsychotic treatment. This study highlights both the clinical effectiveness of antipsychotic medications as well as their ability to restore high-level capacities and function in severely mentally ill populations.

Further affirming their central role in the treatment of schizophrenia, Glick and colleagues[15] offer a comprehensive, data-driven synthesis of the mid- and long-term efficacy of antipsychotic medications. Drawing from extensive evidence of studies with a duration of 3 months or longer, the authors concluded that their findings from controlled and observational long-term studies "closely [parallel] the efficacy observed in short-term controlled studies." Glick and colleagues provided treatment recommendations in support of long-term treatment of schizophrenia. Based on their findings, the literature, and clinical experiences, they emphasized that antipsychotics consistently reduce relapse risk, improve symptom stability, and enhance functional outcomes over the long term, especially when used in a personalized and continuous manner. A personalized model underscores the need to optimize the use of antipsychotics across the illness trajectory and highlights that, when applied thoughtfully, antipsychotic medications confer not only short-term relief but also durable, life-stabilizing benefits in patients with schizophrenia.

Additional support for long-term antipsychotic treatment comes from the systematic review conducted by Takeuchi et al.[16] that examined 14 international clinical practice guidelines and pharmacological treatment algorithms for schizophrenia published after the year 2000. Their review demonstrated a remarkable global consensus: Virtually all authoritative guidelines recommend continued antipsychotic maintenance

therapy for patients stabilized after an acute episode to prevent relapse. The authors noted that while the exact duration of maintenance therapy may be up for debate, no major guideline supports discontinuation within 5 years of illness onset. Furthermore, intermittent or targeted strategies, defined by the National Institute for Health and Care Excellence (NICE)[17] as "the use of antipsychotic medication only during periods of incipient relapse or symptom exacerbation rather than continuously," also was not recommended. Takeuchi et al.'s comprehensive synthesis affirms that long-term pharmacotherapy is not only evidence based, but also internationally endorsed as a standard of care, especially when tailored to individual risk profiles, functional status, and patient preferences.

Additional evidence for the value of long-term treatment of people with schizophrenia with antipsychotics comes from the largest real-world cohort studies examining schizophrenia outcomes by Tiihonen et al.[18,39] and Taipale et al.[19] These studies illustrate that continuous antipsychotic use is associated with reduced relapse rates, lowered mortality, and improved long-term functioning. Specifically, in a nationwide cohort of 29,823 patients with schizophrenia in Finland, Tiihonen and colleagues compared the effectiveness of antipsychotic treatment strategies using observational data and within-individual analyses. The results demonstrated that continuous antipsychotic use was associated with a dramatically reduced risk of hospitalization and all-cause mortality. In particular, this study found that clozapine and long-acting injectables (LAIs) were most effective at preventing hospitalization, with clozapine associated with a 22% lower risk of rehospitalization compared to olanzapine, and with LAIs significantly outperforming their oral counterparts. In the complementary FIN20 study by Taipale et al. – a nationwide longitudinal analysis of over 62,000 patients with schizophrenia and up to two decades of follow-up (median 14.1 years) – the researchers found that long-term antipsychotic use conferred a substantial survival benefit. Compared to no antipsychotic use, "long-term antipsychotic use was associated with substantially lower all-cause, cardiovascular and suicide mortality in people with schizophrenia." Furthermore, in a 20-year nationwide follow-up study,[39] the authors cautioned that the "risk of treatment failure or relapse after discontinuation of antipsychotic use does not decrease during the first 8 years of illness, and that long-term antipsychotic treatment is associated with increased survival." These high-quality, population-level studies provide some of the most convincing evidence that continuous antipsychotic treatment not only prevents relapse, but saves lives.

Collectively, these studies illustrate that long-term antipsychotic treatment is associated with substantial reductions in hospitalization rates and reduced risk of death from all causes, including cardiovascular disease and suicide, among individuals with schizophrenia.

What happens if people with schizophrenia don't take antipsychotic medications for psychosis?

No harm, no foul?

Although antipsychotic medications have demonstrated efficacy in short- and long-term trials in people with schizophrenia, their long-term impact remains a subject of ongoing inquiry: For whom do these benefits persist in the long run, and what happens when patients discontinue treatment or go untreated? Some patient advocates argue that if the short-term trials show only about a 20% reduction in positive symptoms for responders, with minimal improvement in negative symptoms, quality of life, and social functioning, and if not all patients achieve even this modest benefit, then antipsychotic treatment might reasonably be considered optional. Their position is that a patient could always resume medication later and potentially obtain the same symptom relief if they change their mind. They point to evidence that a portion of patients recover without sustained antipsychotic treatment, citing studies that report recovery rates of around 21% without treatment in first-episode schizophrenia[20] and of roughly 11% in patients with multiepisode schizophrenia,[21] suggesting that the costs and side effects of treatment might not be justified for everyone if there is the chance of recovering without it. For example, Harrow and Jobe's observational studies[22,23] demonstrated that a subgroup of individuals with schizophrenia who discontinued antipsychotic medication were less likely to be psychotic and experience more periods of recovery compared to their continuously medicated counterparts. Similarly, Wunderink et al.[24] found that among first-episode patients in remission, dose reduction or discontinuation was associated with improved long-term social recovery at the 7-year mark. Such findings are often cited in debates questioning the need for long-term pharmacologic maintenance. On the other hand, critics of these studies have raised important counterpoints, notably on the study design, patient selection, and illness severity. They highlight that patients who discontinue medication successfully may represent a fundamentally different clinical phenotype, such as those with a milder course of illness and an intrinsically better prognosis or those with greater psychosocial resilience, rather than evidence that medication itself causes poor outcomes. Supporting this, a study more closely generalizable to real-world settings by Robinson et al.[25] prospectively followed patients after their first episode of schizophrenia or schizoaffective disorder and found that patients who discontinued antipsychotic medication had a fivefold higher risk of relapse compared to those who maintained treatment. In their study, 53% of patients who relapsed for the first time after 2 years of stability had discontinued medication use, "suggesting the continued importance of maintenance medication treatment" extending beyond the vulnerable early years following illness onset.

The brain pays the price of relapse

There has been a growing discussion around the impact of intermittent or targeted treatment in patients with partial insight and adherence difficulties, and there have even been some proposals to curtail continuous treatment. However, numerous studies show that each psychotic relapse is neurobiologically costly and contributes to treatment resistance, and that the brain may not fully recover to baseline functioning after repeated such episodes.[2] Emsley[26] emphasized that the factor most strongly correlated with brain volume decline is relapse duration, reinforcing the idea that chronicity of untreated psychosis is neurotoxic. While individualized treatment planning may involve dose reductions or carefully supervised discontinuation in rare cases, unstructured or prolonged refusal of medication should not be misconstrued as benign. The long-term risks, including symptom exacerbation, treatment resistance, suicidality, and functional decline, highlight the need for proactive monitoring and ongoing patient engagement, even after symptom remission. A more realistic and compassionate harm-reduction model may involve minimizing relapse duration, using LAIs when appropriate, and maintaining the lowest effective dose tailored to individual needs.

Taken together, these findings affirm that while schizophrenia is a heterogeneous and complex illness, the vast majority of patients derive significant benefit from sustained pharmacologic treatment. Rather than reject maintenance treatment altogether, these studies underscore the importance of tailoring care to the patient's clinical trajectory, risk profile, and preferences, using shared decision-making grounded in the best available evidence, including assessment of the risk of long-term progressive brain damage worsened by a lack of continuous treatment.

Since schizophrenia is now known to be associated with structural brain abnormalities, including reductions in gray matter volume, particularly in the prefrontal cortex, hippocampus, and temporal lobes,[27,28] a critical debate in the literature concerns whether long-term structural brain changes, especially reductions in gray matter volume, are due to illness or to the treatment. A close examination of the literature reveals a complex yet reassuring picture. The available evidence increasingly supports the view that schizophrenia itself is associated with progressive neuroanatomical deterioration, and that this disease-driven brain toxicity may be mitigated, not worsened, by antipsychotic treatment. Concerns about potential brain volume loss due to antipsychotic medications persist, but these concerns are increasingly counterbalanced by growing evidence suggesting that schizophrenia itself is far more neurotoxic than its treatment. An extensive review by Fountoulakis and Stahl[28] reveals that while some brain changes may be observed in medicated patients, these are often less pronounced than the changes seen in those who remain untreated and are more plausibly linked to illness progression.[28,29] Fountoulakis and Stahl[28] argue that the literature does not support that antipsychotics cause loss of brain volume; rather, it indicates that antipsychotics might exert a protective effect against brain volume loss. Lawrie[30] has also dismantled unfounded fears about antipsychotics, stating that they "probably do not shrink the brain," and that such fears do not have clinical relevance.

More recently, a landmark triple-blind randomized, placebo-controlled magnetic resonance imaging (MRI) study by Chopra et al.[29] further clarified this issue, showing that patients treated with second-generation antipsychotics exhibited less progression of gray matter loss over time and, in some, even a reversal of volume deficits. They concluded that antipsychotic medication might reverse illness-

related volume loss in the pallidum, and they noted that their findings were consistent with earlier studies that suggested a neuroprotective effect of second-generation antipsychotic medication. This aligns with findings from an analysis of 202 patients' MRI data from the Iowa Longitudinal Study of first-episode schizophrenia, in which Emsley[26] found that relapse duration (not the number of relapses) and treatment intensity are associated with "significant reductions in brain volume measures." Although continuous treatment remains ideal for symptom control and relapse prevention, these findings suggest that any antipsychotic exposure, whether consistent or sporadic, may confer neuroprotective benefits at appropriate dosages, preferably at the lowest medication dosage indicated. This paradigm offers hope for patients with adherence challenges, reframing discontinuous treatment as a viable harm-reduction strategy.

The cost to the brain of delay in onset of treatment

Perhaps the most convincing evidence that schizophrenia is associated with progressive structural brain degeneration comes from studies of how long treatment is delayed after the onset of a first psychotic episode. Emerging evidence from neuroimaging, clinical outcomes, and biomarker studies reinforces a critical principle: In schizophrenia, as in stroke or traumatic brain injury, "time is brain." Longer duration of untreated psychosis (DUP), defined as the interval between the onset of psychotic symptoms and the initiation of effective antipsychotic treatment, has been consistently associated with poorer long-term outcomes, reduced functional recovery, and progressive structural brain changes.[3,31,32] In the USA, Kane et al.[33] reported that the average DUP among first-episode patients was 74 weeks, much longer than the under 12-week target recommended by the World Health Organization and the International Early Psychosis Association. This prolonged delay represents a critical window of missed opportunity, during which patients are often deteriorating in the absence of adequate treatment.

Neuroimaging studies have shown that even modest delays in treatment contribute to reductions in gray matter volume, which are most pronounced in the prefrontal cortex, hippocampus, and temporal lobes,[27,28] regions responsible for memory, executive functioning, and emotional regulation. Poor outcomes are associated with prominent hippocampal volume reduction in schizophrenia and with long DUP.[27] These changes may be evident even before the transition to full-blown psychosis, suggesting that neurobiological alterations occur in the prodromal phase.[34] Prolonged DUP has been associated with hippocampal atrophy and decreased gray matter volume in orbitofrontal, parietal,[35] and occipitotemporal regions,[36] reinforcing the hypothesis that untreated psychosis may have neurotoxic effects on several brain structures essential for memory and executive function. Guo et al.[36] aligned with Goff et al.,[27] suggesting that untreated psychosis itself drives structural brain changes and that structural brain abnormalities are associated with poor treatment response and poor long-term outcomes, thereby stressing the importance of early detection and treatment. Stone et al.[32] proposed a dual pathway, whereby both neurodevelopmental vulnerabilities and neurodegenerative processes contribute to cognitive deficits in long-term untreated schizophrenia. In 2020, Kraguljac et al.[37] added to this body of work with a multimodal imaging study showing that first-episode patients already exhibit widespread abnormalities in brain structure, particularly white matter integrity, and glutamatergic metabolism at the time of diagnosis. A major strength of their study was that they recruited participants who were either antipsychotic medication-naive (83%) or had less than or equal to 5 days of antipsychotic exposure in their lifetime. This work contributes efforts to disentangle the controversy over whether these structural changes are caused by antipsychotic drugs or are intrinsic to the psychotic illness itself. Furthermore, their findings indicate that "DUP exerts its effects on treatment response through affecting white matter integrity," adding to a growing body of evidence of white matter integrity as a predictor of treatment response and echoing the importance of early intervention efforts in schizophrenia.

These findings emphasize the urgent need for early identification and intervention in schizophrenia. The longer a patient remains untreated, the more likely they are to experience neuroanatomic deterioration, functional decline, and treatment resistance. Studies[31] show that even short delays of 7 days reduce functional recovery, with the steepest decline occurring within the first month. Recent research by Slovakova et al.[38] added nuance to this: Differences as slight as weeks in DUP translated to worse outcomes 5 years later. For patients with adherence challenges, the evidence increasingly supports harm-reduction strategies, such as low-dose maintenance, mostly due to the fact that relapse duration, not number of relapses, correlates most strongly with brain volume loss.[26]

Timely intervention, lasting recovery: Advancing evidence-based treatment for schizophrenia

The findings we presented throughout this review converge on a central message: The timely and sustained use of antipsychotic medication remains the most effective evidence-based strategy for reducing symptoms, preventing relapse, and optimizing functional outcomes in schizophrenia. While concerns about potential side effects and long-term safety have fueled debate, these must be balanced against the substantial and well-documented risks associated with untreated or inconsistently treated psychosis. It is a myth that there are no consequences to refusing treatment of psychosis with antipsychotics in schizophrenia and that reinstituting treatment at a later date will always work as well as if it had been continuously given.

Rather than a one-size-fits-all approach (i.e., everyone with schizophrenia needs to be treated continuously forever versus everyone with schizophrenia can stop their medications with impunity), contemporary care must reflect the heterogeneity of schizophrenia. Individuals vary in their symptom trajectories, functional goals, treatment tolerance and response, and levels of insight. The goal is not to promote indiscriminate medication use, but rather to emphasize early initiation and thoughtful, individualized treatment as the standard, particularly in light of data showing that treatment delays and interruptions are associated with poorer outcomes. Thus, the all-too-common situation of intermittent or inconsistent treatment remains a serious clinical risk. While harm-reduction approaches may provide flexibility and reduce barriers for some, the cumulative burden of relapse, particularly prolonged episodes, underscores the value of sustained therapeutic engagement. The evidence increasingly supports the notion that every episode of untreated psychosis matters. The longer psychosis is left untreated, the more difficult it becomes to reverse its impact. Moreover, neuroimaging findings and real-world outcomes suggest that untreated schizophrenia is more neurotoxic than appropriately dosed antipsychotic medications. Although ongoing refinement in treatment algorithms and novel medications may be necessary, the pendulum should not swing so far toward skepticism that it obscures reality: Antipsychotic medications remain the cornerstone of recovery for individuals with schizophrenia.

In reframing this conversation, we must promote a nuanced narrative, one that upholds patient autonomy while also acknowledging the realities of a prominent symptom of schizophrenia: lack of insight into the illness. As the field moves forward, integration of biological, clinical, and lived-experience approaches will be essential to informing shared decision-making and to developing more personalized, ethical, compassionate, and effective care strategies for people living with schizophrenia.

References

1. GBD 2016 Disease and Injury Incidence and Prevalence Collaborators. Global, regional, and national incidence, prevalence, and years lived with disability for 328 diseases and injuries for 195 countries, 1990–2016: A systematic analysis for the Global Burden of Disease Study 2016. *Lancet.* 2017;**390**(10100):1211–1259. doi: 10.1016/S01406736(17)32154-2. Erratum in: *Lancet.* 2017;**390**(10106):e38. doi: 10.1016/S0140-6736(17)32647-8.

2. Agid O. Re-evaluating the prognosis of schizophrenia: Tackling the issue of inadequate treatment. *Expert Review of Neurotherapeutics.* 2024;**24**:831–835. doi: 10.1080/14737175.2024.2365943.

3. Penttila M, Jaaskelainen E, Hirvonen N, et al. Duration of untreated psychosis as predictor of long-term outcome in schizophrenia: Systematic review and meta-analysis. *The British Journal of Psychiatry.* 2014;**205**:88–94. doi: 10.1192/bjp.bp.113.127753.

4. Correll CU. From receptor pharmacology to improved outcomes: Individualising the selection, dosing, and switching of antipsychotics. *European Psychiatry.* 2010;**25**(2):S12–S21. doi: 10.1016/S0924-9338(10)71701-6.

5. Correll CU. Do antipsychotics work in people with schizophrenia? A review of outcomes and effect sizes. *CNS Spectrums.* 2025;**30**(1):e59.

6. Kahn RS, Fleischhacker WW, Bother H, et al. Effectiveness of antipsychotic drugs in first-episode schizophrenia and schizophreniform disorder: An open randomised clinical trial. *The Lancet.* 2008;**371**(9618):1085–1097. doi: 10.1016/S0140-6736(08)60486-9.

7. Leucht S, Arbter D, Engel RR, et al. How effective are second-generation antipsychotic drugs? A meta-analysis of placebo-controlled trials. *Molecular Psychiatry.* 2009;**14**(4):429–447. doi: 10.1038/sj.mp.4002136.

8. Leucht S, Tardy M, Komossa K, et al. Antipsychotic drugs versus placebo for relapse prevention in schizophrenia: A systematic review and meta-analysis. *The Lancet.* 2012;**379**(9831):2063–2071. doi: 10.1016/S0140-6736(12)60239-6.

9. Leucht S, Cipriani A, Spineli L, et al. Comparative efficacy and tolerability of 15 antipsychotic drugs in schizophrenia: A multiple-treatment meta analysis. *The Lancet.* 2013;**382**(9896):951–962. doi: 10.1016/S0140-6736(13)60733-3.

10. Leucht S, Leucht C, Huhn M, et al. Sixty years of placebo-controlled antipsychotic drug trials in acute schizophrenia: Systematic review, Bayesian meta-analysis, and meta-regression of efficacy predictors. *American Journal of Psychiatry.* 2017;**174**:927–942. doi: 10.1176/appi.ajp.2017.16121358.

11. Agid O, Siu CO, Potkin SG, et al. Meta-regression analysis of placebo response in antipsychotic trials, 1970–2010. *American Journal of Psychiatry.* 2013;**170**(11):1335–1344.

12. Antipsychotic Trials of Intervention Effectiveness (CATIE) Investigators. Effectiveness of antipsychotic drugs in patients with chronic schizophrenia. *New England Journal of Medicine.* 2005;**353**(12):1209–1223.

13. Haro JM, Edgell ET, Novick D, et al. SOHO Advisory Board. Effectiveness of antipsychotic treatment for schizophrenia: 6-month results of the Pan-European Schizophrenia Outpatient Health Outcomes (SOHO) study. *Acta Psychiatr Scandinavica.* 2005;**111**(3):220–231. doi: 10.1111/j.1600-0447.2004.00450.x.

14. Faizi A, McDermott B, Warburton K. Do antipsychotic medications work? An exploration using competency to stand trial as the functional outcome. *CNS Spectrums.* 2025;**30**(1):e29.

15. Glick ID, Correll CU, Altamura C, et al. Antipsychotic medications for schizophrenia: A data-driven, personalized clinical approach. *Journal of Clinical Psychiatry.* 2011;**72**(12):1616–1627.

16. Takeuchi H, Suzuki T, Uchida H, et al. Antipsychotic treatment for schizophrenia in the maintenance phase: A systematic review of the guidelines and algorithms. *Schizophrenia Research.* 2012;**143**(2–3):219–225. doi: 10.1016/j.schres.2011.11.021.

17. National Institute for Health and Care Excellence. Core interventions in the treatment and management of schizophrenia in primary and secondary care (update). http://guidance.nice.org.uk/CG82/NICEGui dance/pdf/English (2009).

18. Tiihonen J, Mittendorfer-Rutz E, Majak M, et al. Real-world effectiveness of antipsychotic treatments in a nationwide cohort of 29 823 patients with schizophrenia. *JAMA Psychiatry*. 2017;**74**(7):686–693. doi: 10.1001/jamapsychiatry.2017.1322.

19. Taipale H, Tanskanen A, Mehtala J, et al. 20-year follow-up study of physical morbidity and mortality in relationship to antipsychotic treatment in a nationwide cohort of 62, 250 patients with schizophrenia (FIN20). *World Psychiatry*. 2020;**19**:61–68. doi: 10.1002/wps.20699.

20. Hansen HG, Speyer H, Starzer M, et al. Clinical recovery among individuals with a first-episode schizophrenia an updated systematic review and meta-analysis. *Schizophrenia Bulletin*. 2023;**49**(2):297–308. doi: 10.1093/schbul/sbac103.

21. Jaaskelainen E, Juola P, Hirvonen N, et al. A systematic review and meta-analysis of recovery in schizophrenia. *Schizophrenia Bulletin*. 2013;**39**(6):1296–1306. doi: 10.1093/schbul/sbs130.

22. Harrow M, Jobe TH. Does long-term treatment of schizophrenia with antipsychotic medications facilitate recovery? *Schizophrenia Bulletin*. 2013;**36**(5):962–965. doi: 10.1093/schbul/sbt034.

23. Harrow M, Jobe TH, Tong L. Long-term effectiveness of antipsychotics. *Psychological Medicine*. 2023;**53**:1129–1133. doi: 10.1017/S0033291721001732.

24. Wunderink L, Nieboer RM, Wiersma D, et al. Recovery in remitted first-episode psychosis at 7 years of follow-up of an early dose reduction/discontinuation or maintenance treatment strategy: Long-term follow-up of a 2-year randomized clinical trial. *JAMA Psychiatry*. 2013;**70**(9):913–920. doi: 10.1001/jamapsychiatry.2013.19.

25. Robinson D, Woerner MG, Alvir JM, et al. Predictors of relapse following response from a first episode of schizophrenia or schizoaffective disorder. *Archives of General Psychiatry*. 1999;**56**(3):241–247.

26. Emsley R. Antipsychotics and structural brain changes: Could treatment adherence explain the discrepant findings? *Therapeutic Advances in Psychopharmacology*. 2023;**13**:20451253231195258.

27. Goff, D, Zeng B, Ardekani B, et al. Association of hippocampal atrophy with duration of untreated psychosis and molecular biomarkers during initial antipsychotic treatment of first episode psychosis. *JAMA Psychiatry*. 2018;**75**(4):370–378. doi: 10.1001/jamapsychiatry.2017.4595.

28. Fountoulakis KN, Stahl SM. The effect of first- and second-generation antipsychotics on brain morphology in schizophrenia: A systematic review of longitudinal magnetic resonance studies with a randomized allocation to treatment arms. *Journal of Psychopharmacology*. 2022;**36**(4):428–438. doi: 10.1177/02698811221087645.

29. Chopra S, Fornito A, Francey SM, et al. Differentiating the effect of antipsychotic medication and illness on brain volume reductions in first-episode psychosis: A longitudinal, randomized, triple-blind, placebo-controlled MRI study. *Neuropsychopharmacology*. 2021;**46**(8):1494–1501. doi: 10.1038/s41386-021-00980-0.

30. Lawrie SM. Do antipsychotic drugs shrink the brain? Probably not. *Journal of Psychopharmacology*. 2022;**36**(4):425–427. doi: 10.1177/02698811221092252.

31. Drake RJ, Husain N, Marshall M, et al. Effect of delaying treatment of first-episode psychosis on symptoms and social outcomes: A longitudinal analysis and modelling study. *Lancet Psychiatry*. 2020;**7**(7):602–610. doi: 10.1016/S2215-0366(20)30147-4.

32. Stone WS, Cia B, Liu X, et al. Association between the duration of untreated psychosis and selective cognitive performance in community-dwelling individuals with chronic untreated schizophrenia in rural China. *JAMA Psychiatry*. 2020;**77**(11):1116–1126. doi: 10.1001/jamapsychiatry.2020.1619.

33. Kane JM, Robinson DG, Schooler NR, et al. Comprehensive versus usual community care for first-episode psychosis: 2-year outcomes from the NIMH RASIE Early Treatment Program. *American Journal of Psychiatry*. 2016;**173**:362–372.

34. Fusar-Poli P, Radua J, McGuire P, Borgwardt S. Neuroanatomical maps of psychosis onset: Voxel-wise meta-analysis of antipsychotic-naïve VBM studies. *Schizophrenia Bulletin*. 2012;**38**(6):1297–1307. doi: 10.1093/schbul/sbr134.

35. Malla AK, Bodnar M, Joober R, Lepage M. Duration of untreated psychosis is associated with orbital–frontal grey matter volume reductions in first episode psychosis. *Schizophrenia Research*. 2010;**125**:13–20.

36. Guo X, Li J, Wei Q, et al. Duration of untreated psychosis is associated with temporal and occipitotemporal gray matter volume decrease in treatment naïve schizophrenia. *PLoS ONE*. 2013;**8**(12):e83679. doi: 10.1371/journal.pone.0083679.

37. Kraguljac NV, Anthony T, Morgan CJ, et al. White matter integrity, duration of untreated psychosis, and antipsychotic treatment response in medication-naïve first-episode psychosis patients. *Molecular Psychiatry*. 2021;**26**:5347–5356. doi: 10.1038/s41380-020-0765x.

38. Slovakova A, Kudelka J, Skoch A, et al. Time is the enemy: Negative symptoms are related to even slight difference in the duration of untreated psychosis. *Comprehensive Psychiatry*. 2024;**130**:142450. doi: 10.1016/j.comppsych.2024.152450.

39. Tiihonen J, Tanskanen A, Lic PH, Taipale H. 20-year nationwide follow-up study on discontinuation of antipsychotic treatment in first-episode schizophrenia. *American Journal of Psychiatry*. 2018;**175**:8.

Assisted Outpatient Treatment

Are Court-Ordered Antipsychotic Medications Effective?

Sophia Kocher and Marvin Swartz

Introduction

Assisted Outpatient Treatment (AOT) has emerged as a potential, but controversial response to treatment non-adherence, increased symptomatology such as severe hallucinations, and subsequent relapse for individuals with debilitating psychiatric illnesses.[1–6] Several states, including California and New York, have recently promoted the use of AOT to try to address high rates of homelessness among persons with severe mental illness.

The American Psychiatric Association (APA) in its Position Statement on AOT[7] describes AOT as "a civil court procedure wherein a judge orders a person with severe mental illness to adhere to an outpatient treatment plan designed to prevent relapse and dangerous deterioration." It notes that the goal of such programs is to meet the needs of persons with severe mental illness whose complex treatment and human service needs are unmet by community mental health programs. Thus, these programs seek to reduce rates of relapse and hospitalization, the likelihood of dangerous behavior, and incarceration.[7] In doing so, programs must balance the ethical principles of patient autonomy and beneficence, resorting to AOT only when previous treatment options fail. Per the APA, these programs also must be implemented in a nondiscriminatory manner to ensure they are fairly applied and respectful.[7]

The controversies about AOT

Those in favor of AOT argue that it can promote access to treatment for those with severe mental illnesses such as schizophrenia, bipolar disorder, major depression, panic disorder, obsessive compulsive disorder, and post-traumatic stress disorder.[1] The court order not only commits a patient to receive treatment, it also commits the health system to provide that care. While AOT programs may encroach on patient autonomy, mandated outpatient regimens are far less restrictive than hospitalization, homelessness, or incarceration.[4] In addition, proponents of AOT argue that, while AOT-type interventions limit autonomy in the short run, they can restore a more durable autonomy in returning patients to community independence and better functioning.[8,9] As a corollary, they also argue that under the throes of a full-blown psychosis, a person controlled by delusions and hallucinations is not fully autonomous.[8,9] In fact, repeated cycles of involuntary hospitalizations are one of the negative outcomes these programs aim to prevent. Proponents also argue that AOT serves as an earlier point of entry into care systems, including ones for social support, thus reducing prolonged social isolation and suffering. Critics focus on AOT's coercive nature and the social/political/legal ramifications of framing medical non-adherence as a legal matter and subjecting patients to potential criminalization.[10] Still, others criticize AOT programs for not being stringent enough to be effective.[1,5,6]

Central to these critiques is the question of whether AOT can actually "work." Studies of AOT effectiveness have shown mixed results arguably as a result of its implementation.[1,5,6]

Several studies demonstrate positive outcomes, but studies have varied methodologies, inconsistent implementation, different outcome measures, and many lack generalizability. Further implementation of these programs is very situationally dependent, in that they are implemented in varied communities with varied resources and systems of care.[1,2,5,6] For example, several studies conducted in the United States were compared to one in the United Kingdom, which are vastly different systems of care.[6] What the literature *does* demonstrate is that the success of AOT depends on successful implementation, good treatment resources, and an adequate duration of court-ordered treatment.[6] Therefore, when thinking about AOT in relation to other community-based interventions it may be time to shift the question. When caring for individuals with severe mental illness we should be asking: *for whom does court-mandated outpatient treatment work and under what conditions?*

The APA consensus on this question is that AOT can play a significant role in the recovery of individuals with severe mental illness when programs are well-planned, offer intensive and individualized services, and last for a sustained period of time.[7] Centered around intensive outpatient services, these programs can enhance treatment adherence and reduce hospitalization rates; and for a subset of the patient population, they aim to mitigate the likelihood of dangerous behavior. However, AOT should not be seen as a primary tool for preventing violence.[5] Instead, programs should seek to mobilize treatment resources with a focus on preventing patients' severe deterioration.

Assessments of for whom these programs would most benefit should be based on past clinical history of relapse due to treatment non-adherence.[7] AOT is especially vital to assist patients at risk of relapse who are unlikely to seek treatment voluntarily due to their mental illness. In terms of what services programs should offer, the APA cites research showing that comprehensive services, including medication management and psychosocial support, enhance AOT's effectiveness.[6] The APA also recommends thorough psychiatric and physical examinations to address co-occurring medical issues[7] Of note, although psychotropic medication often plays a crucial role in the treatment plan for patients, involuntary administration of medications is not authorized under AOT and requires separate legal authority and approval. That is, patients under AOT are ordered by the court to comply with treatment recommendations but they cannot be forcibly administered medication and legal charges cannot be levied against non-adherent patients. Indeed, the legal sanction for non-adherence is a law enforcement transport for an examination to assess whether a higher level of care is needed.

The APA further recommends that AOT programs be held accountable for implementation in maximizing the success of the court orders.[7] Key factors in success are clinician involvement in treatment planning and engaging patients and families in treatment preferences whenever possible. Even under court-ordered treatment, the APA recommends close collaboration with the patient to select medication

regimens that are tolerated and effective.[7] In addition, the APA stipulates that patients should be provided due process legal protections, similar to those afforded for involuntary hospitalization. Finally, regular evaluations of programs should be conducted to ensure equitable application and to address any disproportionate use among minority groups. Some critics of AOT argue that not only is AOT coercive and ineffective but that the court mandate to adhere to prescribed medications, most often antipsychotic medications, compels AOT recipients to take ineffective and harmful medications. As one opponent said:

> What would you want if you were in this position? Do you want to be forced to take a medication that you feel has really harmful side effects? I want to change the narrative on this and make it about choice.
>
> (Accessed October 30, 2024. https://www.madinamerica.com/2024/05/maryland-enacts-a-draconian-assisted-outpatient-treatment-program/).

Are antipsychotics effective and tolerable?

The treatment of acute schizophrenia and other psychotic disorders does present challenges, one major one being patient adherence to prescribed therapies. Utilizing the court order, AOT can be a potentially effective strategy to ensure consistent adherence to antipsychotic medications. However, mandating antipsychotic treatment is criticized by some physicians, patients, members of the public, and policymakers due to their known side effects and limited effectiveness – suggesting that their use under court order be minimized. The following brief review considers the effectiveness and side effects of antipsychotic medications, informing discussions about their use as part of AOT.

A systematic meta-analysis by Leucht et al. examines the effectiveness of antipsychotic drugs for the treatment of acute exacerbations of schizophrenia compared to placebo responses in clinical trials over the past 60 years.[11] Leucht et al. analyzed 167 double-blind randomized controlled trials, totaling 28,102, mainly chronic, patients. Their work highlights the efficacy of antipsychotic medications, revealing that approximately twice as many patients improved with antipsychotics compared to placebo. They found that 51% of the antipsychotic group experienced at least a "minimal" symptom response, defined as either at least a 20% reduction from baseline on common symptom rating scales (e.g., the PANSS, BPRS, or Clinical Global Impression Scale) indicating at least "slightly improved" or better, compared to 30% response in the placebo group. Still, only a minority experienced a "good" response, though the majority of those who were improved were in the antipsychotic group.[11] These data support arguments that antipsychotic medication as part of the treatment regimen under AOT can enhance treatment effectiveness.

However, the review also reveals that while antipsychotics can be effective, they often have significant side effects. In their meta-analysis, antipsychotic drugs were associated with more movement disorders, more sedation, more weight gain, prolactin increases, and more electrocardiogram (EKG) QT interval prolongation than placebo. In their analysis, effect sizes of side effect differences across different drug types demonstrated significant heterogeneity, reflecting the differences in individual antipsychotics. This difference in side effect profiles was most notable between first (older) and second (newer) generation antipsychotics as both classes were included in the meta-analysis.[11] This variation presents an opportunity for intervention: careful drug choices and modifications of individualized treatment regimens can reduce side effect burdens for patients. The structured programing and prolonged treatment courses of AOT provide a chance for providers to find an efficacious treatment regimen while selecting a specific medication to minimize side effects and promote the best possible outcomes. It is important to note that even when prescribing under court oversight the physician's ethical duty continues to be to the patient, meaning he/she has a duty to find a treatment plan that is tolerable and effective. AOT does not absolve the physician of his/her fidelity to good ethical care.

In their review, Leucht et al. further respond to questions about the efficacy of antipsychotics.[11] Skepticism about whether these drugs actually "work" likely stems from a number of trials in recent years that show older drugs, like haloperidol, failing to outperform placebo. Their meta-analysis identifies an increased placebo response over time as a moderator of drug efficacy, rather than a decrease in drug response itself.[11] This suggests that the apparent decrease in drug efficacy in trials may well be influenced more by improved patient response to placebo rather than a true decline in the effectiveness of the drugs per se. They also note that trends of decreasing

effect size (superiority of drug over placebo) in clinical trials of recent years may be an artifact of study design. More recent studies tend to use standardized criteria for assessment of improvement as well as larger and more diverse samples, both of which can decrease effect sizes.[11] Thus, this trend should not be thought of solely as antipsychotic drugs becoming less efficacious.

In response to potential sources of bias and the perceived integrity of drug treatment, Leucht et al. discuss the significant impact of industry sponsorship on effect sizes.[11] Surprisingly, they found industry sponsorship of drug trials to be associated with smaller effect sizes, which they hypothesize is due to large studies that involve multiple countries and study sites with different populations and multiple raters administrating rating scales. Multiple raters lead to increasing variability in rating scores and increased measurement error. AOT may provide a structured treatment framework that may help reveal the true benefits of these medications in a real-world setting, offering insights that are less influenced by the placebo effects.

Finally, and perhaps most importantly, Leucht's review highlights the improvement of quality of life and social functioning with antipsychotic treatment, even in the short term (6 weeks). AOT has the potential to enhance these benefits by promoting adherence and continuity of care, supporting individuals with severe mental illness in achieving better health outcomes.

Antipsychotics are also the mainstay treatment for long-term maintenance treatment for patients with schizophrenia. In their comprehensive Cochrane review, Ceraso et al. examine whether antipsychotics are effective for relapse prevention, in addition to their ability to reduce acute symptoms of schizophrenia.[12] They reviewed 75 randomized controlled trials involving 9,145 participants to see the effects of maintenance medication compared to stopping antipsychotic agents.

They found that antipsychotics significantly reduced the risk of relapse compared to placebo. This finding was consistent across studies and time frames. Indeed, risk ratios suggest that the likelihood of relapse was nearly three times higher (RR 0.38) for those not on medication maintenance treatment (at 7–12 months). Those in the placebo group were more likely to leave the study early, both for any cause and due to the inefficacy of the intervention. Antipsychotic use was also associated with decreased hospitalization.

Importantly, these effects persisted even when accounting for participants who had been stable for various periods (1–3 months) before the start of a trial.[12] Antipsychotic medication uses still reduced relapse rates (with no difference between the duration of pre-trial stability), demonstrating the robust sustained efficacy of antipsychotics in preventing symptom recurrence over time.

Further, these studies demonstrate that quality of life may be superior for patients treated with antipsychotics. Although fewer studies measured this outcome, there was a clear and statistically significant improvement in quality-of-life measurements for those taking antipsychotics. In their pooled data, they found substantial heterogeneity in the amount of improvement, due in part to the use of different scales across studies, yet all had the same trend toward improvement. Also in their analysis, they found those in the antipsychotic group reported improved social functioning.[12] Medication management had a positive effect on the ability to engage in activities and relationship – they found that those continuing treatment tended to experience higher satisfaction with their life and with their treatment. Of key importance, poor adherence to prescribed antipsychotics and repeated episodes of psychoses clearly impact long-term outcomes of schizophrenia including poorer functioning, higher risk of hospitalization, arrest, violence, victimization, poorer life satisfaction, and greater substance use, and alcohol-related problems.[13] These improvements must be weighed against the side effects of medication therapy. The review found antipsychotic medications, in the long term (>3 months), associated with a greater number of movement disorders (e.g., akathisia, akinesia, dyskinesia, dystonia, tremor), and increased weight gain and sedation.[12] The review was also limited by the duration of follow-up. Studies included in the analyses generally lasted up to 1 year, meaning that further work must be done to assess the long-term morbidity and mortality of these drugs as well as the potential impact of social/environmental factors on remission of symptoms with antipsychotic treatment. Nevertheless, the authors conclude that "stopping treatment [may be] far more harmful than thoughtfully maintaining it."[12]

With regard to the side effects of antipsychotics, the types of adverse effects are diverse. In their systematic review, Young et al. reveal that side effects are common and that their incidence increases with antipsychotic polypharmacy and increased duration.[14] Moreover, different drugs were found to have different side effect profiles. For example, clozapine was more strongly associated with metabolic disturbance and olanzapine was associated with the most weight gain.

Importantly, these side effects can be managed. However, Young et al. found that despite clinical guideline recommendations, there was a disappointing rate of baseline monitoring and follow-up: for lipid monitoring, glucose monitoring, and no evidence of evaluation for sexual dysfunction (the side effect they found to be most common).[14] Because antipsychotic drugs vary in their side effects, increased monitoring would allow for interventions to better manage side effects. Of the studies they reviewed, the ones that assessed the efficacy of adverse effect management strategies found effective non-therapeutic and therapeutic interventions that resulted in improved control of adverse effects. For example, one found significant decreases in weight gain with a program of physical exercise, diet therapy, and group therapy.[15] Another found a significant decrease in cholesterol and triglycerides with statin therapy.[16] Still, Young et al. note that only a minority of patients receive these interventions. One of the studies in their review found that few patients were receiving lipid-lowering therapy and only a minority received antihypertensive medications.[17,18] These findings underscore a need for greater emphasis on managing antipsychotic side effects. This also suggests that courts could play an important role in emphasizing standards of care in prescribing medications.

These reviews underscore that antipsychotic drugs are indeed demonstrably effective in reducing relapse, improving symptoms, and reducing hospitalization. However, antipsychotic drugs do increase the risk of troublesome side effects, including health risks such as weight gain. This puts the responsibility on the physician treating an AOT patient to prescribe wisely and to find the most tolerable medication regimens that reduce risk and maximize benefit. In many ways, this is no different than the role of the physician working with a "voluntary" patient. In either case, treatment adherence is largely driven by collaboratively finding a regimen that is acceptable and tolerable to the patient. And importantly, professional medical ethics demand that the physician honor the physician–patient relationship by finding a treatment regimen that the patient can best tolerate.[18]

Conclusion

These reviews provide solid evidence that antipsychotic regimens are demonstrably effective in treating psychotic symptoms and that maintenance antipsychotic treatment reduces relapse and poor outcomes. Antipsychotics are the consensus treatment of choice for patients with psychotic disorders. These reviews also make clear that there is a substantial side effect burden associated with these medications. Absent careful monitoring and side effect management, certain side effects can have serious long-term effects. As a result, it is incumbent on the treating clinician to monitor side effects carefully and make changes in the medication regimen to find the most tolerable regimen. If AOT required a single fixed and unchanging regimen of medications it would clearly pose an ethical problem for the treating clinicians and be unfair to the patients under AOT. However, that is not the case, AOT clinicians can and are ethically obliged to collaborate with AOT patients to find tolerable and effective medication regimens.

References

1. Cripps SN, Swartz MS. Update on assisted outpatient treatment. *Curr Psychiatry Rep.* 2018;**20**(12):112.

2. Phelan JC, Sinkewicz M, Castille DM, et al. Effectiveness and outcomes of assisted outpatient treatment in New York State. *Psychiatr Serv.* 2010;**61**(2):137–143.

3. Meldrum ML, Kelly EL, Calderon R, Brekke JS, Braslow JT. Implementation status of assisted outpatient treatment programs: a national survey. *Psychiatr Serv.* 2016;**67**(6):630–605.

4. Monahan J, Bonnie RJ, Appelbaum PS, et al. Mandated community treatment: beyond outpatient commitment. *Psychiatr Serv.* 2001;**52**(9):1198–1205.

5. Swartz MS, Bhattacharya S, Robertson AG, Swanson JW. Involuntary outpatient commitment and the elusive pursuit of violence prevention. *Can J Psychiatry.* 2017;**62**(2):102–108.

6. Swanson JW, Swartz MS. Why the evidence for outpatient commitment is good enough. *Psychiatr Serv.* 2014;**65**(6):808–811. doi:10.1176/appi.ps.201300424

7. American Psychiatric Association. Position statement on involuntary outpatient commitment and related programs of assisted outpatient treatment. December 2020. Accessed August 19, 2024. www.psychiatry.org/getattachment/d50db97b-59aa-4dd4-a0ec-d09b4e19112e/Position-Involuntary-Outpatient-Commitment.pdf

8. Hegarty L, Brusasco M. Life, liberty and the therapeutic relationship: examining the place of compulsory treatment in modern psychiatry. *Australas Psychiatry.* 2021;**29**(1):66–68.

9. Glick ID, Shader RI. The problem of medical-psychiatric illness in the homeless and its occurrence in the midst of a viral pandemic: a commentary. *Psychiatry Res.* 2020;**290**:113118.

10. Steinert T. Ethics of coercive treatment and misuse of psychiatry. *Psychiatr Serv.* 2017;**68**(3):291–294.

11. Leucht S, Leucht C, Huhn M, et al. Sixty years of placebo-controlled antipsychotic drug trials in acute schizophrenia: systematic review, Bayesian meta-analysis, and meta-regression of efficacy predictors. *Am J Psychiatry.* 2017;**174**(10):927–942.

12. Ceraso A, Lin JJ, Schneider-Thoma J, et al. Maintenance treatment with antipsychotic drugs for schizophrenia. *Cochrane Database Syst Rev.* 2020;**8**(8):CD008016.

13. Ascher-Svanum H, Faries DE, Zhu B, et al. Medication adherence and long-term functional outcomes in the treatment of schizophrenia in usual care. *J Clin Psychiatry.* 2006;**67**(3):453–460.

14. Young SL, Taylor M, Lawrie SM. "First do no harm." A systematic review of the prevalence and management of antipsychotic adverse effects. *J Psychopharmacol.* 2015;**29**(4):353–362.

15. Attux C, Martini LC, Araújo CM, et al. The effectiveness of a non-pharmacological intervention for weight gain management in severe mental disorders: results from a national multicentric study. *Braz J Psychiatry.* 2011;**33**(2):117–121.

16. Hanssens L, De Hert M, Kalnicka D, et al. Pharmacological treatment of severe dyslipidaemia in patients with schizophrenia. *Int Clin Psychopharmacol.* 2007;**22**(1):43–49.

17. Mackin P, Bishop DR, Watkinson HM. A prospective study of monitoring practices for metabolic disease in antipsychotic-treated community psychiatric patients. *BMC Psychiatry.* 2007;**7**:28.

18. Mackin P, Bishop D, Watkinson H, Gallagher P, Ferrier IN. Metabolic disease and cardiovascular risk in people treated with antipsychotics in the community. *Br J Psychiatry.* 2007;**191**:23–29.

Chapter

12

Forensic Assertive Community Treatment
An Emerging Best Practice

J. Steven Lamberti and Robert L. Weisman

Introduction

Prior to the 1950s, people with serious mental illness (SMI) such as schizophrenia, schizoaffective disorder, and bipolar disorder were primarily served by large state psychiatric hospitals. Between 1955 and 1976, approximately 70% of state and county psychiatric hospital inpatients were discharged into communities across America,[1] many of which lacked the necessary services to care for them in community settings. To address the special needs of formerly institutionalized patients with SMI, the assertive community treatment (ACT) model was developed in the 1970s in Madison, Wisconsin following the downsizing of Mendota State Hospital.[2] Unlike traditional outpatient treatment which requires individuals to travel to clinics for care, ACT teams engage and serve people in their preferred community settings. In addition to providing outreach, several characteristics distinguish ACT teams from traditional clinic-based mental health teams. ACT teams are intensively staffed, with a service provider-to-recipient ratio of approximately 1:10. These teams typically include a psychiatrist, nurses, social workers, and a licensed chemical dependency counselor, with many teams also including peer providers, housing specialists, family specialists, and/or vocational specialists. Given the comprehensive scope of ACT services, the ACT model is sometimes referred to as "a hospital without walls".[3] To promote ACT model dissemination, core ACT criteria were identified and incorporated into standardized fidelity scales including the Dartmouth Assertive Community Treatment Scale (DACTS)[4] and the Tool for Measurement of Assertive Community Treatment (TMACT).[5] Research showed that high fidelity ACT teams were effective at preventing psychiatric hospitalization, reducing homelessness, and improving engagement in treatment.[6–8] Subsequent research studies, however, consistently showed that ACT teams were not effective at preventing arrest or incarceration.[9–13]

FACT origins

Despite questions about ACT's effectiveness in addressing criminal justice outcomes, some ACT team clinicians continued applying and adapting the ACT model to better serve justice-involved individuals who were enrolled in their ACT teams. By the mid-1990s, published reports began to emerge from ACT teams that exclusively served clients with criminal histories,[14,15] a clear departure from the original ACT model. Some of these teams began calling themselves *FACT* teams,[16] but it remained unclear whether or how these teams differed from standard ACT teams. One early FACT team was Project Link which began in Rochester, NY, following the downsizing of the local state hospital, Rochester Psychiatric Center (RPC).[17] As RPC's census declined, county officials began documenting an alarming increase of people with SMI entering the county jail. To address this issue, the authors obtained county funding in 1995 to begin Project Link, a mobile treatment team that provided in-reach to incarcerated adults with SMI to engage them in care. All referrals to Project Link came from the county jail and court system, so team clinicians began working closely with judges, court staff, and probation officers to prevent their service recipients' re-arrest. Analysis of pre-post enrollment data showed significant reductions in both incarceration and hospitalization, along with improved community functioning.[18] Project Link received the American Psychiatric Association's Services Achievement Gold Award in 1999 as an innovative service delivery model.[19] These experiences prompted the authors to consider whether similar teams were operating in other states.

To address this question, the authors conducted a national survey study in collaboration with the National Association of County Behavioral Health Directors (NACBHD). Over 300 NACBHD members were surveyed to identify ACT teams that (1) served only justice-involved patients, (2) had a criminal justice agency as their primary referral source, and (3) partnered with criminal justice agencies to perform jail diversion. Team members were subsequently interviewed to ensure that their teams met both ACT fidelity criteria and FACT study criteria. A total of 16 FACT teams in nine states were identified, but significant differences were noted in their structure and daily operations. The authors concluded that FACT was an emerging model of care, and that research was needed to better define the model and test its effectiveness. The resulting paper was published in 2004 as the first formal study of FACT, coining the term "forensic assertive community treatment" in the literature.[16,20] The authors published a follow-up national survey study in 2011 and noted that the number of FACT teams had nearly doubled by that time.[21] Most recently, findings from a 2024 national ACT survey study indicate that FACT may now be present in 19 states.[22]

The number of FACT teams currently operating in the United States is unknown, but the number is likely to be significant. According to state officials, for example, 20 FACT teams are currently operating in the states of New York and Ohio alone.[23,24] In addition, research reports have described the application of ACT to forensic and justice-involved populations in Canada,[25] the Netherlands,[26] New Zealand,[27] and Belgium.[28] These reports have continued to raise basic questions about the nature of FACT and its effectiveness in serving justice-involved adults with SMI.

What do we know (and not know) about FACT operation and effectiveness?

At least four randomized controlled trials of FACT effectiveness have been conducted to date. First, in a 2-year study comparing FACT with treatment as usual in 235 individuals with SMI facing either misdemeanor or felony charges, FACT patients spent fewer days in jail but the difference was not significant.[29] The FACT group also had significantly more bookings, likely due to a combination of sanctions and new crimes, and no differences in convictions for new crimes between FACT and usual care. Second, in a 2-year study comparing FACT with treatment as usual in 134 incarcerated adults with SMI, FACT patients had fewer bookings, fewer psychiatric hospital days, and more outpatient treatment contacts.[30] The FACT group also had fewer jail days but the difference was not significant, and no differences in convictions were found. Increased outpatient costs were partially offset by decreased hospital and jail costs, but no significant differences were found in overall costs between FACT and usual care. Third, a 1-year NIMH-funded study compared FACT with outpatient clinic treatment plus intensive case management in a group of 70 adults with psychotic disorders who were arrested for misdemeanor crimes.[31] Patients receiving FACT had significantly fewer days in jail, fewer convictions for new crimes, and fewer days in the hospital along with significantly increased engagement in outpatient mental health services. A subsequent return-on-investment analysis of outcome data found a $1.50 return for every $1 spent on FACT treatment.[32] Lastly, in 2019 the authors conducted a randomized controlled trial of two FACT teams in Minneapolis and St. Paul, MN. Recruitment was halted early due to COVID-19 and riots following George Floyd's murder, and data were analyzed on the remaining 40 study participants. Although limited by the small sample size, preliminary data analysis suggested that FACT intervention was associated with 88% fewer days in jail and prison compared to standard care which included an ACT option.[33]

Three comprehensive literature reviews have also examined FACT effectiveness. The first, a 2016 review by Marquant et al., revealed "limited yet promising evidence in support of the effectiveness of forensic ACT for forensic outcome measures".[34] The authors also stated that the evidence for FACT's effectiveness in achieving non-forensic outcomes such as reduction of hospitalization "is even more limited." A second literature review was published in 2020 by Cuddeback and colleagues.[35] It concluded that "studies of FACT to date provide moderate evidence to support FACT's effectiveness toward reducing recidivism among justice involved persons with severe mental illness." This review also suggested that FACT is effective at promoting greater use of outpatient mental health services and at reducing hospital days. Most recently, a systematic review and meta-analysis of the FACT literature was published by Goulet et al. in 2022 and examined both forensic and health-related outcomes.[36] The authors reported that forensic outcomes were positive and primarily driven by reductions in jail days. Positive results were also noted for utilization of outpatient mental health services, but mixed results were noted for hospitalization and health-related outcomes.

One reason why FACT reviews and studies have reported inconsistent findings is that FACT teams vary widely in their structure and operations. Simply put, it is not possible to draw definitive conclusions about the FACT model's effectiveness in the absence of a definitive FACT model. In the absence of a standardized model, there continues to be uncertainty about FACT effectiveness and how FACT differs from ACT, if at all. For example, some authors have described FACT as a "first generation" intervention that aims to prevent criminal recidivism primarily by treating mental illness.[37–39] This view suggests that FACT consists of little more than enrolling justice-involved clients into standard ACT programs, a view that was evident in New York's implementation of forensic ACT in 2016.[40,41] In contrast, other authors have described FACT as a criminologically informed hybrid that incorporates crime prevention principles into clinical team operations.[42,43]

To address this issue, the Substance Abuse and Mental Health Service Administration (SAMHSA) published a guideline in 2019 which listed seven "Key Components of FACT".[44] Three, however, pertained to ACT (e.g., high ACT fidelity, around-the-clock access, and flexible funding and implementation support). The four remaining components were (1) serving clients with histories of multiple incarcerations, (2) addressing criminogenic risks and needs, (3) having criminal justice specialists on the team, and (4) cross-system mental health and criminal justice team member training. Despite the publication of the SAMHSA guideline in 2019, subsequent reviews have suggested that FACT teams continue to vary widely in their structure and daily operations.[35,36,45] This ongoing problem raises basic questions about how FACT differs from ACT, who FACT teams should treat, and which elements of program design and operation are necessary for FACT effectiveness.

What are the key components of FACT?

To help address these questions, the authors published a 2021 review entitled "Essential Elements of Forensic Assertive Community Treatment",[45] based on their experience serving as FACT clinicians, researchers, and consultants. That paper presented key components of FACT which are updated and summarized as follows:

1. **A high fidelity ACT team.** Because FACT is based on the ACT model, FACT teams should meet ACT fidelity criteria with the understanding that ACT alone is generally not sufficient to prevent the arrest and incarceration of service recipients. High fidelity is recommended because high fidelity ACT teams outperform low fidelity ACT teams in preventing hospitalization, homelessness, and substance use, outcomes that are also important to FACT teams.[45] In hiring FACT team members, it should be recognized that persons of color are highly over-represented within correctional settings.[46] To help overcome cultural and language barriers to their engagement, FACT teams should make extra efforts to hire staff members whose racial/ethnic demography resembles that of their service recipients. Engagement of justice-involved clients can also be facilitated by hiring forensic peer specialists. Lastly, FACT teams should create a forensic liaison position to serve as a single point of contact for criminal justice professionals who provide legal oversight to FACT service recipients. Forensic liaisons can also play a key role in FACT teams by helping to screen referrals, and by conducting risk/need assessments as discussed below.

2. **Dual admission criteria.** Because FACT service recipients are involved in both the mental health and criminal justice systems, admission decisions must consider criteria within each system. FACT's mental health criteria are identical to those used by ACT teams (e.g., presence of a serious mental disorder, evidence of functional impairment, frequent use of emergency room and hospital services, and lack of engagement with standard outpatient treatment). Criminal justice admission criteria, however, can vary depending on local needs. For example, they can include the history of arrest or incarceration, or current involvement in probation, parole, or a mental health court. A note of caution is warranted in considering criminal justice criteria: Some authorities assume that because FACT serves individuals with the most severe mental disorders, then it should also serve clients with the highest recidivism risk. However, individuals with the highest recidivism risk have been found to respond less well to FACT intervention compared to other FACT service recipients.[31,47] To illustrate these points, Figure 12.1 introduces a framework that presents the relationship between psychiatric diagnosis and recidivism risk (as determined by standardized

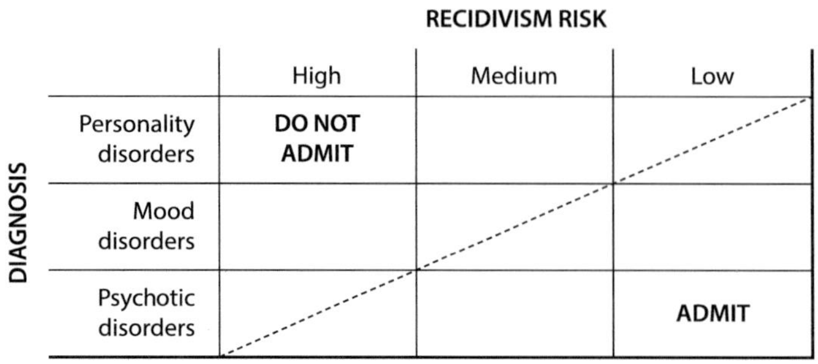

Figure 12.1 FACT enrollment framework.

assessment tools discussed below) with respect to appropriateness for FACT enrollment. The framework presents diagnostic and risk characteristics that are most appropriate for FACT enrollment toward the lower right corner and those that are least appropriate toward the upper left corner. Enrollment decisions for individuals with diagnostic and risk characteristics near the middle of Figure 12.1, as represented by a dotted diagonal line, should be determined individually based on careful evaluation. For example, a high-risk client accurately diagnosed with bipolar disorder would be appropriate for admission, while a high-risk client with a questionable bipolar diagnosis may not be. Within this framework, it might be argued that prioritizing the enrollment of individuals with a low or even a moderate risk for criminal recidivism is not an appropriate use of FACT resources. The counterargument, however, is that these individuals are suffering from untreated serious mental disorders and have typically failed to engage in outpatient mental health services including ACT. Although trapped in a harmful and costly "revolving door" cycle of repeated hospitalization, homelessness, and arrest, they are more likely to benefit from FACT than individuals with high degrees of criminality.

3. **Risk/need assessment.** According to the Risk-Need Responsivity (RNR) model, the predominant approach to crime prevention today, preventing arrest and incarceration among justice-involved individuals, requires engaging them in interventions that target the risk factors driving their involvement.[48] These risk factors, also called "criminogenic needs," are criminal history, antisocial personality, antisocial cognition, social support for crime, family problems, work and school problems, lack of healthy leisure pursuits,

and substance use. Research has consistently shown that the presence of these risk factors increases the likelihood of arrest and that addressing these risk factors effectively reduces the likelihood of arrest.[48,49] Criminogenic needs can be identified through the use of standardized risk/need assessment tools such as the Level of Service/Case Management Inventory (LS/CMI),[50] the Ohio Risk Assessment System (ORAS),[51] or the Correctional Assessment and Intervention System (CAIS).[52] Once they are identified, criminogenic needs must then be addressed through incorporation into FACT service recipients' problem lists and treatment plans.

4. **Criminal justice collaboration.** Collaborating with criminal justice professionals enables shared problem-solving between mental health and criminal justice service providers, laying a foundation for the use of therapeutic alternatives to punishment.[53,54] In addition, the collaboration also enables the use of legal authority to help engage individuals with untreated SMI as discussed below. It should be noted that effective collaboration requires communication as well as shared goals and values. Collaborating with criminal justice staff who value the use of punishment over problem-solving, for example, can result in increased rather than decreased arrest rates among FACT service recipients.[55,56] Ideal criminal justice partners potentially include mental health court judges and specialty (i.e., mental health) probation and parole officers because they are experienced in serving people with SMI. Also, they can provide legal oversight of treatment in community settings (i.e., legal leverage).

5. **Legal leverage.** Legal leverage is the use of legal authority to promote engagement in necessary

treatments and services. It is based on the practice of therapeutic jurisprudence, or the use of law as a therapeutic instrument.[57] Examples of legal leverage include a judge offering treatment as an alternative to incarceration, or stipulating treatment as a condition of probation. Legal leverage is an essential element because FACT service recipients usually have long histories of refusing treatment, thus leaving themselves and their families to suffer the potentially catastrophic consequences of untreated SMI. Most people with SMI can be engaged by consistently providing services that are person-centered, trauma-informed, and culturally attuned. Despite clinicians' best efforts, however, some people with SMI remain unable or unwilling to accept treatment. Many suffer from anosognosia, or unawareness of illness, and are simply not aware they are ill.[58] To minimize perceived coercion (i.e., internal perception of being treated unfairly), it is important to utilize legal leverage in a manner described by Dr. Edward Latessa as "respectful guidance toward compliance" rather than using threats to force compliance.[49] Offering treatment as an alternative to punishment can initiate the process of *recovery*, whereby clients may move beyond feeling forced into treatment to eventually becoming active participants in their own self-care.[59,60]

6. **Informed choice.** Although justice-involved adults with SMI may be offered FACT as an alternative to punishment, they must still choose whether to accept FACT versus opting to receive punitive legal consequences for their behaviors. Those who agree to FACT enrollment without having an adequate understanding of FACT services and requirements, however, may be more likely to drop out once the responsibilities of participation become clear. Extra efforts should be made to provide clear information about FACT participation and alternatives, especially given the limited literacy, motivational impairments, and cognitive limitations commonly associated with serious mental disorders.

7. **Evidence-based mental health and substance use intervention.** Legal leverage is only as effective as the treatments and services that individuals are leveraged to receive. Three deserve special mention here. First, integrated dual diagnosis treatment (IDDT) is a part of both ACT and FACT.[61] In the authors' experience, however, the availability and quality of chemical dependency treatment services varies widely among ACT and FACT teams alike. In addition, co-occurring substance use may be the single strongest driver of arrest and incarceration among FACT service recipients.[62] It is therefore imperative that FACT teams provide the highest quality addiction treatment services possible. Second, in addition to having high rates of co-occurring substance use disorders, justice-involved adults with SMI typically have high rates of both treatment refusal and drug-refractory psychosis. To address these issues, FACT teams must make extra efforts to ensure that long-acting injectable medications and clozapine, respectively, are offered whenever they are clinically indicated.[63] Ensuring optimal pharmacotherapy is particularly important for FACT teams given compelling evidence that pharmacotherapy of psychosis and mania can reduce criminal justice system involvement.[62] Lastly, FACT teams should be prepared to offer cognitive-behavioral therapies that are designed to address antisocial cognitions and behaviors.[45,64]

8. **Evidence-based criminal justice intervention.** For optimal effectiveness, FACT clinicians and their collaborating criminal justice partners must each bring their respective "A games" to the table. In the field of community corrections, for example, the use of evidence-based practices is emphasized in training programs including Effective Practices in Community Supervision (EPICS),[65] Staff Training Aimed at Reducing Rearrest (STARR),[66] and the Proactive Community Supervision model (PCS).[67] Generally speaking, effective correctional interventions share three key features. They target criminogenic needs, they require individuals to demonstrate appropriate behaviors, and they shape behavior by extinguishing inappropriate behaviors and reinforcing appropriate ones. The principles of effective correctional intervention and associated best practices are collectively known as "what works" within the field of community corrections.[49]

9. **Shared training.** Shared training is an essential element because FACT involves collaboration between mental health and criminal justice

professionals, a process that requires partnership between service providers with distinctly different values, priorities, cultures, and practices. Criminal justice staff, for example, value justice and prioritize public safety while focusing on fighting crime. Clinicians, on the other hand, value wellness and prioritize patient health while focusing on fighting illness. Shared training can take many forms including attendance at training events and cross-training, a process whereby collaborating partners teach each other about their respective service systems and practices. In addition to training, hosting informal "open house" get-togethers where FACT clinicians and their criminal justice partners can become acquainted can go a long way toward building mutual trust and cooperation.

Current challenges for FACT model development and implementation

FACT teams continue to emerge across the United States. As of this writing, new FACT implementation initiatives are underway in several states including California, Kentucky, New York, North Carolina, and Pennsylvania. Lack of a widely accepted FACT model, however, continues to serve as a major barrier to both program implementation and outcome assessment. Steps have been taken toward FACT model standardization, most notably SAMHA's 2019 guideline,[44] but further efforts are needed. An important next step is to develop a valid and reliable FACT fidelity scale. The authors published an experimental FACT fidelity scale as part of their NIMH study in 2017,[31] and they published a revised and expanded scale called the Rochester Forensic Assertive Community Treatment Scale (RFACTS) in 2021.[45] The reliability and validity of the RFACTS, however, have yet to be tested.

Another challenge for FACT model development pertains to the question of how to define and implement "criminal justice collaboration." Collaboration with criminal justice service providers is widely viewed as essential in serving justice-involved adults with SMI.[68,69] Yet questions remain about the nature and extent of such collaboration. A key question is whether FACT teams should plan to collaborate with a single versus multiple criminal justice agencies. Collaborating with multiple agencies (i.e., *multipoint collaboration*) can ensure a steady stream of referrals, but it can also limit collaboration effectiveness due to the demands of interfacing with multiple agencies. Working in primary partnership with a single criminal justice agency such as a mental health court or a parole department (i.e., *single-point collaboration*) can potentially enable the most efficient and effective collaboration. A single agency, however, may not be able to provide an adequate number of referrals.

An additional challenge for FACT model development and implementation is to determine FACT's target population. This is a critical question because whichever population a FACT team decides to serve will have a major impact on the team's outcomes. FACT serves justice-involved clients, and so FACT teams can potentially receive referrals from a variety of criminal justice sources. One source that has emerged in recent years concerns individuals who have been found incompetent to stand trial (IST) and are awaiting competency restoration. Due to a lack of resources, many such individuals languish in jail for months, risking victimization and self-injurious behaviors while placing state governments at risk for civil actions. Although FACT teams can potentially provide community-based competency restoration, this approach presents the challenges of managing violence and escape risk in unstructured community settings.[70] To minimize such risks, FACT teams that accept IST defendants should prioritize those with clear histories of SMI and without histories of repeated violent crimes.

Recommendations for FACT research

The challenges facing FACT model development highlight the need for research in several areas. These include research to develop a reliable and valid FACT fidelity scale, to determine which individuals are most appropriate for FACT enrollment, and to identify the most critical elements of FACT design and operation. In particular, research is needed to compare the effectiveness of single-point versus multipoint collaboration designs, and to compare the impact of various forms of legal leverage versus no legal oversight on client outcomes. Lastly, given that substance use is an especially strong driver of arrest among people with serious mental disorders, research and policy-level efforts are needed to develop effective approaches to addiction treatment for FACT service recipients.

References

1. Mechanic D, Rochefort DA. Deinstitutionalization: An appraisal of reform. *Annu Rev Sociol*. 1990;**16**:301–327.

2. Stein LI, Santos AB. *Assertive Community Treatment of Persons With Severe Mental Illness*. WW Norton & Company; 1998.

3. Boust SJ, Kuhns MC, Studer L. Assertive community treatment. In: Stout CE, Hayes RA, eds. *The Evidence-Based Practice: Methods, Models and Tools for Mental Health Professionals*. Wiley and Sons; 2005.

4. Teague GB, Bond GR, Drake RE. Program fidelity in assertive community treatment: Development and use of a measure. *Am J Orthopsychiatry*. 1998;**68**:216–232.

5. Monroe-DeVita M, Teague GB, Moser LL. The TMACT: a new tool for measuring fidelity to assertive community treatment. *J Am Psychiatr Nurses Assoc*. 2011;**17**:17–29.

6. Bond GR, Salyers MP. Prediction of outcome from the Dartmouth assertive community treatment fidelity scale. *CNS Spectr*. 2004;**9**:937–942.

7. McHugo GJ, Drake RE, Teague GB, Xie H. Fidelity to assertive community treatment and client outcomes in the New Hampshire dual disorders study. *Psychiatr Serv*. 1999;**50**:818–824.

8. Latimer EA. Economic impacts of assertive community treatment: a review of the literature. *Can J Psychiatry*. 1999;**44**:443–454.

9. Bond GR, Drake RE, Mueser KT, Latimer E. Assertive community treatment for people with severe mental illness: Critical ingredients and impact on patients. *Disease Manage Health Outcomes*. 2001;**9**:141–159.

10. Calsyn RJ, Yonker RD, Lemming MR, Morse GA, Klinkenberg WD. Impact of assertive community treatment and client characteristics on criminal justice outcomes in dual disorder homeless individuals. *Crim Behav Men Health*. 2005;**15**:236–248.

11. Jennings JL. Does assertive community treatment work with forensic populations? Review and recommendations. *Open Psychiatry J*. 2009;**3**:13–19.

12. Cuddeback GS, Morrissey JP, Domino ME, et al. Fidelity to recovery-oriented ACT practices and consumer out- comes. *Psychiatr Serv*. 2013;**64**:318–323.

13. Domino ME, Gertner A, Grabert B, et al. Do timely mental health services reduce re-incarceration among prison releasees with severe mental illness? *Health Serv Res*. 2019;**54**:592–602.

14. Inciardi JA, Isenberg H, Lockwood D, Martin SS, Scarpitti FR. Assertive community treatment with a parolee population: an extension of case management. *NIDA Res Monogr*. 1992;**127**:350–367.

15. Wilson D, Tien G, Eaves D. Increasing the community tenure of mentally disordered offenders: An assertive case management program. *Int J Law Psychiatry*. 1995;**18**:61–69.

16. Lamberti JS, Weisman R, Faden DI. Forensic assertive community treatment: Preventing incarceration of adults with severe mental illness. *Psychiatr Serv*. 2004;**55**:1285–1293.

17. Lamberti JS, Weisman RL. Preventing incarceration of adults with severe mental illness: Project Link. In: Landsberg G, Rock M, Berg LKW, Smiley A, eds. *Serving Mentally Ill Offenders: Opportunities for Mental Health Professionals*. Springer Publishing Company; 2002.

18. Lamberti JS, Weisman RL, Schwarzkopf SB, et al. The mentally ill in jails and prisons: Towards an integrated model of prevention. *Psychiatr Q*. 2001;**72**:63–77.

19. Lamberti, JS. Project link: Department of Psychiatry, University of Rochester, Rochester, NY. Gold Award: prevention of jail and hospital recidivism among persons with severe mental illness. *Psychiatr Serv*. 1999;**50**:1477–1480.

20. Landess J, Holoyda B. Mental health courts and forensic assertive community treatment teams as correctional diversion programs. *Behav Sci Law*. 2017;**35**:501–511.

21. Lamberti JS, Deem A, Weisman RL, LaDuke C. The role of probation in forensic assertive community treatment. *Psychiatr Serv*. 2011;**62**:418–421.

22. Moser LL. *Findings from the National ACT Study*. University of North Carolina; 2024 unpublished.

23. Sullivan A. Commissioner, New York State Office of Mental Health 2024, personal communication.

24. Kruszynski R. Director, Case Western Reserve University Center for Evidence-Based Practices 2024, personal communication.

25. Aubry T, Goering P, Veldhuizen S, et al. A multiple-city RCT of housing first with assertive community treatment for homeless Canadians with serious mental illness. *Psychiatr Serv*. 2016;**67**:275–281.

26. Kusters I, Van Horn JE, Cnossen TEA. Forensic (F) ACT: a study exploring indication, risk assessment and recidivism. *Tijdschr Psychiatr*. 2018;**60**:672–681.

27. McKenna B, Skipworth J, Tapsell R, et al. Impact of an assertive community treatment model of care on the treatment of prisoners with a serious mental illness. *Australas Psychiatry*. 2018;**26**:285–289.

28. Marquant T, Goethals K. Results of forensic assertive community treatment in Belgium after 33 months. *Eur Psychiatr*. 2016;**33**(S1):S460–S461.

29. Cosden M, Ellens J, Schnell J, Yamini-Diouf Y. Efficacy of a mental health treatment court with assertive

community treatment. *Behav Sci Law*. 2005;**23**:199–214.

30. Cusack KJ, Morrissey JP, Cuddeback GS, Prins A, Williams DM. Criminal justice involvement, behavioral health service use, and costs of forensic assertive community treatment: A randomized trial. *Community Ment Health J*. 2010;**46**:356–363.

31. Lamberti J, Weisman R, Cerulli C, et al. A randomized controlled trial of the Rochester forensic assertive community treatment model. *Psychiatr Serv*. 2017;**68**:1016–1024.

32. Maeng D, Tsun Z-Y, Lesch E, et al. Affordability of forensic assertive community treatment programs: A return-on-investment analysis. *Psychiatr Serv*. 2023;**74**:358–364.

33. Lamberti JS, Weisman RL, Jacobowitz DJ, Chapman B. A randomized controlled trial of the Rochester FACT model in Minnesota (unpublished).

34. Marquant T, Sabbe B, Van Nuffel M, Goethals K. Forensic assertive community treatment: a review of the literature. *Community Ment Health J*. 2016;**52**:873–881.

35. Cuddeback GS, Simpson JM, Wu JC. A comprehensive literature review of Forensic Assertive Community Treatment (FACT): Directions for practice, policy and research. *Int J Ment Health*. 2020;**49**:106–127.

36. Goulet M-H, Dellazizzo L, Lessard-Deschênes C, et al. Effectiveness of forensic assertive community treatment on forensic and health outcomes: a systematic review and meta-analysis. *Crim Just Behav*. 2022;**49**:838–852.

37. Wolff N, Frueh BC, Huening J, et al. Practice informs the next generation of behavioral health and criminal justice interventions. *Int J Law Psychiatry*. 2013;**36**:1–10.

38. Epperson MW, Wolff N, Morgan RD, et al. Envisioning the next generation of behavioral health and criminal justice interventions. *Int J Law Psychiatry*. 2014;**37**:427–438.

39. Bonfine N, Wilson AB, Munetz MR. Meeting the needs of justice-involved people with serious mental illness within community behavioral health systems. *Psychiatr Serv*. 2020;**71**:355–363.

40. Lamberti J. *Project ACT: Developing a Forensic Assertive Community Treatment (FACT) Collaboration with Mental Health Court University of Rochester Medical Center Grand Rounds Presentation*. March 9, 2022.

41. Forensic Assertive Community Treatment (FACT): Guidelines Addendum. New York State Office of Mental Health. 2024. https://omh.ny.gov/omhweb/act/forensic-act-program-addendum.pdf

42. Weisman RL, Lamberti J, Price N. Integrating criminal justice, community healthcare, and support services for adults with severe mental disorders. *Psychiatr Q*. 2004;**75**:71–85.

43. DeLuca JS, O'Connor LK, Yanos PT. Assertive community treatment with people with combined mental illness and criminal justice involvement. In: Calkins C, Jeglik EL, eds. *New Frontiers in Offender Treatment*. Springer Publishing Company; 2018.

44. SAMHSA. Forensic assertive community treatment (FACT). A service delivery model for individuals with serious mental illness involved in the criminal justice system. PEP19-FACT-BR. SAMHSA, 1–8. 2019

45. Lamberti JS, Weisman RL. Essential elements of forensic assertive community treatment. *Harv Rev Psychiatry*. 2021;**29**:278–297.

46. Kovera MB. Racial disparities in the criminal justice system: Prevalence, causes, and a search for solutions. *J Soc Issues*. 2019;**75**:1139–1164.

47. Erickson SK, Lamberti JS, Weisman R, et al. Predictors of arrest during forensic assertive community treatment. *Psychiatr Serv*. 2009;**60**:834–837.

48. Andrews D, Bonta J. *The Psychology of Criminal Conduct*. 7th ed. Routledge: 2024.

49. Latessa EJ, Johnson SL, Koetzle D. *What Works (and Doesn't) in Reducing Recidivism*. Routledge: 2020.

50. Andrews DA, Bonta J, Wormith S. *Level of Service/Case Management Inventory: LS/CMI*. Multi-Health Systems Toronto; 2000.

51. Latessa EJ, Lemke R, Makarios M, Smith P. The creation and validation of the Ohio Risk Assessment System (ORAS). *Fed Probat*. 2010;**74**:16–22.

52. Baird C. The CAIS/JAIS approach to assessment. In: *Handbook of Recidivism Risk/Needs Assessment Tools* John Wiley & Sons. Wiley Online Library; 2018:31–47.

53. Kamin D, Weisman RL, Lamberti JS. Promoting mental health and criminal justice collaboration through system-level partnerships. *Front Psychiatry*. 2022;**13**:1–8.

54. Lamberti JS. Preventing criminal recidivism through mental health and criminal justice collaboration. *Psychiatr Serv*. 2016;**67**:1206–1212.

55. Draine J, Solomon P. Threats of incarceration in a psychiatric probation and parole service. *Am J Orthopsychiatry*. 2001;**71**:262–267.

56. Solomon P, Draine J. One-year outcomes of a randomized trial of case management with seriously mentally ill clients leaving jail. *Eval Rev*. 1995;**19**(3):256–273.

57. Wexler DB. Two decades of therapeutic jurisprudence. *Touro Law Rev*. 2008;**24**:1–14.

58. Lehrer DS, Lorenz J. Anosognosia in schizophrenia: hidden in plain sight. *Innov Clin Neurosci.* 2014;**11**:10–17.

59. Lamberti JS, Russ A, Cerulli C, et al. Patient experiences of autonomy and coercion while receiving legal leverage in forensic assertive community treatment. *Harv Rev Psychiatry.* 2014;**22**:222–230.

60. Anthony WA. Recovery from mental illness: the guiding vision of the mental health service system in the 1990s. *Psychiatr Rehabil J.* 1993;**16**:11–23.

61. Kikkert M, Goudriaan A, De Waal M, Peen J, Dekker J. Effectiveness of Integrated Dual Diagnosis Treatment (IDDT) in severe mental illness outpatients with a co-occurring substance use disorder. *J Subst Abuse Treat.* 2018;**95**:35–42.

62. Lamberti JS, Katsetos V, Jacobowitz DB, Weisman RL. Psychosis, mania and criminal recidivism: associations and implications for prevention. *Harv Rev Psychiatry.* 2020;**28**:179–202.

63. Torrey EF, Lieberman J. The underuse of clozapine and long-acting injectable antipsychotics. *Psychiatr Serv.* 2025;**76**:90–92.

64. Tafrate RC, Mitchell D (eds.). *Forensic CBT: A Handbook for Clinical Practice.* John Wiley & Sons; 2014.

65. Smith P, Schweitzer M, Labrecque RM, Latessa EJ. Improving probation officers' supervision skills: An evaluation of the EPICS model. *J Crim Justice.* 2012;**35**:189–199.

66. Clodfelter TA, Holcomb JE, Alexander MA, Marcum CD, Richards TN. A case study of the implementation of Staff Training Aimed at Reducing Rearrest (STARR). *Fed Probat.* 2016;**80**:30–38.

67. Taxman FS, Yancey C, Bilanin JE. Proactive community supervision in Maryland: Changing offender outcomes. *Citeseer* MD: Maryland Division of Parole and Probation; 2006:1–33.

68. Morrissey JP, Fagan JA, Cocozza JJ. New models of collaboration between criminal justice and mental health systems. *Am J Psychiatry.* 2009;**166**:1211–1214.

69. Parker A, Scantlebury A, Booth A, et al. Interagency collaboration models for people with mental ill health in contact with the police: a systematic scoping review. *BMJ Open.* 2018;**8**:1–13.

70. Danzer GS, Wheeler EM, Alexander AA, Wasser TD. Competency restoration for adult defendants in different treatment environments. *J Am Acad Psychiatry Law.* 2019;**47**(1):68–81.

Does Compulsory Community Treatment for Discharged Forensic Hospital Patients Work?
The Recent Evidence Base

Melinda DiCiro, Melanie Scott, and Sean Sterling

Over the decades, research has demonstrated the efficacy of Conditional Release Programs (CONREP) and Compulsory community treatment for forensic patients following discharge from inpatient commitment. Since a forensic commitment is based on criminal behavior, the primary concern is the risk of criminal and violent behavior. While secure forensic hospitalization can constrain criminal and violent behavior, there are drawbacks, including the criminalization of mental illness, high costs, and undermining patient autonomy and functioning. Furthermore, the principles of treatment in the least restrictive alternative (*Olmstead v. LC*, 1999) and Risk, Need, Responsivity (RNR) support community treatment when feasible and effective. Therefore, continued study of these programs and their utility is essential for establishing best practices.

Additionally, understanding the factors influencing recidivism for patients released from forensic hospitals informs policies necessary for public safety, while reducing the criminalization of mental illness. The growing focus on community treatment for forensic populations highlights the need to identify factors contributing to success. As such, this article synthesizes current knowledge on Compulsory community treatment's impact on recidivism among discharged forensic patients, highlighting its role in improved outcomes and safety for individuals and the community. In doing so, we review findings from a 2024 California Department of State Hospitals (DSH) report, from our perspectives as study researchers (Drs. DiCiro and Sterling) and as an overseer of CONREP (Dr. Scott).

CONREP and Compulsory court supervision

Depending on the jurisdiction, CONREP and Compulsory court supervision are mechanisms wherein a court or administrative law hearing can mandate outpatient treatment and supervision for forensic patients released from a forensic hospital. The goals of these programs are to (1) provide necessary treatment and support for those with severe and persistent mental health disorders, (2) ensure a successful transition to the community, and (3) mitigate potential dangerousness and protect public safety.[1,2]

Most CONREP and similar programs include housing support, case management, individual and group therapy, medication management, substance use screening and treatment, home visits, and other services tailored to individual needs and risk levels. When necessary, CONREP programs can temporarily rehospitalize a patient who decompensates, shows signs of dangerousness, or violates the terms and conditions of release. In addition, a court can revoke CONREP treatment for unsuccessful programming or committing a new offense. Supervised outpatient treatment through CONREP has consistently been shown to effectively reduce criminal recidivism and improve forensic patient outcomes in the United States and internationally.

Recidivism rates for direct hospital discharges

The literature has consistently demonstrated that patients unconditionally released or directly discharged from forensic hospitals evidence poor treatment outcomes and significantly higher rates of recidivism. Such outcomes were demonstrated in a study by Fazel et al.,[3] which analyzed 6,520 patients discharged from psychiatric hospitals in Sweden between 1973 and 2009, wherein 69% were rehospitalized, and 40% were convicted for a violent offense after discharge. Likewise, Wolf et al.[4] followed 2,248 patients directly discharged from forensic hospitals in Sweden between 1992 and 2013 and found that 6.9%

violently recidivated within 12 months and 10.9% within 24 months; the strongest predictors of violent recidivism were previous violent crime and male gender. They also noted that longer lengths of stay reduced recidivism for those tied to Compulsory outpatient treatment after hospital discharge.

Siddiqui et al.[5] examined post-discharge recidivism among 66 patients directly discharged from a forensic psychiatric service in Saudi Arabia between 2005 and 2020. Results found that 68.18% were rehospitalized during the 15-year study period, and 16.66% violently offended after discharge. Ojansuu[6] found similar results in exploring criminal and violent recidivism among 501 patients directly discharged from forensic hospitals in Finland between 1999 and 2018. On average, patients spent 10 years committed within the forensic hospital, and 16.6% re-offended after discharge (mean time to conviction of 3.8 years). Furthermore, the re-offense was considered violent in 9.6% of the sample. Sample characteristics showed that the patients were primarily diagnosed with schizophrenia (91%) and that more than half had a co-occurring substance use disorder (63.5%). Additionally, a longer treatment duration was associated with a reduced likelihood of general recidivism.

Recidivism rates for discharge to CONREP

Overwhelmingly, the literature has also shown that patients discharged from a forensic hospital to CONREP consistently have lower recidivism rates than those directly discharged from forensic hospitals without CONREP treatment. Reynolds[7] highlights this using a sample of 110 patients released into CONREP from the Missouri Department of Mental Health. Results showed only a 1% recidivism rate and a 7% revocation rate after a 3-year follow-up. Similarly, Parker[8] found that for an Assertive Community Treatment program that supervised 83 Not Guilty by Reason of Insanity (NGRI) patients in CONREP, after a 5-year follow-up, only 5 of the 83 patients were rearrested. This pattern of low recidivism rates was also found at the Oregon CONREP, where, in a sample of 238 patients with NGRI, recidivism rates were less than 1%, with only moderate revocation rates ($n = 81$, 33.6%).[9]

In a California study by McDermott et al.,[1] the authors tracked 93 NGRI patients discharged from a California state hospital (2002–2013) for 4.83 years, comparing those unconditionally discharged directly from the state hospital with those discharged to CONREP treatment in the community. Results found that nearly half of those unconditionally discharged (43.8%) were rearrested during the study period compared to those released under CONREP (8.2%). Additionally, those who were NGRI but restored to sanity and unconditionally released also had higher arrest rates (25%). While time to rearrest did not differ among groups, those released to the community without CONREP were nearly nine times more likely to re-offend than those released with CONREP. Patient characteristics showed that CONREP patients were more often White, with a diagnosis of schizophrenia, while those unconditionally discharged were often diagnosed with a personality disorder. Overall, the results showed that court-mandated treatment (CONREP) had the most potent effect on preventing arrests. From 2008 to 2015, Rossetto et al.[10] examined female forensic patients rehospitalized after conditional or unconditional discharge from Italian Residences for the Execution of the Security Measure (REMs)—small, local treatment centers that replaced forensic hospitals and are integrated with community psychiatry resources. Follow-up was conducted through 2018. Overall, the results found that for patients conditionally released, 70.8% did not require readmission or rehospitalization. Key predictors of rehospitalization were having a substance use disorder, having a personality disorder, being unconditionally discharged, younger age, and having a shorter inpatient stay. The diagnosis of schizophrenia was unrelated. The authors posited that readmission most depended on whether the person was discharged on conditional release or not. Also, in a Swedish study, Noland and Strandh[11] used a survival analysis to examine 1,150 forensic patients discharged from forensic hospitals between 2009 and 2018. Outcomes showed that older age at discharge was associated with a lower likelihood of recidivism, while having a substance use disorder, a history of crime before the index offense, or a diagnosed personality disorder without psychosis was associated with a higher likelihood of recidivism.

Treatment outcomes without CONREP or Compulsory outpatient treatment

Not all states utilize CONREP or Compulsory outpatient treatment upon discharge from forensic hospitals. For example, in England, Westhead et al.[12] followed a group of 843 patients – 70.3% of whom were admitted from prison to a medium secure psychiatric facility between July 1983 and June 2013. The patients were discharged to prisons, high, medium, low, and nonsecure hospital facilities, as well as the community. Of the 843 discharged patients, 43.8% were convicted of a new offense within the first 5 years of release. The conviction rate for "serious offenses" (defined as offenses warranting a life sentence) was 3.1%. Additionally, 61.6% of the patients were readmitted to a psychiatric inpatient service (though not necessarily to a forensic hospital). There was also a higher long-term risk of premature mortality. Of those released directly to the community, two-thirds were readmitted to a psychiatric service, with 31.8% readmitted within the first year. The authors emphasized the need for treatment and supervision after hospital discharge to assist in reintegration.

Similarly, in examining release without CONREP, Haroon et al.[13] examined post-release outcomes of insanity acquittees discharged from state hospitals in North Carolina between 1996 and 2020. North Carolina is unique because it is one of eight states that lack an enforceable court monitoring program for released state hospital patients. The follow-up period ranged from 1 year to almost 23 years. Overall, the authors assert that conditionally released patients have lower rates of rearrest and rehospitalization compared to those unconditionally discharged. Specifically, the median time to rehospitalization for unconditionally released patients was 1.8 years, and 27.9% of acquittees were rehospitalized after unconditional release. Additionally, 14.8% had re-offended and were convicted of a new crime within a median period of 2 years. Furthermore, the authors compared recidivism in North Carolina to that of different states using CONREP. They concluded that insanity acquittees in North Carolina have higher rates of criminal recidivism than acquittees in other states due to lack of CONREP.

Reynolds[14] provided a commentary on the study by Haroon et al.[13] and championed the value of CONREP. He noted that the reconviction rate in the Haroon et al. study parallels that of unsupervised (i.e., directly discharged) forensic patients in other states but substantially exceeds that of court-supervised CONREP. Citing his experience in the Missouri and Colorado systems, Reynolds agreed with Haroon et al. that the absence of court supervision accounts for higher recidivism rates. Reynolds highlighted the benefits of court authority to monitor patients and address conditional release violations through early detection and intervention, thereby reducing unnecessarily long hospitalizations and supporting better outcomes while lowering costs.

Finally, regarding sexually violent persons on supervised release, Ambroziak et al.[15] explored re-offense recidivism for 205 sexually violent persons on supervised release from a state forensic hospital over the years. Although this patient population did not evidence high rates of severe mental illness compared with other post-release recidivism populations, the results revealed the value of community supervision. The authors found a 1.5% rate of new sex offense charges in the supervised release sample, whereas a comparable group of offenders released directly from prison to the community (with fewer restrictions and less oversight) recidivated at nearly double that rate (2.9%), despite a more conservative outcome variable (convictions).

The 2024 California DSH CONREP effectiveness study

In California, CONREP programs provide oversight, structure, and treatment and serve as a step-down for reintegration into the community. The statute includes a mechanism for rehospitalization when patients show signs of decompensation or violate the conditions of their release. A court can also revoke the CONREP status. Patients are released to CONREP when a court deems them able to meet the program's terms and conditions and can be treated safely and effectively in the community. Alternatively, patients may be directly discharged from the hospital to the community when a court finds they no longer meet commitment criteria. Comparing CONREP-treated and directly discharged patients reveals the value of ongoing, court-supervised treatment for forensic patients.

CONREP comprises patients from the following five primary commitment schemes: Not Guilty by Reason of Insanity (NGI, also known as insanity acquittees); Incompetent to Stand Trial (IST); Offenders with Mental Health Disorders (OMD-Parole), a postprison civil commitment scheme as a condition of parole for those who remain dangerous due to their mental disorder; Offenders with Mental Health Disorders (OMD-Civil), a civil commitment scheme for those who remain dangerous beyond the parole period; and Sexually Violent

Predator (SVP), a postprison civil commitment scheme for individuals whose mental disorders render them predisposed to commit predatory sex offenses.

Between 1990 and 2002, the California DSH conducted five evaluations of its CONREP, consistently demonstrating the program's effectiveness in reducing recidivism. The initial 1990 study of 710 patients showed that CONREP participants had significantly lower rearrest rates than those directly discharged patients (6.7% vs. 27.3%). Subsequent studies in 1993, 1998, 1999, and 2002 confirmed these positive outcomes, with the 2002 analysis of 2,101 patients showing an overall rearrest rate of 8.9% for CONREP participants. Throughout these studies, CONREP patients demonstrated improved social functioning and lower recidivism rates across all commitment categories, although rates varied by legal classification. The program's success was attributed to enhanced patient functioning during treatment and the ability to temporarily rehospitalize struggling patients. Notably, CONREP consistently proved to be more cost-effective, operating at approximately 20% of the state hospital's costs while maintaining better outcomes.

Following a hiatus after the 2002 report, a July 2024 report confirmed earlier California findings, reinforcing CONREP's role in enhancing patient outcomes and public safety. The 2024 California DSH CONREP Effectiveness Study compared outcomes between patients directly discharged from state hospitals and those released through CONREP (CONREP-treated). This report provides compelling evidence for the program's effectiveness in patient treatment, reintegration, and public safety. As the primary researchers for this study, we summarize the most salient outcomes and conclusions, augmenting our summary with statistical analyses and details not explicated in the government report.

Methods Used in this Study

We analyzed rearrests for general and violent crime and other relevant variables for 2,613 patients who were either discharged directly to the community ($N =$ 2,011) or discharged to CONREP ($N = 602$) from California state hospitals between 2012 and 2017. Follow-up through 2018 permitted at least 1 year in the community for all patients studied. The study population included individuals in four of the five commitment categories described above. This study

used the first identified arrest event as the recidivism outcome variable. We chose available variables with established relationships to recidivism and violence in populations with severe mental illness (Bonta et al.,[16] Harris et al.,[17] among others), including commitment category, mental health diagnoses, and lengths of stay. We also examined the time of arrest.

Data were collected through the California DSH and CONREP tracking systems, linked with California Department of Justice (DOJ) arrest and prosecution records. The project was approved by the California Committee for the Protection of Human Subjects, which waived informed consent due to the retrospective, data-based nature of the study. We followed DSH deidentification protocols, and the results were deemed to be at low risk of identifying individual patients. Statistical analyses were performed using SPSS Version 23.

The study revealed dramatically lower fixed recidivism rates for any arrest among CONREP-treated patients compared to directly discharged patients across 1-, 3-, and 5-year time frames. Directly discharged patients were seven times more likely to be rearrested within 1 year and four and a half times more likely within 3 years. CONREP-treated patients maintained a significantly lower probability of rearrest at 5 years (five times lower). Note: Known deaths were removed from the calculation for the corresponding interval. The DSH CONREP Effectiveness Study (2024) also examined rearrests for sex offenses as well as other variables not discussed in this article. Statistical analyses (using chi-square tests on 2×2 contingency tables) revealed significant differences in recidivism rates, as shown in Figure 13.1 and Tables 13.1–13.3.

Table 13.1 One-year fixed recidivism for any arrest

	Direct discharge	CONREP treated
$N =$ with at least 365 days (1 year) post discharge	2003	596
$N =$ arrested within 365 days	427	18
Recidivism rate	21.23%	3.02%

Note: Odds ratio 8.70; .95 CI 5.37 to 14.07; Phi = +.2 χ^2 Pearson 109.38; $p < .0001$.

Table 13.2 Three-year fixed recidivism for any arrest

	Direct discharge	CONREP treated
N = with at least 1095 days (3 years) post discharge	1207	350
N = arrested within 1095 days for this group	502	33
Recidivism rate	41.59%	9.43%

Note: Odds ratio 6.84; .95 CI 4.69 to 9.96; Phi = +.28 χ2 Pearson 124.44; p < .0001.

Table 13.3 Five-year fixed recidivism for any arrest

	Direct discharge	CONREP treated
N = with at least 1825 days (5 years) post discharge	463	125
N = arrested within 1825 days for this group	228	12
Recidivism rate	49.24%	9.60%

Note: Odds ratio 9.13; .95 CI 4.90 to 17.02; Phi = +33 χ2 Pearson 64.04; p < .0001.

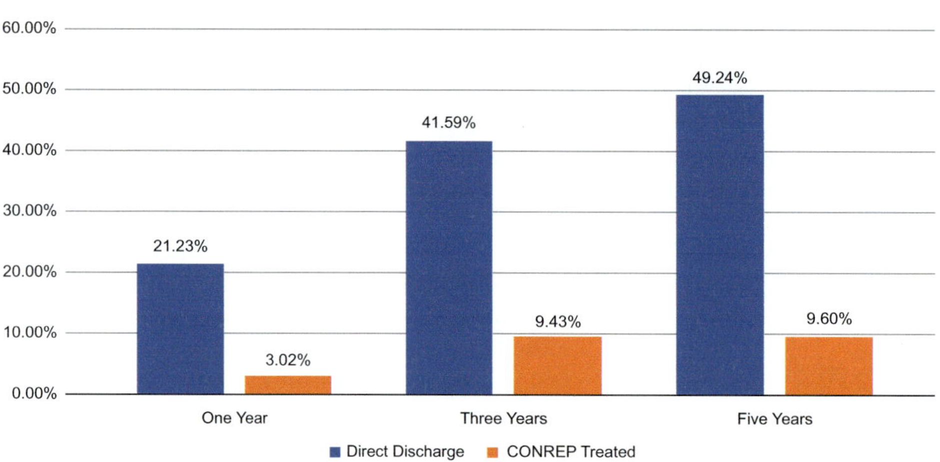

Figure 13.1 Fixed recidivism rates by treatment status. Reprinted from the California Department of State Hospitals CONREP Effectiveness Study (2024).

Violent recidivism

Results revealed dramatically lower fixed recidivism rates for violent arrests among CONREP-treated patients compared with directly discharged patients across 1-, 3-, and 5-year time frames. Violent offenses were defined as those leading to or posing a threat of physical injury or death, contact sex offenses, and actual or implied threats of violence. Directly discharged patients were nearly nine times more likely to be rearrested for a violent offense within 1 year, five times more likely within 3 years, and almost nine times more likely within 5 years. As shown in Figure 13.2 and Tables 13.4–13.6, statistical analysis shows significant differences in violent recidivism rates.

Tables 13.4–13.6 compare fixed recidivism rates for violent offense arrests.

A Cox regression analysis determined that, for those arrested, half of the CONREP-treated patients were arrested at approximately 500 days versus approximately 400 days for directly discharged patients ($\chi2$ = 10.942, df = 2, p < .004). Further analysis revealed that three-quarters of the arrested CONREP-treated patients were arrested within the first 18 months. Longer lengths of stay in CONREP correlated with lower recidivism (point biserial correlation; Pearson r = −.082; p = .026, one-tailed test).

We also found distinct differences between CONREP-treated patients and those directly discharged. CONREP participants tended to be older (mean age 45.48 vs. 42.11 years), had more extended hospital stays (mean 1895.67 vs. 797.7 days), and included more female patients (23.8% vs. 5.1%). Additionally, CONREP patients were more likely to have psychotic disorders and less likely to have previous state hospital commitments or personality disorders. Because the literature consistently associates these factors with lower recidivism, these group differences likely partially account for their lower recidivism rates. Table 13.7 shows the differences between the groups.

We conducted a logistic regression analysis of potentially impactful variables to examine the impact of factors affecting rearrest. The most potent contributor to rearrest was being directly discharged, followed by a younger age, having more state hospital commitments, lower commitment offense severity, OMD commitment, and male gender. Ethnicity, psychotic disorder diagnosis, and personality disorder diagnosis were not significantly related to rearrest. Hospital LOS approached significance. The logistic regression model showed a significant association between variables and recidivism (shared variance of 22%), with good specificity (83% correctly classified as non-recidivating) but poor sensitivity (41% correctly

Table 13.4 One-year fixed recidivism rates for a violent offense

	Direct discharge	CONREP treated
N = with at least 365 days (1 year) post discharge	2003	596
N = arrested within 365 days	306	12
Violent recidivism rate	15.27%	2.0%

Note: Odds ratio 8.77; .95 CI 4.89 to 15.74; Phi = + .17, χ2 Pearson 75.25; p < .0001.

Table 13.5 Three-year fixed recidivism rates for a violent offense

	Direct discharge	CONREP treated
N = with at least 1095 days (3 years) post discharge	1207	350
N = arrested within 1095 days for this group	356	25
Violent recidivism rate	29.49%	7.14%

Note: Odds ratio 5.43; .95 CI 3.55 to 8.32; Phi = +.22, χ2 Pearson 73.34; p < .0001.

Table 13.6 Five-year fixed recidivism rates for a violent offense

	Direct discharge	CONREP treated
N = with at least 1825 days (5 years) post discharge	463	125
N = arrested within 1825 days for this group	159	<11[a]
Violent recidivism rate	34.34%	~6.0%[b]

Note: Odds ratio 8.81; .95 CI is 4.01 to 19.35; Phi = +.26 χ2 Pearson 40.13; *p* < .0001. *N* arrested within 1825 days: direct discharge = 159; CONREP treated = 7. Violent recidivism rate: direct discharge = 34.34%; CONREP treated = 5.60%.Odds ratio: 8.81; 95% CI 4.01 to 19.35; Phi = +.26; χ2 Pearson = 40.13; *p* < .0001.

[a] Numbers <11 not published for data deidentification.

[b] Approximate percentage for deidentification.

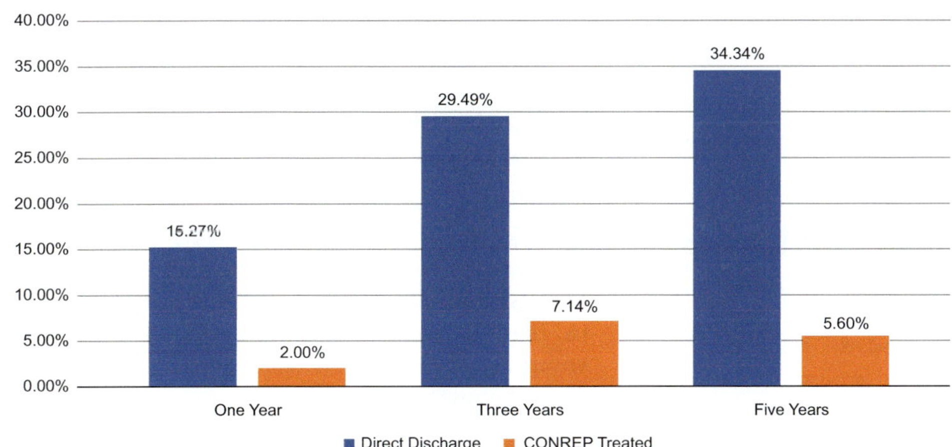

Figure 13.2 Fixed recidivism rate for violent offenses by treatment status. Reprinted from the California Department of State Hospitals CONREP Effectiveness Study (2024).

Table 13.7 Group differences between directly discharged and CONREP-treated patients

Variable	Group difference and direction	Significance
Gender	Those in the directly discharged group were **more** likely to be male.	Odds ratio 5.98; Phi +.27 χ2 Pearson 192.02 $p < .0001$
Age at discharge	The CONREP-treated group was **older** than the directly discharged groups.	An independent samples t-test Results: $t = 6.050$ (df) $= 990.944$; $p = .000$ two-tailed test.
Race-ethnicity	Those in the directly discharged group were	–
	Less likely to be White	Odds ratio .68; Phi -.08 χ2 Pearson 17.41 $p < .0001$
	More likely to be Black.	Odds ratio 1.31 Phi+.05 χ2 Pearson 6.11 p < .01
	More likely to be Hispanic.	Odds ratio 1.31 Phi+.05 χ2 Pearson 6.11 $p < .01$
	Less likely to be Asian	Odds ratio .55 Phi+.06 χ2 Pearson 8.58 $p < .003$
Hospital LOS	CONREP-treated patients had **longer** lengths of stay in the hospital than did directly discharged patients.	Independent samples t-test: $t = 16.274$ (df) =775.53; $p = <.000$ two-tailed test.
Commitment offense category	Directly discharged patients were less likely to have a violent commitment offense.	Odds ratio .48; Phi -.11 χ2 Pearson 32.8 $p < .0001$
	Directly discharged patients were significantly more likely to have a sex offense.	Odds ratio 2.64 Phi +.1 χ2 Pearson 25.5 $p < .0001$
Commitment offense severity	The mean commitment offense severity for the CONREP-treated group was **higher** than that of the directly discharged groups.	An independent samples t-test: $t = 8.3426$. (df) =975.788; $p < .000$ two-tailed test.
Commitment type	Directly discharged patients were **more** likely to be OMD parole.	Odds ratio 19.11 Phi -.51 χ2 Pearson 1. 96 688 $p < .0001$
	Less likely to be OMD civil.	Odds ratio .68 Phi -.06 χ2 Pearson 9.69 $p < .0001$
	Less likely to be NGI	Odds ratio .05 Phi -.59 χ2 Pearson 896.3 $p < .0001$ Odds ratio 21.32 Phi -.59 χ2 Pearson 912. 94 $p < .0001$
	More likely to be SVP.	Odds ratio 2.83 Phi −06 χ2 Pearson 9.81 $p < .0001$
Number commitments	–	Odds ratio 5.1 Phi +.06 χ 2 Pearson 71.3 $p < .0001$
Diagnostic category	Directly discharged patients were **less** likely to have a psychotic disorder.	Odds ratio .60 Phi .1 χ 2 Pearson 223.7 p < .0001
	More likely to have a paraphilic disorder.	Odds ratio 3.4 Phi +.11 χ 2 Pearson 24.57 p < .0001
	More likely to have a depressive disorder.	Odds ratio 1.53 Phi +.04 χ 2 Pearson 3.61 p < .057
	About **equally** likely to have a substance use disorder	Odds ratio .91 Phi .002 χ 2 Pearson .76 p = .38 ns
	More likely to have ASPD	OR 3.27 Phi +.09 χ 2 Pearson 19.5 p < .0001

classified as recidivating), resulting in an overall correct classification rate of 71%. Table 13.8 displays the logistic regression model.

Duration of treatment effectiveness

The research demonstrated that CONREP's impact extended beyond the active treatment phase. Only 4% of the patients were arrested during treatment and only 7% recidivated after program completion. Notably, longer CONREP stays were correlated with better outcomes, suggesting a dose–response relationship between treatment duration and success.

Comparison to a similar California population

Because rearrest rates for OMD commitment categories (those committed to a state hospital after serving a prison sentence) were higher than those for NGI (those committed directly to a state hospital in lieu of a conviction and prison term), we compared the OMD rates to recidivism in an analogous population. Specifically, we compared the rearrest rates of directly discharged and CONREP-treated groups for the entire sample—and the OMD-Parole and OMD-Civil categories—to the

Table 13.8 Logistic regression: factors impacting rearrest

			Predicted			
				Recidivism		
	Observed			No	Yes	Percentage correct
Step 1	Recidivism	No		1388	287	82.9
		Yes		548	378	40.8
	Overall percentage					67.9

a. The cut value is .500

		Variables in the equation						95% CI for EXP(B)	
		B	S.E.	Wald	df	Sig.	Exp(B)	Lower	Upper
Step 1	Age at discharge	−.025	.004	35.554	1	.000	.975	.967	.983
	Gender	.397	.191	4.334	1	.037	1.488	1.094	2.163
	Length of stay in hospital	.000	.000	3.277	1	.070	1.000	1.000	1.000
	Number of commitments	.637	.110	33.855	1	.000	1.891	1.528	2.344
	OMD	.732	.154	22.605	1	.000	2.080	1.538	2.812
	Any personality disorder	.110	.162	.457	1	.499	1.116	.812	1.533
	Any psychotic disorder	−.045	.104	.193	1	.661	0.956	.78	1.171
	Commitment offense severity	−0.116	.024	24.373	1	000	0.890	.85	.932
	CONCEPT treated	−1.118	.161	47.967	1	000	0.327	.239	.449
	Work ethic	−.46	.093	.247	1	.619	0.955	.798	1.145
	Constant	−.281	.540	.270	1	.603	0.755		

reconviction rates of individuals from the California Department of Corrections and Rehabilitation (CDCR) who were enrolled in the Enhanced Outpatient Program (EOP) upon prison release (EOP is an intensive outpatient psychiatric treatment program in California Prisons). CDCR EOP reconviction rates were 22.90% at 1 year and 51.80% at 3 years. In comparison, rearrest rates in this study were 21.32% for directly discharged and 3.02% for CONREP-treated patients at 1 year, and 41.59% versus 9.43% at 3 years.[19] For the OMD-Parole group, directly discharged patients had rearrest rates of 25.55% (1 year) and 47.64% (3 years), while CONREP-treated patients had rates of 7.14% (1 year) and 14.29% (3 years). For the OMD-Civil group, directly discharged rates were 19.19% (1 year) and 39.89% (3 years) versus 5.45% (1 year) and 13.85% (3 years) for CONREP-treated patients. Reconviction rates for the CDCR EOP group were consistently higher than the rearrest rates from the state hospitals, aside from a slightly higher rearrest rate for the OMD-Parole group after 1 year. Actual recidivism differences between the CDCR and DSH groups are likely higher, given that arrest is a more sensitive outcome variable than conviction. Figure 13.3 visually displays these differences.

These outcomes suggest that Compulsory treatment post-release may reduce recidivism for incarcerated individuals with severe mental health disorders, although further exploration is warranted, given potential confounding factors. Furthermore, before 2024, a high number of OMD-Parole patients were decertified by the Superior Court and released from the state hospital directly into the community within 5 days, leaving little time for care coordination. This gap may have contributed to the comparatively high rate for the OMD-Parole commitment category. Since 2024, the state hospital has been permitted up to 30 days to coordinate release plans, which could reduce the risk of recidivism.

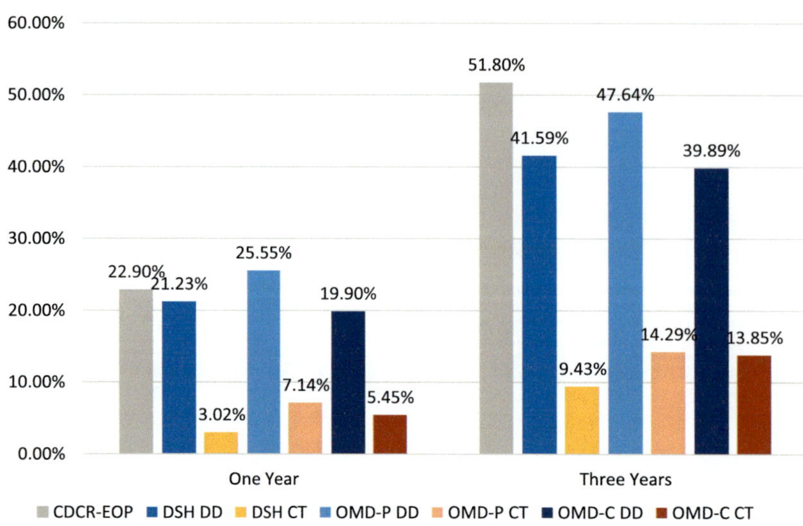

Figure 13.3 Reconviction rates for CDCR EOP prison releases and rearrest rates for OMD-P and OMD-C commitment DSH direct discharge and CONREP-treated patients.

Discussion

The results show that CONREP's approach to graduated community reintegration of forensic patients provides substantial benefits. CONREP has the legal authority to ensure treatment compliance, including medication compliance and the required monitoring and support. Even though group differences complicate isolating CONREP-specific effects, the magnitude of the differences in outcomes strongly supports the conclusion that CONREP treatment contributes to reduced criminal and violent recidivism for forensic patients with severe mental illnesses. Consistent positive outcomes across groups – even those with higher rates of known risk factors – further attest to these benefits. Moreover, low-risk patients can be readily identified and classified. Specifically, CONREP may be a more appropriate setting than continued inpatient hospitalization for older patients with severe mental illness, particularly those with more extended hospital stays, those who belong to the NGI commitment category, and those who have psychotic disorder diagnoses without co-occurring personality or substance use disorders. Such placement is consistent with RNR principles in managing low-risk patients.

Conclusions from the 2024 California DSH CONREP effectiveness report

The findings support the expansion of CONREP services – a California effort begun in 2021. The data suggest that broadening program access could reduce recidivism even among higher-risk populations. Although the directly discharged group had more risk factors, these did not account for the dramatically higher recidivism rates; logistic regression revealed that direct discharge was the most impactful predictor of rearrest. Furthermore, the model correctly classified 83% of the non-recidivists, suggesting that low-risk patients can be accurately identified and better served in the community. Expanding CONREP would allow more patients access to community reintegration programs and support, enabling treatment in the least restrictive environment and consistent with the RNR principles.

Several limitations should be acknowledged, including the reliance on arrest data as the primary outcome measure, potential data inconsistencies and inaccuracies, limited analysis of variable interactions, and incomplete death record access. Nevertheless, our conclusions are based on a substantial sample (2,613 patients) over a meaningful period (2012–2017, with follow-up through 2018), and the differences between directly discharged and CONREP-treated patients support firm conclusions about the program's effectiveness.

Differences in rearrest rates compared with the McDermott et al. study[1] may be attributed to differences in time frames, means of controlling for time effects, population differences, data sources (e.g., Google search for convictions vs. DOJ data), and legislative changes, such as California's Proposition 47 in 2014. In contrast to McDermott et al.'s findings, our study found that the effect of CONREP treatment persisted after program completion. This study also included forensic patients with multiple commitment types.

This comprehensive evaluation adds to the growing body of evidence supporting supervised outpatient treatment as an effective approach for managing forensic patients in the community while maintaining public safety and promoting successful rehabilitation.

Conclusions from effectiveness of supervised community release programs for forensic patients

Compulsory community treatment of discharged forensic hospital patients does indeed work. These recent findings are congruent with decades of earlier research and show that forensic patients with psychotic illnesses and lower criminality can be safely and effectively treated in the community. CONREP, with its guardrails and incentives, provides an off-ramp from carceral settings, allowing safe reintegration and solidifying treatment gains. Recent studies confirm that Compulsory community treatment substantially reduces further justice involvement for forensic patients following their release from forensic hospitals. Despite the challenge of drawing generalizable conclusions from studies with varying outcome measures (e.g., reconviction vs. rearrest vs. rehospitalization), patient characteristics, commitment schemes, follow-up durations, treatment protocols, comparison group types, and legal/social contexts, the overall evidence demonstrates that risk factors for recidivism – such as lack of community treatment, substance use disorders, personality disorders, male gender, and younger age with higher index offense severity (an inverse relationship to recidivism per Laskorunsky[18]) – are significantly mitigated by supervised community treatment programs.

The empirical evidence demonstrates that such programs significantly reduce recidivism among forensic patients following psychiatric hospitalization, with the California CONREP study showing a fourfold to sevenfold reduction. This effect is consistent across diverse jurisdictions and legal frameworks. Longer treatment durations correlate with better outcomes, although the relationship between initial hospital stay and recidivism is complex. Moreover, racial disparities in forensic mental health systems underscore structural barriers and potential biases that warrant further examination.

Overall, the data provide compelling evidence that adequately structured, Compulsory community treatment is safe and effective. Reduced recidivism via CONREP and other court-supervised programs enhances patient autonomy and functioning and improves public safety. Future program development should focus on expanding access, addressing systemic disparities, and ensuring adequate resources for sustained implementation.

References

1. McDermott BE, Ventura MI, Juranek I, Scott CL. Role of mandated community treatment for justice-involved individuals with serious mental illness. *Psychiatr Serv.* 2020;71(7):656–662.

2. California Department of State Hospitals. *Conditional Release Program (CONREP) effectiveness study.* California Department of State Hospitals; 2024.

3. Fazel S, Fimińska Z, Cocks C, Coid J. Patient outcomes following discharge from secure psychiatric hospitals: Systematic review and meta-analysis. *Br J Psychiatry.* 2016;208(1):17–25.

4. Wolf A, Fanshawe TR, Sariaslan A, et al. Prediction of violent crime on discharge from secure psychiatric hospitals: A clinical prediction rule (FoVOx). *Eur Psychiatry.* 2018;47:88–93.

5. Siddiqui JA, Qureshi SF, Alzahrani A. Recidivism rate among patients discharged from long care unit in forensic psychiatry program at Mental Health Hospital, Taif, Saudi Arabia. *Indian J Ment Health.* 2021;8(2):173–180.

6. Ojansuu I, Latvala A, Kautiainen H, et al. General and violent recidivism of former forensic psychiatric patients in Finland. *Front Psychiatry.* 2023;14:1157171.

7. Reynolds JB. A description of the forensic monitoring system of the Missouri Department of Mental Health. *Behav Sci Law.* 2016;34(2–3):378–395.

8. Parker GF. Outcomes of assertive community treatment in an NGRI conditional release program. *J Am Acad Psychiatry Law.* 2004;32(3):291–303.

9. Vitacco MJ, Tabernik HE, Zavodny D, Bailey K, Waggoner C. Reconsidering risk assessment with insanity acquittees. *Law Hum Behav.* 2018;42(5):403–412.

10. Rossetto S, Franconi F, Piccione M, De Girolamo G. Differences between readmitted and non-readmitted women in Italian Forensic Unit: A retrospective study. *Front Psychology.* 2021;12:1–10.

11. Noland E, Strandh M. Historical, clinical and situational risk factors for post-discharge recidivism in forensic psychiatric patients: A Swedish registry study. *Int J Law Psychiatry*. 2021;79:101749.

12. Westhead J, Gibbon S, McCarthy L, Hatcher R, Clarke M. Long-term outcomes after discharge from medium secure care: Still a cause for concern? *J Forensic Psychiatry Psychol*. 2023;34(2):166–178.

13. Haroon H, Wolfe N, Feizi S, Barboriak P. Assessing two decades of insanity acquittee release from the North Carolina forensic program. *J Am Acad Psychiatry Law*. 2023;51(3):342–352.

14. Reynolds JB. The value of conditional release for insanity acquittees. *J Am Acad Psychiatry Law Online*. 2023;51(3):353–356.

15. Ambroziak G, Vincent S, Kahn R, Mundt J, Thornton D. Recidivism and violations among sexually violent persons on supervised release. *Psych Pub Policy and Law*. 2023;29(1):93–105.

16. Bonta J, Blais J, Wilson HA. A theoretically informed meta-analysis of the risk for general and violent recidivism for mentally disordered offenders. *Aggress Violent Behav*. 2014;19(3):278–287.

17. Harris G, Rice M, Quincey V, Cormier C. Mentally disordered and other violent offenders. In: Harris G, Rice M, Quincey V, Cormier C, eds. *Violent Offenders: Appraising and Managing Risk*. 3rd ed. Washington DC: American Psychological Association; 2015;63–91.

18. Laskorunsky J. *Minnesota Criminal History Score Recidivism Project*. Minneapolis. MN: Unit of Minnesota Robina Institute of Crim Law and Crim Justice; 2018.

19. California Department of Corrections and Rehabilitation Outcome Evaluation Report; 2017.

Early Intervention for Schizophrenia
A Pathway to Improved Clinical Outcomes

Takesha Cooper

Clinical vignette: The life and loss of "Roger"

Roger was a 60-year-old man living with both HIV and schizophrenia who was admitted to the hospital for treatment of a chronic obstructive pulmonary disease (COPD) exacerbation. He was referred to the psychiatry consultation-liaison team due to persistent psychotic symptoms that had not responded to multiple antipsychotic trials. Roger's psychiatric history revealed a diagnosis of schizophrenia in early adulthood, marked by hallucinations and delusions of grandeur. Over the next four decades, he cycled through jails, prisons, shelters, and periods of homelessness. Though intermittently connected with outpatient care, his illness remained poorly controlled.

At age 55, after being deemed not competent to stand trial following an assault, Roger was sent to the state hospital. During that stay, he assaulted a nurse while experiencing active psychosis and was subsequently transferred to jail, where he served a short sentence.

After his release, he returned to homelessness, and was later found emaciated and struggling to breathe on the street. Findings upon hospital admission included: oxygen saturation at 88% on room air, HIV viral load of 100,000 copies/mL (previously undetectable when treated) and significant leukopenia.

While Roger's pulmonary and infectious disease conditions improved over a month-long hospitalization, his psychosis remained unremitting despite treatment with several antipsychotics, including both oral and long-acting injectable formulations of typical and atypical agents (e.g., haloperidol, risperidone, quetiapine, prolixin). He continued to exhibit complex delusions, including the belief that Jesus had impregnated him and infected him with HIV. Despite this, Roger was deeply engaging and responsive to compassionate care. The treatment team advocated for his continued hospitalization, even after his medical issues had stabilized, due to the lack of a psychiatric inpatient unit willing to manage his HIV and history of aggression.

Although clozapine had never been trialed – likely due to concerns about neutropenia in the context of HIV – this option was eventually pursued following repeated denials from skilled nursing facilities and complex discharge planning challenges. Within three weeks of clozapine initiation and titration to 350 mg daily, Roger showed marked improvements in aggression, psychosis, and adherence to his HIV medications. Placement was finally secured at a facility out of state for individuals with complex psychiatric and medical comorbidities. Tragically, Roger died in the hospital before transfer could occur. An autopsy is pending.

The psychiatric team expressed gratitude that Roger did not die alone on the street – but mourned the missed opportunities throughout his life. His story underscores the urgent need for systemic change.

Introduction

Schizophrenia is a chronic and severe mental disorder that affects approximately 1% of the global population. Characterized by profound disruptions in thinking, perception, and behavior, it often leads to significant impairments in social and occupational functioning. Traditionally, schizophrenia has been associated with a deteriorating course; however, contemporary research underscores the potential for improved outcomes through early intervention strategies. This chapter explores the rationale, components, and benefits of early intervention, emphasizing its critical role in enhancing prognosis and recovery (McGorry, Killackey, & Yung, 2008).

Epidemiology, onset and early intervention

Schizophrenia typically manifests in late adolescence to early adulthood, with a median age of onset in the early to mid-20s for males and late 20s for females (American Psychiatric Association, 2013). The period preceding the first psychotic episode – the prodromal phase – is marked by subtle changes in cognition, mood, and behavior.

Individuals may experience social withdrawal, unusual thoughts, and a decline in daily functioning. The duration of untreated psychosis (DUP) – the time from symptom onset to initiation of treatment – is often prolonged. A longer DUP has been consistently associated with poorer clinical and functional outcomes (Marshall et al., 2005). Early interventions can fundamentally alter the trajectory of schizophrenia and are most effective when they are multidisciplinary, personalized, and sustained over time. Reducing DUP improves symptomatic and functional outcomes, including better medication adherence, fewer relapses, and higher quality of life (Penttilä, Jääskeläinen, Hirvonen, Isohanni, & Miettunen, 2014). There is also neurobiological evidence suggesting that early intervention may preserve brain structure and function by leveraging neuroplasticity during a critical developmental window (Birchwood, Todd, & Jackson, 1998) (Cooper, Seigler, & Stahl, 2023). As a result, early-phase treatment may be more effective and better tolerated. The most effective early intervention programs are designed to address the full spectrum of needs that arise in early psychosis, including symptom management, functional recovery, family engagement, and social reintegration.

Models of care and program examples

Several international and U.S.-based care models provide frameworks for early intervention services, demonstrating replicable success across diverse healthcare systems. At their core, early intervention programs for schizophrenia typically offer a comprehensive, multidisciplinary approach designed to address both clinical and functional recovery. Core components include low-dose antipsychotic medication, individual and group psychotherapy (often using cognitive behavioral therapy), family education and support, case management, and assistance with school, work, and social reintegration when ready. These services are developmentally tailored and delivered in a coordinated manner, often in community or outpatient settings, with a strong emphasis on engaging both the patient and their family early in the course of illness.

Coordinated Specialty Care (CSC) is the leading model in the United States and was validated through the NIMH-funded Recovery After an Initial Schizophrenia Episode (RAISE) study. CSC teams include psychiatrists, therapists, employment and education specialists, case managers, and peer support specialists. This model emphasizes shared decision-making, individualized care plans, and community integration (Kane et al., 2016). Services are usually delivered in outpatient settings and tailored to developmental stages, recognizing the unique challenges of psychosis in adolescence and early adulthood.

The Early Psychosis Prevention and Intervention Centre (EPPIC) in Melbourne, Australia, represents one of the earliest and most influential international models. EPPIC offers time-limited but intensive services for youth aged 15 to 24, integrating medical, psychological, vocational, and social interventions. Its success has catalyzed similar programs across Europe and Asia, reinforcing the scalability and global relevance of early psychosis care (McGorry et al., 2002).

Assertive Community Treatment (ACT), while not specific to early intervention, is often integrated into early psychosis services for individuals with high acuity or co-occurring conditions. ACT provides multidisciplinary, community-based care with 24/7 availability, minimizing the need for hospitalization and addressing both clinical and social determinants of health (Dieterich et al., 2017). When combined with CSC principles, ACT can be particularly effective for individuals with housing instability, trauma histories, or frequent psychiatric hospitalizations. These three models share a commitment to early, assertive, and sustained intervention that prioritizes recovery and community reintegration. The key to success lies in accessibility, coordination, and person-centered care.

Medication and therapy

Medication remains a foundational element, with low-dose, second-generation antipsychotics typically recommended for first-episode psychosis to minimize side effects and maximize adherence (Kahn et al., 2008). Medication choice is guided by clinical presentation, patient preference, side effect profile, and family history. The goal is not merely symptom suppression but optimizing tolerability to promote sustained engagement. Clozapine is also approved to reduce the risk of recurrent suicidal behavior in patients with schizophrenia or schizoaffective disorder who are considered at chronic risk for reexperiencing suicidal behavior (FDA, 2010). On February 24, 2025, the FDA officially ended the mandatory requirements associated with the Clozapine Risk Evaluation and Mitigation Strategy (REMS) program. This followed a recommendation from the Psychopharmacologic Drugs Advisory Committee, which concluded that the REMS no longer contributed significantly to the safe use of clozapine and was an unnecessary barrier to access (FDA, 2024). In addition to medication, psychotherapeutic interventions are critical. Cognitive behavioral therapy (CBT) has demonstrated efficacy in reducing positive symptoms, enhancing coping strategies, and delaying or preventing relapse (Bighelli et al., 2021). Family psychoeducation equips caregivers with the tools to support recovery while reducing expressed emotion —an identified predictor of relapse (Dixon et al., 2001).

Barriers to early intervention

Despite the demonstrated effectiveness of early intervention programs, multiple barriers hinder their widespread implementation. These barriers span structural, clinical, cultural, and policy domains, contributing to delays in diagnosis and treatment.

Stigma continues to be one of the most significant barriers to accessing mental health care. Many individuals and families hesitate to seek support due to fears of being labeled, facing discrimination, or experiencing internalized shame. This challenge is especially pronounced among youth and young adults, who may misinterpret early symptoms or intentionally hide them from caregivers and health professionals (Corrigan, 2004).

Misconceptions persist, including the belief that mental illness is not as legitimate as physical illness, and that individuals should simply "try harder" to overcome conditions like depression. To address these harmful attitudes, coordinated public and provider education efforts are essential to normalize help-seeking behaviors and reduce stigma-related delays in care.

Misdiagnosis and under-recognition frequently occur, especially in primary care and educational settings. Early signs of psychosis – such as social withdrawal, anxiety, or mild paranoia – can be misattributed to typical adolescent behavior, mood disorders, or substance use. As a result, many individuals remain undiagnosed until symptoms become severe, missing the opportunity for preventive intervention (Singh & Grange, 2006).

Access limitations, including geographic disparities and insurance coverage gaps, further restrict timely intervention. Rural areas often lack specialized early psychosis programs, forcing families to travel long distances or settle for fragmented care. Financial barriers, particularly in underinsured or uninsured populations, compound these challenges.

Cultural and systemic inequities exacerbate disparities in access and quality of care. Black, Indigenous, and People of Color (BIPOC) are disproportionately subject to coercive pathways to care, including involuntary hospitalization and involvement with law enforcement, rather than voluntary, recovery-oriented services (Oluwoye et al., 2021).

Language barriers, lack of accountability for past harms by medical institutions, and lack of culturally informed providers further alienate marginalized communities.

Addressing these barriers requires a multifaceted approach that includes workforce development, policy advocacy, and the expansion of culturally responsive care. Without deliberate strategies to close these gaps, early intervention will remain inaccessible to those who might benefit most.

Reflections on missed opportunities

Roger's life could have unfolded very differently had our healthcare, social, and legal systems been better equipped to respond to severe mental illness with urgency, compassion, and evidence-based care. If he had received early intervention at the time of his first psychotic break – rather than entering a decades-long cycle of incarceration, homelessness, and episodic treatment – he may have enjoyed stability, independence, and connection. Instead of being criminalized for behavior rooted in psychosis, he could have received coordinated, community-based care that addressed both his mental health and social needs.

Importantly, Roger never received a trial of clozapine, the gold standard for treatment-resistant schizophrenia, until the final months of his life – even after multiple medication failures over several decades. This delay was likely due to systemic inertia and concerns about side effects in the context of comorbid HIV, despite evidence that clozapine can be safely administered in such cases with proper monitoring. His case exemplifies the consequences of failing to follow evidence-based treatment algorithms and illustrates the profound costs of fragmented care.

In a more humane and responsive system – one that values early identification, comprehensive intervention, and respect for the dignity of those living with schizophrenia – Roger's outcome could have been drastically different. His story challenges us to confront the moral and structural failures that allow individuals with treatable illnesses to fall through the cracks. It is a sobering reminder that early intervention is not merely a clinical strategy – it is a call to action rooted in equity, ethics, and compassion.

References

American Psychiatric Association. *Diagnostic and Statistical Manual of Mental Disorders*. 5th ed. American Psychiatric Publishing; 2013.

Bighelli I, Rodolico A, García-Mieres H, et al. Psychosocial and psychological interventions for relapse prevention in schizophrenia: A systematic review and network meta-analysis. *Lancet Psychiatry*. 2021;**8**(11):969–980. doi:10.1016/S2215- 0366(21)00243-1

Birchwood M, Todd P, Jackson C. Early intervention in psychosis: The critical period hypothesis. *Br J Psychiatry*. 1998;**172**(33):53–59. doi:10.1192/S000712500029768

Cooper T, Seigler MD, Stahl S. Rapid onset brain plasticity at novel pharmacologic targets hypothetically drives innovations for rapid onset antidepressant actions. *J Psychopharmacol*. 2023;**37**(3):242–247. doi:10.1177/02698811231161243

Corrigan PW. How stigma interferes with mental health care. *Am Psychol*. 2004;**59**(7):614–625. doi:10.1037/0003-066X.59.7.614

Dieterich M, Irving CB, Park B, Marshall M. Intensive case management for severe mental illness. *Cochrane Database Syst Rev*. 2017;**1**:CD007906. doi:10.1002/14651858.CD007906.pub3

Dixon L, McFarlane WR, Lefley H, et al. Evidence-based practices for services to families of people with psychiatric disabilities. *Psychiatr Serv*. 2001;**52**(7):903–910. doi:10.1176/appi.ps.52.7.903

Kahn RS, Fleischhacker WW, Boter H, et al. Effectiveness of antipsychotic drugs in first-episode schizophrenia and schizophreniform disorder: An open randomized clinical trial. *Lancet*. 2008;**371**(9618):1085–1097. doi:10.1016/S0140-6736(08)60486-9

Kane JM, Robinson DG, Schooler NR, et al. Comprehensive versus usual community care for first-episode psychosis: 2-year outcomes from the NIMH RAISE Early Treatment Program. *Am J Psychiatry*. 2016;**173**(4):362–372. doi:10.1176/appi.ajp.2015.15050632

Marshall M, Lewis S, Lockwood A, et al. Association between duration of untreated psychosis and outcome in cohorts of first-episode patients: A systematic review. *Arch Gen Psychiatry*. 2005;**62**(9):975–983. doi:10.1001/archpsyc.62.9.975

McGorry PD, Killackey E, Yung AR. Early intervention in psychosis: Concepts, evidence and future directions. *World Psychiatry*. 2008;**7**(3):148–156.

McGorry PD, Yung AR, Phillips LJ. The "close-in" or ultra high-risk model: A safe and effective strategy for research and clinical intervention in prepsychotic mental disorder. *Schizophr Bull*. 2002;**28**(3):485–496. doi:10.1093/oxfordjournals.schbul.a006989

Oluwoye O, Kriegel LS, Alcover KC, McDonell MG. Racial and ethnic disparities in first-episode psychosis: A review of the literature. *Psychiatr Serv*. 2021;**72**(5):567–577. doi:10.1176/appi.ps.202000353

Penttilä M, Jääskeläinen E, Hirvonen N, Isohanni M, Miettunen J. Duration of untreated psychosis as a predictor of long-term outcome in schizophrenia: Systematic review and meta-analysis. *Br J Psychiatry*. 2014;**205**(2):88–94. doi:10.1192/bjp.bp.113.127753

Singh SP, Grange T. Measuring pathways to care in first-episode psychosis: A systematic review. *Schizophr Res*. 2006;**81**(1):75–82. doi:10.1016/j.schres.2005.09.018

U.S. Food and Drug Administration. Clozaril [Prescribing Information]. 2010. www.accessdata.fda.gov/drugsatfda_docs/label/2010/019758s062lbl.pdf

U.S. Food and Drug Administration. Frequently asked questions about the Clozapine REMS modification. Published December 21, 2024. Accessed April 30, 2025. www.fda.gov/drugs/postmarket-drug-safety-information-patients-and-providers/frequently-asked-questions-clozapine-rems-modification

Cardiometabolic Disorders in Persons Living with Schizophrenia
The Right to Equality

Roger S. McIntyre, Liyang Yin, and Christine E. Dri

The nomenclature describing schizophrenia has changed over the centuries. Contemporary psychiatry began approximately in the late 1800s. The moniker "dementia praecox" was not only a name proposed to describe schizophrenia at the time, but also a typology to disambiguate persons with progressive functional loss from those with episodic functional change and less overall social deterioration. Eugen Bleuler coined the term "schizophrenia" in 1908 and placed a significant emphasis on the centrality of profound social and cognitive disturbances as part of the disease formulation (i.e., the four As of schizophrenia: affect, association, ambivalence, autism; Arantes-Gonçalves et al. 2018; Ashok et al. 2012).

From its original iteration in 1952, the Diagnostic and Statistical Manual of Mental Disorders (DSM) has embraced the nomenclature of Bleuler, as well as the defining characteristic of the condition as being a profound, severe, persistent, and progressive functional loss (Tandon et al. 2013). Over the past seven decades the conceptualization of schizophrenia has been updated to include not only profound neurodevelopmental and neurodegenerative brain changes, but also multisystemic organ involvement. A significant reconceptualization of schizophrenia has occurred over the past several decades wherein this disorder is now also considered a multisystemic disease state wherein multiple organ systems in the person with this lived experience are affected and contribute to the loss of human capital (i.e., education attainment, annual earnings, etc.).

Academic endeavors that have broadly sought to estimate and precisely enumerate the types and frequencies of medical comorbidities in schizophrenia have produced a highly replicated finding that adults living with schizophrenia are differentially affected by obesity, severe obesity, abdominal obesity, impaired glucose tolerance, type 2 diabetes mellitus (T2DM), International Diabetes Federation (IDF) and National Cholesterol Education Program (NCEP) Adult Treatment Panel III (NCEP-ATP III)-defined metabolic syndrome, metabolic liver diseases, and cardiovascular disease (e.g., metabolic dysfunction associated with steatotic liver disease; Afzal et al. 2021; Dong et al. 2024; De Hert et al. 2009; Jawad et al. 2023). In addition to contributing to overall illness burden and morbidity, the aforementioned diseases further exacerbate the underlying brain disturbance in schizophrenia, worsening the psychopathological presentation (Hagi et al. 2021). Moreover, each of the cardiometabolic conditions summarized herein contributes to excess and premature mortality, with cardiovascular disease being the single largest cause of premature death in this affected population (Peritogiannis et al. 2022; Ringen et al. 2014).

This chapter is a clarion call for achieving equality in schizophrenia with respect to physical, mental, and social well-being by contemporaneously prioritizing mental health and physical health (World Health Organization n.d.). The premise of this chapter is that individuals living with schizophrenia, in addition to having a serious brain-related disorder, are also affected by multiple medical conditions that, unless simultaneously addressed, will continue to disadvantage people with lived experience and belie their ability to achieve wellness, according to the World Health Organization. A derivative of this clarion call is not only to contemplate this topic, but also to encourage the development of frameworks of care and prevention, supported by adequate funding and access to timely, high-quality care, so that persons with schizophrenia are not further discriminated against by inadequately addressing conditions that are highly treatable and erode the quality and duration of their lives.

Cardiometabolic disorders in persons living with schizophrenia and related disorders

For several decades, original research reports largely from high-income but also low- and middle-income countries have documented an elevated prevalence of cardiometabolic disorders in persons living with schizophrenia (Zhao et al. 2023). It is also well established that, globally, a pandemic of cardiometabolic disorders is occurring, with a large and elevated prevalence of these conditions regardless of national gross domestic product (GDP) and/or health care system.

The rates of overweight/obesity and abdominal obesity have been reported to be significantly higher in persons with schizophrenia. For example, a synthesis of 120 studies from 43 countries (of which the majority were high-income countries, although Sub-Saharan African, South Asian, and Middle Eastern countries were also included) reported that persons with schizophrenia and severe mental illness had a combined pooled prevalence of overweight/obesity of approximately 60%, with persons living in the Middle East exhibiting the highest prevalence (Afzal et al. 2021). Taken together, the rate of obesity was approximately three times greater in the mentally ill population studied compared to the general population (Afzal et al. 2021). This relatively high rate of severe obesity is a nuanced observation and underscores the separate but related finding that excess weight in persons with schizophrenia is more severe when compared to the general population. A related finding that has often been replicated is that women living with schizophrenia are approximately 1.5 times more likely than men to be living with obesity (Afzal et al. 2021).

The rates of impaired glucose tolerance and T2DM are also significantly elevated in persons with schizophrenia compared to the general population. In addition, the age of onset for T2DM in persons with schizophrenia appears to be lower relative to the general population (Dong et al. 2024). Pooling the extant literature, the T2DM is approximately twofold more likely in persons with schizophrenia than in the general population (e.g., odds ratio [OR] = 2.15; Dong et al. 2024). Similar to the gender distribution of obesity, females living with schizophrenia also have a higher rate of T2DM than males (Dong et al. 2024).

The rates of T2DM are also higher in persons with schizophrenia with longer illness duration.

In addition to the estimated higher rates of obesity and T2DM, the rates of metabolic syndrome are significantly elevated in schizophrenia. Multiple definitions of metabolic syndrome have been proposed, with that of the IDF and the NCEP-ATP III being the most commonly cited (Expert Panel on Detection, Evaluation, and Treatment of High Blood Cholesterol in Adults 2001). Although definitions of metabolic syndrome differ, they are relatively similar insofar as they all include dysglycemia, dyslipidemia, hypertension, and abdominal obesity. There is significant heterogeneity in the estimated prevalence of metabolic syndrome in persons with schizophrenia. Nevertheless, a pooled prevalence of approximately 40% has been generally reported, with there being a higher prevalence in some Western countries (approximately 80%) and lower prevalence in select Asian countries (approximately 20%; Salari et al. 2024).

Metabolic liver diseases are a group of conditions that include simple steatosis, fibrosis, and cirrhosis. Metabolic liver diseases exact their own forms of morbidity and are risk factors for premature mortality. Moreover, metabolic liver diseases represent a risk for hepatocellular carcinoma, and in many regions globally they are becoming the most common reason for liver transplantation (Eslam et al. 2020; Simon et al. 2021). The estimated global prevalence of metabolic liver diseases in the general population is approximately 25% (Feng et al. 2025). Higher rates of metabolic liver diseases in the general population are observed in persons living with obesity (i.e. 25–40%) and T2DM (i.e., 35–45%; Chiang and McCullough 2014).

Individuals living with schizophrenia also have a rate of metabolic liver diseases that, at the very least, is similar to rates reported in the general population (Jawad et al. 2023). A more recent estimate of the rates of metabolic liver diseases in persons with schizophrenia suggests that the overall risk of metabolic liver diseases may be higher than in the general population (Gangopadhyay et al. 2022; Rus et al. 2022). In addition to metabolic liver diseases, persons with schizophrenia are also differentially affected by other types of liver diseases, including infectious (e.g., hepatitis A, B, C) as well as alcohol-related liver diseases (Grant et al. 2022).

Each of the aforementioned metabolic diseases is a risk factor for cardiovascular disease. In addition, persons who live with schizophrenia are significantly less likely to receive primary or preventive treatments for cardiovascular disease risk factors and are considerably less likely to receive cardiovascular interventions to reduce major adverse cardiovascular events (Polcwiartek et al. 2024). Moreover, persons with schizophrenia are more likely to engage in unhealthy behaviors (e.g., tobacco smoking), contributing further to their cardiovascular risk (Sagud et al. 2019). A consensus exists that inequities in health care, along with housing, economic and health care insecurity, are significant contributors to the elevated cardiovascular risk in persons living with schizophrenia.

Taken together, the results from both epidemiological and cross-sectional research provide a convergent and alarming finding that rates of treatable and preventable cardiometabolic disorders are significantly elevated in persons with schizophrenia relative to the general population (Ringen et al. 2014). The increased risk in this population is a consequence of social and economic determinants of health, as well as inadequate access to primary and preventative health care, higher rates of trauma, unhealthy behaviors, exposure to weight- and metabolic-disrupting psychotropic drugs, and neurobiological aspects intrinsic to schizophrenia (e.g., increased immuno-inflammatory activation; McIntyre et al. 2024).

Premature mortality

In addition to having a shorter health span, individuals with schizophrenia have a significantly shorter lifespan. Although death by suicide is significantly higher in persons with schizophrenia relative to the general population, as well as being a contributor to unnatural causes of death, the most common reason for premature and excess mortality in persons with schizophrenia is cardiovascular disease (Peritogiannis et al. 2022). For example, the number of years lost due to schizophrenia has been reported to be approximately 10–25 years (Hjorthøj et al. 2017). The reduced life expectancy in schizophrenia and the mortality gap relative to the general population has been reported in studies conducted in Africa, Asia, Australia, Europe, and North America. It has also been consistently reported that premature mortality rates are higher in men with schizophrenia, and that the average life expectancy is lower for men relative to women (Hjorthøj et al. 2017).

Medical training and care models in schizophrenia have appropriately emphasized the importance of rapid alleviation of the psychopathological features that define schizophrenia. In addition, prioritizing risk assessment as it relates to suicide is emphasized in training and in the clinical encounter when managing people living with schizophrenia. In contradistinction to the emphasis on mortality risk due to suicide, there has been relatively less attention allocated to the risk of premature mortality due to cardiovascular disease, despite this being the single largest contributor to the lower life expectancy and higher mortality in the schizophrenia population. The majority of people with schizophrenia do not receive comprehensive, systematic, routine counseling, education, or treatment as it relates to risk factor modification for cardiometabolic disorders (Ali et al. 2023; Galderisi et al. 2021).

Health in schizophrenia will not be achieved unless persons with lived experience receive integrated care emphasizing in both mental health and physical health domains

The studies that are briefly summarized herein convincingly establish the elevated and growing prevalence of cardiometabolic disorders in persons living with schizophrenia (Salari et al. 2024). In addition to being highly replicated, this rate increase is almost universally observed across studies conducted in different countries, regardless of socioeconomics, race, ethnicity, and health care system. A separate but also highly replicated finding is the increase in premature mortality with decreased life expectancy due to cardiovascular diseases (Correll, Solmi, et al. 2017). The reduction in health span and lifespan due to cardiometabolic disorders is modifiable and, in many cases, preventable.

The increased prevalence of cardiometabolic disorders reflects inequities in health care access as well as health care systems that do not provide integrated or parity of care to persons with serious mental illness (Correll, Ng-Mak, et al. 2017). More specifically, persons with serious mental illness are more likely to receive suboptimal primary and preventive health care for chronic noncommunicable disorders. All persons with schizophrenia, as with all marginalized and economically disadvantaged groups, should have equal access to primary and preventive high-quality longitudinal care. The available evidence indicates that, in the schizophrenia population, having access to such care models reduces overall medical burden (Fond et al. 2023; McIntyre et al. 2024).

Precarity with respect to housing, economics, physical safety due to living in high-crime neighborhoods, and access to meaningful social engagements are all known to be relevant to one's risk of cardiometabolic disorders. The higher prevalence of cardiometabolic disorders in persons with schizophrenia is accounted for to a significant extent by a lack of policies that prioritize the safety and security of marginalized groups, notably people with serious mental illness (Kyle and Dunn 2008). Interventions that target social or economic and/or spatial determinants of health have been shown to improve health outcomes in persons living with schizophrenia.

In addition, the clinical encounter for persons with schizophrenia who have access to the health care system rarely includes adequate attention being given to medical risk factor modification. Occam's razor explains in part the inadequacy of care for medical-related matters in schizophrenia in light of the complexity of the psychopathology of this illness (Solmi et al. 2021). In addition, organizational and systems-level disincentives exist in some jurisdictions due to the need to provide adequate resources to care for persons' medical needs along with their psychiatric needs (McGinty et al. 2021). Despite the introduction of parity laws in some jurisdictions, whether care models have been commensurate with best practices for persons with serious mental illness is less well established.

The overrepresentation of metabolic disorders in persons with schizophrenia is not only a consequence of socioeconomic and spatial determinants, as well as deficiencies and fairness in policy and health care implementation, but also reflects the intricate neurobiological risk of schizophrenia, as well as adverse events related to some psychiatric medications. For example, it is known that persons with schizophrenia exhibit alterations in glucose regulatory signaling and immune inflammatory functioning as part of the pathophysiology of the illness (Kancsev et al. 2025). These factors are well-known contributors to cardiometabolic risk, as well as contributing to the pathophysiology of schizophrenia. Separately, it has been reported for over a century that unaffected first-degree relatives of persons living with schizophrenia are also at high risk of cardiometabolic disorders, underscoring overlapping environmental causes as well as genetic factors (Mothi et al. 2015).

In summary, the elevated rate of cardiometabolic disorders in schizophrenia is not only a clinical priority but also represents a public health concern with respect to the impacts that these disorders have on this often-marginalized and economically disadvantaged group. Much of the risk of cardiometabolic disorders is preventable, modifiable, and fully treatable. In addition to providing frameworks of care as well as access to appropriate resources to improve the symptomatic presentation of schizophrenia, it is equally imperative to target those aspects of the illness that significantly reduce the health span and lifespan of persons with lived experience of this condition. The stigma of schizophrenia is well known, and campaigns that aim to reduce stigma and discrimination not only should attempt to improve understanding of the brain-based manifestations of this illness, but also should recognize that this population is more likely to have increased mortality and loss of life expectancy due to cardiovascular diseases (McIntyre et al. 2007). Such a campaign, if successful, would increase the likelihood that people living with schizophrenia will gain equality in their physical, mental, and social well-being.

References

Afzal, Medhia, Najma Siddiqi, Bilal Ahmad, Nida Afsheen, Faiza Aslam, Ayaz Ali, Rubab Ayesha, et al. 2021. "Prevalence of Overweight and Obesity in People with Severe Mental Illness: Systematic Review and Meta-Analysis." *Frontiers in Endocrinology* 12:769309.

Ali, S., D. Santomauro, A. J. Ferrari, and F. Charlson. 2023. "Schizophrenia as a Risk Factor for Cardiovascular and Metabolic Health Outcomes: A Comparative Risk Assessment." *Epidemiology and Psychiatric Sciences* 32: e8.

Arantes-Gonçalves, Filipe, João Gama Marques, and Diogo Telles-Correia. 2018. "Bleuler's Psychopathological Perspective on Schizophrenia Delusions: Towards New Tools in Psychotherapy Treatment." *Frontiers in Psychiatry* 9:306.

Ashok, Ahbishekh Hulegar, John Baugh, and Vikram K. Yeragani. 2012. "Paul Eugen Bleuler and the Origin of the Term Schizophrenia (*Schizopreniegruppe*)." *Indian Journal of Psychiatry* 54(1):95–96.

Chiang, Dian J., and Arthur J. McCullough. 2014. "The Impact of Obesity and Metabolic Syndrome on Alcoholic Liver Disease." *Clinics in Liver Disease* 18(1):157–163.

Correll, Christoph U., Daisy S. Ng-Mak, Dana Stafkey-Mailey, Eileen Farrelly, Krithika Rajagopalan, and Antony Loebel. 2017. "Cardiometabolic Comorbidities, Readmission, and Costs in Schizophrenia and Bipolar Disorder: A Real-World Analysis." *Annals of General Psychiatry* 16(1):9.

Correll, Christoph U., Marco Solmi, Nicola Veronese, Beatrice Bortolato, Stella Rosson, Paolo Santonastaso, Nita Thapa-Chhetri, et al. 2017. "Prevalence, Incidence and Mortality from Cardiovascular Disease in Patients with Pooled and Specific Severe Mental Illness: A Large-Scale Meta-Analysis of 3,211,768 Patients and 113,383,368 Controls." *World Psychiatry* 16(2):163–180.

De Hert, Marc, Vincent Schreurs, Davy Vancampfort, and Ruud Van Winkel. 2009. "Metabolic Syndrome in People with Schizophrenia: A Review." *World Psychiatry* 8(1):15–22.

Dong, Kai, Shenghai Wang, Chunhui Qu, Kewei Zheng, and Ping Sun. 2024. "Schizophrenia and Type 2 Diabetes Risk: A Systematic Review and Meta-Analysis." *Frontiers in Endocrinology* 15:1395771.

Eslam, Mohammed, Arun J. Sanyal, Jacob George, and International Consensus Panel. 2020. "MAFLD: A Consensus-Driven Proposed Nomenclature for Metabolic Associated Fatty Liver Disease." *Gastroenterology* 158(7):1999–2014.e1.

Expert Panel on Detection, Evaluation, and Treatment of High Blood Cholesterol in Adults. 2001. "Executive Summary of the Third Report of the National Cholesterol Education Program (NCEP) Expert Panel on Detection, Evaluation, and Treatment of High Blood Cholesterol in Adults (adult Treatment Panel III)." *JAMA* 285(19):2486–2497.

Feng, Gong, Giovanni Targher, Christopher D. Byrne, Yusuf Yilmaz, Vincent Wai-Sun Wong, Cosmas Rinaldi Adithya Lesmana, Leon A. Adams, et al. 2025. "Global Burden of Metabolic Dysfunction-Associated Steatotic Liver Disease, 2010 to 2021." *JHEP Reports: Innovation in Hepatology* 7(3): 101271.

Fond, Guillaume B., Dong Keon Yon, Bach Tran, Jasmina Mallet, Mathieu Urbach, Sylvain Leignier, Romain Rey, et al. 2023. "Poverty and Inequality in Real-World Schizophrenia: A National Study." *Frontiers in Public Health* 11:1182441.

Galderisi, Silvana, Marc De Hert, Stefano Del Prato, Andrea Fagiolini, Philip Gorwood, Stefan Leucht, Aldo Pietro Maggioni, Armida Mucci, and Celso Arango. 2021. "Identification and Management of Cardiometabolic Risk in Subjects with Schizophrenia Spectrum Disorders: A Delphi Expert Consensus Study." *European Psychiatry* 64(1):e7.

Gangopadhyay, Anwesha, Radwa Ibrahim, Karli Theberge, Meghan May, and Karen L. Houseknecht. 2022. "Non-Alcoholic Fatty Liver Disease (NAFLD) and Mental Illness: Mechanisms Linking Mood, Metabolism and Medicines." *Frontiers in Neuroscience* 16:1042442.

Grant, Rebecca K., William M. Brindle, Mhairi C. Donnelly, Pauline M. McConville, Thomas G. Stroud, Lorenzo Bandieri, and John N. Plevris. 2022. "Gastrointestinal and Liver Disease in Patients with Schizophrenia: A Narrative Review." *World Journal of Gastroenterology* 28(38):5515–5529.

Hagi, Katsuhiko, Tadashi Nosaka, Dwight Dickinson, Jean Pierre Lindenmayer, Jimmy Lee, Joseph Friedman, Laurent Boyer, et al. 2021. "Association between Cardiovascular Risk Factors and Cognitive Impairment in People with Schizophrenia: A Systematic Review and Meta-Analysis." *JAMA Psychiatry* 78(5):510–518.

Hjorthøj, Carsten, Anne Emilie Stürup, John J. McGrath, and Merete Nordentoft. 2017. "Years of Potential Life Lost and Life Expectancy in Schizophrenia: A Systematic Review and Meta-Analysis." *The Lancet: Psychiatry* 4(4):295–301.

Jawad, Muhammad Youshay, Shakila Meshkat, Aniqa Tabassum, Andrea Mckenzie, Joshua D. Di Vincenzo, Ziji Guo, Nabiha Batool Musavi, et al. 2023. "The Bidirectional Association of Nonalcoholic Fatty Liver Disease with Depression, Bipolar Disorder, and Schizophrenia." *CNS Spectrums* 28(5):541–560.

Kancsev, Alexander, Eszter Éva Virág-Tulassay, Marie Anne Engh, Szilvia Kiss-Dala, András Attila Horváth, Péter Hegyi, and Szabolcs Kéri. 2025. "Glucose Homeostasis and Cognitive Functions in Schizophrenia: A Systematic Review and Meta-Analysis." *Scientific Reports* 15(1):22898.

Kyle, Tania, and James R. Dunn. 2008. "Effects of Housing Circumstances on Health, Quality of Life and Healthcare Use for People with Severe Mental Illness: A Review: Effects of Housing Circumstances on the Health of People with Severe Mental Illness." *Health & Social Care in the Community* 16(1):1–15.

McGinty, Emma E., Rachel Presskreischer, Joshua Breslau, Jonathan D. Brown, Marisa Elena Domino, Benjamin G. Druss, Marcela Horvitz-Lennon, et al. 2021. "Improving Physical Health among People with Serious Mental Illness: The Role of the Specialty Mental Health Sector." *Psychiatric Services* 72(11):1301–1310.

McIntyre, Roger S., Angela T. H. Kwan, Joshua D. Rosenblat, Kayla M. Teopiz, and Rodrigo B. Mansur. 2024. "Psychotropic Drug-Related Weight Gain and Its Treatment." *The American Journal of Psychiatry* 181(1):26–38.

McIntyre, Roger S., Joanna K. Soczynska, Jakub Z. Konarski, Hanna O. Woldeyohannes, Candy W. Y. Law, Andrew Miranda, Don Fulgosi, and Sidney H. Kennedy. 2007. "Should Depressive Syndromes Be Reclassified as 'Metabolic Syndrome Type II'?" *Annals of Clinical Psychiatry* 19(4):257–264.

Mothi, Suraj Sarvode, Neeraj Tandon, Jaya Padmanabhan, Ian T. Mathew, Brett Clementz, Carol Tamminga,

Godfrey Pearlson, John Sweeney, and Matcheri S. Keshavan. 2015. "Increased Cardiometabolic Dysfunction in First-Degree Relatives of Patients with Psychotic Disorders." *Schizophrenia Research* **165**(1):103–107.

Peritogiannis, Vaios, Angeliki Ninou, and Maria Samakouri. 2022. "Mortality in Schizophrenia-Spectrum Disorders: Recent Advances in Understanding and Management." *Healthcare (Basel, Switzerland)* **10**(12):2366.

Polcwiartek, Christoffer, Kevin O'Gallagher, Daniel J. Friedman, Christoph U. Correll, Marco Solmi, Svend Eggert Jensen, and René Ernst Nielsen. 2024. "Severe Mental Illness: Cardiovascular Risk Assessment and Management." *European Heart Journal* **45**(12):987–997.

Ringen, Petter Andreas, John A. Engh, Astrid B. Birkenaes, Ingrid Dieset, and Ole A. Andreassen. 2014. "Increased Mortality in Schizophrenia due to Cardiovascular Disease â€" A Non-Systematic Review of Epidemiology, Possible Causes, and Interventions." *Frontiers in Psychiatry* **5**:137.

Rus, Sara Galiano, Víctor Ortiz García de la Foz, María Teresa Arias-Loste, Paula Iruzubieta, Marcos Gómez-Revuelta, María Juncal-Ruiz, Javier Crespo, et al. 2022. "Elevated Risk of Liver Steatosis in First-Episode Psychosis Patients: Results from a 3-Year Prospective Study." *Schizophrenia Research* **246**:30–38.

Sagud, Marina, Alma Mihaljevic Peles, and Nela Pivac. 2019. "Smoking in Schizophrenia: Recent Findings about an Old Problem." *Current Opinion in Psychiatry* **32**(5):402–408.

Salari, Nader, Nima Maghami, Theo Ammari, Hadis Mosafer, Reza Abdullahi, Shabnam Rasoulpoor, et al. 2024. "Global Prevalence of Metabolic Syndrome in Schizophrenia Patients: A Systematic Review and Meta-Analysis." *Journal of Prevention* **45**(6):973–986.

Simon, Tracey G., Bjorn Roelstraete, Hamed Khalili, Hannes Hagström, and Jonas F. Ludvigsson. 2021. "Mortality in Biopsy-Confirmed Nonalcoholic Fatty Liver Disease: Results from a Nationwide Cohort." *Gut* **70**(7):1375–1382.

Solmi, Marco, Jess Fiedorowicz, Laura Poddighe, Marco Delogu, Alessandro Miola, Anne Høye, Ina H. Heiberg, et al. 2021. "Disparities in Screening and Treatment of Cardiovascular Diseases in Patients with Mental Disorders across the World: Systematic Review and Meta-Analysis of 47 Observational Studies." *The American Journal of Psychiatry* **178**(9):793–803.

Tandon, Rajiv, Wolfgang Gaebel, Deanna M. Barch, Juan Bustillo, Raquel E. Gur, Stephan Heckers, Dolores Malaspina, et al. 2013. "Definition and Description of Schizophrenia in the DSM-5." *Schizophrenia Research* **150**(1):3–10.

World Health Organization. n.d. "Constitution of the World Health Organization." Accessed July 18, 2025. www.who.int/about/governance/constitution

Zhao, Chenxu, Tesfa Dejenie Habtewold, Elnaz Naderi, Edith J. Liemburg, GROUP Investigators, Richard Bruggeman, and Behrooz Z. Alizadeh. 2023. "Association of Clinical Symptoms and Cardiometabolic Dysregulations in Patients with Schizophrenia Spectrum Disorders." *European Psychiatry* **67**(1):e7.

Failure to Treat
An American Policy Perspective

Katherine Warburton

Introduction

The cyclical failure of mental health policy in the United States can be best articulated by those who contemporaneously documented it. In the 1840s, reformer Dorothea Linde Dix described the conditions of the insane to the Massachusetts Legislature with these words: "In cages, closets, cellars, stalls, pens! Chained, naked, beaten with rods, and lashed into obedience." Dix's subsequent efforts led to a vast expansion of moral treatment, delivered in bucolic state asylums throughout the United States.[1-4] The proponents of the asylum movement expressed great confidence that the problem of injustice for the mentally ill had been solved.[5]

Roughly a century later, in 1951, journalist Albert Q. Maisel documented the now deteriorated conditions in Dix's asylums in this manner: "We feed thousands a starvation diet [. . .] we jam-pack men, women and sometimes even children into hundred-year-old firetraps in wards so crowded that the floors cannot be seen between the rickety cots, while thousands more sleep on ticks, on blankets or on the bare floors [. . .] hundreds – of my own knowledge and sight – spend 24 hours a day in stark and filthy nakedness."[6] Media exposés such as Maisel's precipitated the deinstitutionalization movement.

Unfortunately, deinstitutionalization in the United States ultimately led to the transinstitutionalization of people with psychotic illness into jails and prisons. Just last year, in 2023, journalist Meg O'Connor gave an update on how people with mental illness were faring in the United States: "During the few hours that people with mental illness are allowed out of their cells [. . .] they are shackled to tables. Some don't have real clothing [. . .] others smear feces on the walls of their cells. Flooded toilets are a regular occurrence. People scream and pace back and forth. Cells overflow with garbage. In certain housing units, mesh screens line the railings of the upper levels to prevent people from jumping."[7]

The lack of progress is evident. What is less obvious are the factors driving the cyclical failure of well-intentioned policies. This policy history is complex, and the failures are multifactorial. Many accounts are reductive and fail to reflect the nuances inherent in large-scale policy reform. However, there is a common theme: a lack of accountability over the process of implementation.

The first attempt

In the United States prior to the mid-1800s, people with severe psychotic disorders were generally chained, caged, and beaten. They were kept in squalid conditions in jails, in almshouses, or locked away in a family home. Within these conditions, people with psychotic disorders were often naked, cold, and/or in the dark. Their symptoms of hallucinations, delusions, and disorganization were attributed to moral failings or religious deviance, rather than illness.[8-10]

This situation began to change significantly in 1843, when Dorothea Dix wrote a report to the Massachusetts State Legislature documenting the misery she had observed upon touring the state. Dix had recently returned from England, where she met Samuel Tuke of the York Retreat. She was influenced by the advent of moral treatment championed by Philippe Pinel in France. The Massachusetts Legislature responded to her report and provided funding for improved conditions. Dix went on to replicate this approach in other states and was ultimately credited with the construction of over 30 asylums throughout the country.[1-4]

In the mid- to the late 1800s, the term "asylum" had a positive connotation. Mental Health asylums during this period most often resembled gothic castles built in the Kirkbride style, named for the psychiatrist-turned architect Thomas Story Kirkbride. These castles were installed on large, beautiful tracts of land. Here, patients could garden, exercise, and enjoy nature on self-sustaining campuses.[9–11] An 1898 report from the asylum at Napa, California listed the copious amount of produce harvested from that campus as a key outcome for the year.[12] Staff and patients lived together on campus. The treatment modality, known as moral treatment, was focused on kindness, compassion, and spiritual nourishment.

Moral treatment, and the asylums that delivered it, fell apart over the next century. Those castles championed by Dix grew overcrowded, understaffed, and neglected. A lack of judicial accountability in the form of vague involuntary detention laws led to unchecked growth. A lack of legislative accountability failed to fund infrastructure and resources to contend with that growth. No administrative accountability meant a lack of oversight provided to ensure humane conditions. The asylums became repositories for any person for whom society did not have a place. This dumping ground effect went beyond typical psychiatric illnesses and included such things as dependent elderly adults and patients with tertiary syphilis.[9,10] In a Life magazine article titled *Bedlam 1946*, Albert Maisel reported, "thousands who might be restored to society linger in manmade hells for a release that comes more quickly only because death comes faster to the abused, the beaten, the drugged, the starved and the neglected."[6]

Hence, the cruel, filthy, and inhumane conditions of the middle of the 1800s were manifest once again 100 years later. The descriptions by Maisel echoed those of Dix, and the origin of the problem was less about whether the patient was in the community or in an institution, and more about the lack of accountability for the humane treatment of patients with psychotic illness evidenced by the society. Conceptually, the reform of moral treatment in asylums was not the fundamental factor driving inhumane conditions. The blame lay in a lack of accountability and oversight.

The second attempt

A federal response followed the state asylum failures. The National Mental Health Act was passed in 1943, which was quickly followed by the establishment of the National Institute of Mental Health (NIMH) in 1949. NIMH, and subsequently the Joint Commission on Mental Illness and Health, went to work exploring federally funded community alternatives to institutionalization. These efforts culminated in the Community Mental Health Act (CMHA) of 1963, which sought to provide federal funding for the resources needed to care for patients with psychosis in their communities. The creation of Medicaid and Medicare in 1965 provided federal funding.[10, 13-16]

States slowly began to seize upon the opportunity to shift the cost of caring for this population to the federal government. Promising new treatments, such as the discovery of chlorpromazine, provided hope that this disease was treatable. The prohibitive potential costs of rehabilitating the state hospitals, combined with outrage at the civil liberties abuses resulting from indiscriminate institutionalization provided the political will to make change. These factors culminated in the process of deinstitutionalization, kicked off at the state level in California with the passage of the Lanterman–Petris–Short (LPS) Act. Lanterman was a conservative lawmaker concerned about the fiscal liability posed by the dilapidated state hospitals; Petris was a liberal lawmaker who was not convinced that schizophrenia was a real disease and who furthermore was intent upon restoring civil liberties to this population. It was a perfect political storm.[8, 13-17]

The LPS act was signed into law in 1967 by California Governor Ronald Reagan and came into effect on July 1, 1969. This was the first state legislative attempt to limit psychiatric institutionalization. Referred to as the "Magna Carta" of mental health legislation, it facilitated deinstitutionalization by raising the bar for involuntary hospitalization to a very high "dangerousness standard." To be involuntary hospitalized, a psychotic person had to be imminently dangerous to themselves or others, or so gravely disabled that they were essentially a danger to themselves. The nation followed suit, and the second round of mental health policy reform in the United States was well underway by the 1970s.[17, 18]

Unfortunately, the federal dollars flowed into local governments without an accountability mechanism. There was no system in place to ensure program services would be developed specifically for deinstitutionalized people with psychotic illnesses. State governments, that continued to run the institutions, were effectively cut out of the funding stream. This created a problem that persists today, wherein the local recipient of federal funding lacks a fiscal incentive to prevent state institutionalization or incarceration. Additionally, the federal government ultimately failed to provide funding in the amount necessary to fully implement the CMHA. Local governments failed to focus the funding to support programs designed for deinstitutionalized persons.[15] Rather, the money was used for patients with less severe conditions or was squandered altogether. In one case, for example, federal CMHA dollars were used to build athletic facilities.[13] Community Mental Health Centers largely provided psychotherapy to middle-class patients without psychotic illnesses.[8, 13, 15, 19] This fractured and irresponsible system of funding resulted, once again, in those most in need falling through the cracks into homelessness and incarceration.[20–27]

A federal report noted in 1977 that "CMHCs attracted a new type of patient who was not very ill and was not a candidate for hospitalization in a state institution." [22,27] The precious federal dollars intended to support people with schizophrenia as they transitioned to community treatment were used to build tennis courts and swimming pools and hire lifeguards.[13] The federal government was not held accountable to fund community programs in the manner promised, and the local governments were not held accountable to spend what money was coming in on the deinstitutionalized populations.

The result is that state institutions are now rapidly filling up with people suffering from schizophrenia, this time through a specific criminal commitment.

Today: The incompetent to stand trial debacle

In 1960, the US Supreme Court held, in basic terms, that it is unconstitutional to try someone for a crime if they are too psychotic to understand trial processes or to rationally assist in their defense.[28] Since deinstitutionalization, there has been an increasing trend of people with schizophrenia being arrested and found to be incompetent to stand trial (IST), which culminated following the Great Recession of 2009.[29–31] The skyrocketing IST population has overwhelmed state hospitals, resulting in patients waiting excessive periods of time in jails to be admitted for restoration. This crisis, happening in most states today, has reached the ironic level of civil liberties groups suing states in federal court to institutionalize people for restoration, so that they may be sent to trial on criminal charges. An examination of the crisis illustrates the mechanics of implementation failure.

In 1972, a psychiatrist named Marc Abramson published a paper in the academic journal *Hospital and Community Psychiatry*. In it, he points out that the standard for involuntary treatment pre-LPS rested on the need for hospitalization, and post-LPS rested on dangerousness. This change resulted in a lack of consideration of psychiatric assessment for the latter standard. He noted a 100% increase in patients found IST in his county the year following the implementation of the LPS Act. He ends the paper by postulating that, "It would indeed be ironic if the Magna Carta of the mentally ill in California led to their criminal stigmatization and incarceration in jails and prisons, where little or no mental health treatment is provided."[32] Abramson's concern about increasing IST commitments would prove prescient – 50 years after the publication of his paper, the use of the IST commitment to institutionalize people with psychotic symptoms would be described as a national crisis.[29] Six years later, in 1978, a Berkeley public policy student named Larry Sosowsky published a paper in *The American Journal of Psychiatry*. This study evaluated arrests for a cohort of 301 state hospital patients for 3 ½ years prior to LPS and 4 ½ years post LPS. The author documented a marked increase in arrests for this population post LPS implementation. He also looked at post-LPS arrest rates for the cohort compared to the general population and was able to demonstrate that the state hospital cohort was nine times more likely to be arrested than the general population.[33]

An April 15, 1979, a story in the *Washington Post* noted that in California, "Crowding within the state's financially strapped system has grown to the point where some mental patients, unable to find a hospital bed, are being arrested and placed in county jails for their own safety. Some have spent as long as a month in prison waiting for a mental hospital bed [. . .] At the Los Angeles County jail there are sometimes as many as 50 mentally disabled persons locked up as long as a month waiting for a bed in the state hospital system."[34]

In 1988, Thomas Arvanites of Villanova University published a paper in the journal *Criminology* looking at IST populations across three states. IST commitments increased post-deinstitutionalization by an average of 20%. The increase in IST admissions, as a percentage of all hospitalizations, was positively correlated to the rate of deinstitutionalization (r = 0.93). Arvanites noted, "An examination of the nature and operation of an IST commitment reveals its potential to emerge as an alternative to civil hospitalization."[35]

In 2010, E. Fuller Torrey provided a review of many of the studies documenting the recriminalization of psychotic illness. Torrey conducted research concluding that there were three times more seriously mentally ill persons in jails and prisons than in hospitals. This work led to the oft-cited observation that the institutions housing the most patients with serious mental illness (SMI) in the United States were Riker's Island jail in New York City, Cooks County jail in Chicago, and Twin Towers jail in Los Angeles. Torrey concluded, "It is thus fact, not hyperbole, that America's jails and prisons have become our new mental hospitals."[36]

In a 2018 retrospective analysis by the National Association of State Mental Health Program Directors Research Institute, Amanda Wik et al. documented a 72% increase in IST patients in state hospitals from 1999 to 2014[30] A separate survey conducted around this time identified that 82% of the states were experiencing a recent surge in IST patients, with a significant percentage facing litigation due to an inability to admit this increasing population in a timely fashion. In this survey, the reasons identified by the states centered on a lack of community mental health services as the primary driver of the crisis in their state.[29] Research conducted by Barbara McDermott at the University of California Davis demonstrated that the majority of IST patients had schizophrenia spectrum disorders. Fully 47% were completely unsheltered, living on the open streets, and two-thirds were experiencing some type of homelessness at the time of their arrest on felony charges. Half had received no mental health services prior to their arrest, and those who did were largely seen in emergency settings.[37]

The IST crisis has produced a cyclical pattern of blame. Federal lawsuits blame states for failing to provide timely admission to swelling populations of patients found IST. States blame local authorities for failing to adequately care for these patients in the community. Local authorities blame a lack of federal reimbursement to provide the type of care needed to wrap around and house these complex patients.

The IST crisis illustrates the consequences of failing to hold systems accountable for the care of people living with schizophrenia. Conditions have reverted to those found by Dorothea Dix 200 years ago – people with psychotic illness are kept in cages (in the form of jail cells) or left on the streets to die. They have once again been abandoned by society. Rather than achieving the desired goal of true deinstitutionalization, the lack of fiscal accountability inherent in the deinstitutionalization movement has instead resulted in the reinstitutionalization of people with psychotic illnesses in jails and forensic hospitals, through a circuit of homelessness, neglect, and criminal justice involvement. The civil liberties protection envisioned by the dangerousness standard has enabled the mental health system to turn away these patients who do not know that they are ill [38-40] and who are often homeless, hungry, and tortured by their symptoms because "they don't want treatment" and they are not evidencing the extreme dangerousness made necessary by the LPS act five decades ago.

Italy as a model

The wheels of policy reform are starting to turn again. This time, there is an existing model providing hope. Reforms in Italy have succeeded proving that when systems are held accountable, people living with psychotic illness can lead meaningful lives in their community. Italy has all but eliminated both the institutionalization and criminalization of schizophrenia, through accountability in community funding combined with the elimination of the dangerousness standard for treating people who lack medical decision-making capacity.[41, 42] Italian psychiatrists have reported that, "Policymakers and healthcare providers should note that closing psychiatric hospitals was not the main objective of the Italian reform; rather, it was to ensure that citizens with mental disorders would be treated just as other patients. This principle has revolutionized the role and focus of psychiatry in Italy, from custody, coercion, and segregation to treatment and care."[41]

Contrast this with the United States, where fractured funding and inadequate infrastructure, combined with a lack of accountability on systems for poor outcomes, are undoubtedly the primary culprits in the current crisis. The all-too-common outcomes of homelessness, incarceration, forensic institutionalization, and early death are enabled by the impossibility of obtaining informed consent from someone who does not understand that they are ill. The requirement that a person who lacks medical decision-making capacity must become dangerous in order to receive evidence-based care results in trauma, victimization, homelessness, brain damage, incarceration, and death. In other words, current civil liberties protections unintentionally provide a shield from accountability for failing to treat the sickest patients in our society, people who do not comprehend that they are ill and who are prisoners of their own psychotic thoughts. Italy has demonstrated that aligning informed consent practices to those used for every other medical condition, in concert with adequately funding a community mental health system, works. Italian policies have resulted in vastly decreased involuntary commitments, nominal numbers of people with SMI in carceral settings, and the successful closure of all state and forensic hospitals nationwide.[42]

Conclusion

To catch up with more advanced nations, the United States needs to delineate systems, policies, measures, and funding mechanisms specifically for schizophrenia spectrum disorders. Grouping psychotic disorders under the larger SMI umbrella enables systems to focus on other disease states to the exclusion of psychotic illness.

Public policy reform must eliminate funding incentives that reward the neglect of people living with psychotic disorders. One option is the creation of funding mechanisms that force the same system that fails patients in the community to pay for the much more expensive institutional care. Accountability can be baked into funding streams by tracking the primary outcomes of arrest, homelessness, incarceration, institutionalization, and death, and predicating funding on performance against these outcomes.

US reforms have started to align the informed consent process for schizophrenia with the process for every other disease, specifically by utilizing the standard medical decision-making model.[43] This prevents the current paradox of trying to obtain informed consent from a person who lacks medical decision-making capacity, and denying treatment when this impossible task is not accomplished.

Reforms should provide targeted, specific funding for a continuum of care for schizophrenia spectrum disorders, including early intervention, family psychoeducation and support, assertive community treatment, robust psychopharmacology, vocational and peer support, and a housing continuum that includes staffed supportive housing. These services should be individualized, and trauma informed.

Both the asylum and deinstitutionalization movements were born of noble intentions, and both failed in implementation in the context of inadequate funding and a lack of accountability. As the horrific conditions on our streets and in our carceral settings begin to drive change, there is no excuse to fail again.

References

1. Nelson EA. Dorothea Dix's liberation movement and why it matters today. *American Journal of Psychiatry Residents' Journal* 2021;**17**(2):8–9.

2. Parry MS. "I tell what I have seen"—The reports of asylum reformer Dorothea Dix. 1843. *American Journal of Public Health* 2006;**96**(4):622–625.

3. Lightner DL. *Asylum, Prison, and Poorhouse: The Writings and Reform Work of Dorothea Dix in Illinois.* Southern Illinois University Press; 1999.

4. Deutsch A. Dorothea Lynde Dix: Apostle of the insane. *The American Journal of Nursing* 1936;**36**(10):987–999.

5. Browne WAF. *What Asylums Were, Are and Ought to Be: Being the Substance of Five Lectures Delivered before the Managers of the Montrose Royal Lunatic Asylum.* A. & C. Black; 1837.

6. Maisel AQ. Bedlam 1946: Most U.S. mental hospitals are a shame and a disgrace. *Life Magazine.* 1946.

7. O'Conner M. In LA Jails, mentally ill people are chained to tables and rarely get psychiatric care. *The Appeal.* https://theappeal.org/los-angeles-county-jails-mental-health-care-conditions. Accessed on April 5, 2024.

8. George P, Jones N, Goldman H, Rosenblatt A. Cycles of reform in the history of psychosis treatment in the United States. *SSM Mental Health* 2023;**3**:100205.

9. Scull A. *Madness in Civilization: A Cultural History of Insanity, from the Bible to Freud, from the Madhouse to Modern Medicine.* Princeton University Press; 2015.

10. Grob GN. *The Mad Among Us: A History of the Care of America's Mentally Ill.* Free Press; 2011.

11. Shorter E. *A History of Psychiatry: From the Era of the Asylum to the Age of Prozac.* Wiley; 1998.

12. State Commission in Lunacy. *First Biennial Report.* Superintendent State Printing; 1899.

13. Torrey EF. *American Psychosis: How the Federal Government Destroyed the Mental Illness Treatment System.* Oxford University Press; 2014.

14. Slate RN, Frailing K, Johnson WW, Buffington-Vollum JK. *The Criminalization of Mental Illness: Crisis and Opportunity for the Justice System.* Carolina Academic Press; 2021.

15. Mechanic D, Grob GN. Rhetoric, realities, and the plight of the mentally ill in America. In: R Apple, JA Golden, eds., *History and Health Policy in the United States.* De Gruyter Brill; 2006:229–249.

16. Erickson B. Deinstitutionalization through optimism: The Community Mental Health Act of 1963. *American Journal of Psychiatry Residents' Journal* 2021;**16**(4):6–7.

17. Barnard AV. *Conservatorship*. Columbia University Press; 2023.

18. Torrey EF. *The Insanity Offense: How America's Failure to Treat the Seriously Mentally Ill Endangers Its Citizens*. W.W. Norton; 2012.

19. Frank RG, Glied S. *Better but Not Well: Mental Health Policy in the United States since 1950*. The Johns Hopkins University Press; 2006.

20. Aderibigbe YA. Deinstitutionalization and criminalization: Tinkering in the interstices. *Forensic Science International* 1997;**85**(2): 127–134.

21. Whitmer GE. From hospitals to jails: The fate of California's deinstitutionalized mentally ill. *The American Journal of Orthopsychiatry* 1980;**50** (1):65–75.

22. Isaac RJ, Armat VC. *Madness in the Streets: How Psychiatry and the Law Abandoned the Mentally Ill*. Treatment Advocacy Center; 2000.

23. Teplin A. Keeping the peace: Police discretion and mentally ill persons. *National Institute of Justice Journal* 2000;7:8–15.

24. Torrey EF. *Nowhere to Go*. HarperCollins Publishers; 1988.

25. Rossi PH. *Down and out in America*. University of Chicago Press; 2013.

26. Lamb HR, Weinberger LE. Deinstitutionalization and other factors in the criminalization of persons with serious mental illness and how it is being addressed. *CNS Spectrums* 2019;**25**(2):1–8.

27. Nursing home care in the United States: Failure in public policy. Subcommittee on long-term care of the special committee on aging United States Senate. 1976; No 7.

28. *Dusky v. United States*, 362 U.S. 402.

29. Warburton K, McDermott BE, Gale A, Stahl SM. A survey of national trends in psychiatric patients found incompetent to stand trial: Reasons for the reinstitutionalization of people with serious mental illness in the United States. *CNS Spectrums* 2020;**25** (2):245–251.

30. Wik A, Hollen V, Fisher WH. Forensic patients in state psychiatric hospitals: 1999–2016. *CNS Spectrums* 2019;**25**(2):196–206.

31. Fitch WL. *Forensic Mental Health Services in the United States*. National Association of State Mental Health Program Directors; 2014.

32. Abramson MF. The criminalization of mentally disordered behavior. *Psychiatric Services* 1972;**23**(4):101–105.

33. Sosowsky L. Crime and violence among mental patients reconsidered in view of the new legal relationship between the state and the mentally ill. *The American Journal of Psychiatry* 1978;**135**(1): 33–42.

34. www.washingtonpost.com/archive/politics/1979/04/1 6/crisis-grows-in-calif-mental-hospitals/d89c73f5-7d7 5-45e2-8c60-db8622dd01a6/. Accessed June 6, 2024.

35. Arvanites TM. The impact of state mental hospital deinstitutionalization on commitments for incompetency to stand trial. *Criminology* 1988;**26**:307–320.

36. Torrey EF, Kennard, AD, Eslinger D, et al. More Mentally Ill Persons Are in Jails and Prisons Than Hospitals: A Survey of the States. 2010.

37. Warburton, K. The New Forensic Patient. Lecture presented at the Neuroscience Education Institute, Colorado Springs. November 2020.

38. Amador XF, Flaum M, Andreasen NC, et al. Awareness of illness in schizophrenia and schizoaffective and mood disorders. *Archives of General Psychiatry* 1994;**51** (10):826–836.

39. Buckley PF, Wirshing DA, Bhushan P, et al. Lack of insight in schizophrenia: Impact on treatment adherence. *CNS Drugs* 2007;**21**(2):129–141.

40. Czobor P, Van Dorn RA, Citrome L, et al. Treatment adherence in schizophrenia: A patient-level meta-analysis of combined CATIE and EUFEST studies. *European Neuropsychopharmacology* 2015;**25** (8):1158–1166.

41. Barbui C, Papola D, Saraceno B. The Italian mental health-care reform: Public health lessons. *Bulletin of the World Health Organization* 2018;**96**(11):731A.

42. Parente L, Carabellese F. The Italian general psychiatry and forensic psychiatry treatment model: A unique story. *CNS Spectrums*. 2025;**30**(1):e1.

43. https://leginfo.legislature.ca.gov/faces/billNavClient.x html?bill_id=202320240SB35

The Italian General Psychiatry and Forensic Psychiatry Treatment Model
A Unique Story

Felice F. Carabellese and Lia Parente

Introduction

Law number 180 is the first and only framework law that imposed the closure of mental hospitals in Italy and regulated compulsory health care treatment, establishing public mental health services. This law made Italy the first country in the world to have abolished psychiatric hospitals.

Law 180 of 1978 is known as the Basaglia law, from the name of the psychiatrist and director of Ospedale Psichiatrico (OP) of Gorizia. Dr. Basaglia underlined the pathogenic effect of long hospitalizations in OP and suggested a different approach to severe mental illness, oriented toward community psychiatry and the rehabilitation of the patient to be implemented in his or her context of origin.

Law 180 then became part of the subsequent Law number 833 of 1978, which established a unique public National Health Care System (Sistema Sanitario Nazionale [SSN]), which in Italy guarantees free and high-quality health care to all citizens for hospital admissions, emergency treatments, services of general practitioners, and pediatrics choice. The SSN represents the center of health care in Italy and it is also fundamental to meet the health protection requirements provided by the Italian Constitution.[a]

The Law number 180 and subsequent Law number 833 substantially provided freedom from compulsory care to patients with mental illness, following international bioethical guidelines that identified the inviolable rights of patients to autonomy and self-determination.[1] Even a patient with severe schizophrenia spectrum disorder could usually accept or refuse the treatments, just like any other patient, according to the Italian Constitutional rights.[b]

The Law number 833 of 1978, in fact, guaranteed to psychiatric patients, freedom and right to give or deny consent to treatment. This freedom conferred on the patient eliminated any presumption according to which the state of "suffering from a mental disorder" automatically entailed the inability to give consent to treatment. In essence, the right to self-determination was returned to the psychiatric patient.

The Law number 883 radically changed mental health care in Italy, providing for the transition to a small open community treatment model entrusted to the public psychiatric services, instead of an asylum model. During this transition period, thousands of patients were discharged from Italian OPs.[c]

The law was followed by ~20 years of transition. "During this transition time, thousands of patients were discharged from the OPs and step by step they returned home to their families whenever possible, otherwise they were transferred to smaller residential therapeutic communities. At the same time, a new public therapeutic model was established to support the reintegration of mentally ill patients back into their family and society".[2] After this transition period, OPs became completely inactive due to cultural, scientific, and maybe economic resistances.

Little by little, they went back home to their families whenever possible, otherwise they were transferred to smaller general psychiatric facilities, based on the community model. These are small communities situated in the urban context with a variable number of patients (from 3 to 15, mostly 10), who live together and take care of all daily chores. These patients, depending on their level of functional autonomy, are assisted by a variable number of health

---

[a] Italian Constitution, Article 32, I paragraph: "the Republic protects health as a fundamental right of the individual and in the interest of the community."
[b] Italian Constitution, Article 13: "Personal freedom is inviolable" and Italian Constitution, article 32, II paragraph: "No one can be forced to a certain medical treatment if not for provision of law."
[c] In 1978, when the 98 Italian OPs closed, there were ~89, 000 patients inside them.

care professionals. If needed, this care is provided throughout the day and at night (for those patients with a lower level of functional autonomy). For others, the care is only for a few hours a day.

Patients placed in communities gradually acquire as greater levels of functional autonomy as possible and in the most favorable cases live in small groups of two or three patients, provide for all their daily needs independently, assisted for a few hours a day by caregivers, and are included in protected work activities. In the less favorable cases, they remain in a community of 10 to 15 patients assisted throughout the day by health professionals, free to carry out rehabilitation, leisure and cultural activities, to see their family members, and to freely frequent the places of interest to them.[3]

During this time, a new public therapeutic model was established to support the reintegration of patients with severe mental illness back into their families and original social context.

From that period onwards, Italian psychiatrists refined their therapeutic rehabilitation practices for patients and family support, developing an increasingly widespread outpatient care system in the local area. These outpatient care systems are multidisciplinary, freely accessible, and focused on the patient's needs and their level of functionality.

The relationship that the psychiatrist and other health professionals build with the patient day after day has become the true therapeutic lever of the treatment, intending to restore personal dignity. Voluntary treatment is the respected priority. Therapeutic relationships are aimed at collaboratively obtaining from the patient consent to the treatment.

Therefore, patients with severe mental disorders, including schizophrenia spectrum disorders, have attained greater economic autonomy, greater housing autonomy, welfare, and material support for their family. Additionally, patients have easy access to outpatient facilities that are open throughout the day, every day, to guarantee continuity of therapy and assistance.

Open services have been created, where patients socialize with each other and carry out a series of creative and playful activities. Policies now protect the patients, take care of their economic and personal interests, and support them in their choices.

Much has been done since then and much remains to be done, of course.

From asylum treatment to community treatment

Before 1978, the threshold for involuntary treatment was based on the dangerousness standard, similar to standards still in practice in other Western countries today.

Royal Law no. 36 of 1904 allowed the hospitalization of mentally ill subjects into an OP indefinitely, when the patient was declared "dangerous to themselves or others" by any doctor or by a police officer. The dangerousness determination and consequent hospitalization in an OP was a police measure, not a health service practice.

Once involuntarily hospitalized in an OP, the OP's Director automatically became the patient's legal guardian and had the sole legal power to decide if and when to discharge the patient.

Therefore, upon admission to the OP, the patient lost all personal rights for an indefinite period: the patient could not make a will, could not receive an inheritance, could not vote, and could not marry. If the patient had sexual intercourse with another person, the latter automatically was considered guilty as a sexual offender by Italian penal code. The patient essentially had no right to his own sexual life.

The subsequent Law number 431 of March 14, 1968, introduced partial modifications to the previous policy, to improve patient rights and protected autonomy; however, it was Law number 833 that restored the will of self-determination and the competence to consent to treatment for mentally ill patients as for all other citizens.

When examining how policy impacts outcomes, an important aspect of the modifications to Italian law in 1978 is the change in the criteria for determining involuntary treatment.

The involuntary hospitalization procedure was changed in fact by Law number 833 from a dangerousness standard (like that currently in use in western countries such as the United States) to a medical standard. A police measure was previously used to order mentally ill individuals considered to be "dangerous to themselves or others" to indefinite hospitalization in an OP.

The Italian regulation for civil commitment no longer considered danger to oneself or others as a prerequisite, going beyond the Royal Decree 36 of 14 February 1904, which allowed the admission to OPs of those said to be of "sick mind" and dangerous to themselves or others was changed by Law 833 of 1978. Under this new law, involuntary hospitalization became an exclusively health care act authorized by a magistrate and it could only be ordered when all of the following three conditions are met and recognized by at least two medical doctors: the need for emergency care, a treatment that required hospitalization, and incompetence to give valid consent to medical treatment due to the patient's severe illness. This aligned the standard for involuntary treatment in schizophrenia with that for other medical conditions, away from a need for dangerousness and toward an evaluation of medical necessity and medical competence to give consent to treatment.

The involuntary hospitalization has a default duration (maximum 7 days, renewable once or twice for 7 more days at a time, subject to the approval of the same magistrate and at the request of the psychiatrist for valid medical reasons). During the entire duration of the involuntary hospitalization, the hospitalized patient is protected and safeguarded in all rights and prerogatives by a special magistrate. In both cases (voluntary and involuntary), hospitalization can occur only in a general hospital, not in an OP, with newly created psychiatry wards in general hospitals consisting of small treatment units with up to 16 beds.

The transition to a medical necessity model for involuntary hospitalization, rather than a dangerousness model, has not resulted in abuses. For example, in Italy in 2021, only 7.6% of all hospital admissions were involuntary. The mean duration of hospitalizations was 12.8 days. Approximately 30% of patients admitted at discharge had a diagnosis of schizophrenic disorder. However, more than 70% of patients who receive three or more lifetime involuntary hospitalizations have schizophrenia spectrum disorders (Ministry of Health source). This is a problem of adherence to treatment which, as is known, makes the course of schizophrenic disorders problematic.

The policy change was also followed by a profound change of the psychiatrist's professional roles and responsibilities. Initially, their tasks mainly involved patient monitoring. After the Law number 833 of 1978, their therapeutic activity became more focused on the support and strengthening of the patient's functional autonomy and social reintegration. In this manner, Italian psychiatrists act in accordance with the fundamental constitutional rights, which were fully restored for the mentally ill patients too by the

new law.[d] It revealed that Italian psychiatrists strongly rejected the previous role of social control required by the dangerousness standard.

The refusal of Italian psychiatrists to be agents of social control was evident in reform, which decreed the closure of Italian High Security Hospitals (Ospedale Psichiatrico Giudiziario [OPG]) in 2015.

Before that, on April 1, 2008, the Decree of the Italian Prime Minister implemented the prior Decree-Law (Number 230)[e] on June 22, 1999, which transferred the responsibility of treating an OPG's patients and the mentally ill prisoners from the Department of Justice to the Department of Health. By June 30, 2010, there were 1,457 men and 95 women who were socially dangerous inpatients in the six Italian OPGs.

The following Decree Law issued on December 20, 2011, number 211, provided for the transfer of the OPGs' patients to the community facilities located in each of Italy's 20 regions, named Residence for Execution of Security Measure (REMS), pending the closure of the OPGs initially expected by February 1, 2013.

REMS is mental health community facility under Mental Health Department (DSM) coordination each with 20 beds, suitable for the accommodation and treatment of socially "dangerous" offenders found Not Guilty by Reason of Insanity (NGRI) with a higher level of social dangerousness. REMS resemble small security hospitals, locked, secure facilities that provide inpatient treatment.

The Decree Law of March 25, 2013, postponed the closure of the OPGs until April 1, 2014. The Decree Law of March 31, 2014 (Number 52), which was modified and came into effect on May 30, 2014 (Number 81), set the final closing date of the OPGs and the discharge of all inpatients as April 1, 2015. With the law of May 30, 2014, Number 81, Italy passed from a forensic psychiatric model based on

---

[d] Italian Constitution, Article 2: "The Republic recognizes and guarantees the inviolable human rights." Note that the Law 833 abolished the automatic recourse to legal protection for a mentally ill subject at his entry into the OP.

[e] Decree of the Prime Minister: Procedure and criteria for the transfer of health function to the National Health Care Service, work relationships, financial resources, and equipment and instruments in matters of correctional health (General Series no. 126 of May 30, 2008). This decree established and described the transfer of all treatment of mentally ill prisoners in Italy from the Department of Justice to the Department of Health.

Table 17.1 Main innovative laws on psychiatric care in Italy

Italian mental health care laws	System structure	Patient's condition
Presence of mental asylums in Italy since the 1400s, but regulated by:	–	People were interned in OPs:
- Royal Decree no. 36 of 1904, "Provisions on mental asylums and the mentally ill" (OP management by Italian provincial). - Royal Decree no. 615 of 1909 "Regulations on mental asylums and the mentally ill" (OP management by Italian provincial).	- In 1904 there were 98 OPs in Italy - In all 98 OPs there were 89 000 patients	- Without consent - Dangerousness standard - With a police measure - Internment for indefinite time - Losing all rights - OP's director automatically became the patient's legal guardian
- Law no. 431 of March 14, 1968	- Creation of provincial day hospitals - Each OP divided into sections with 125 beds - No automatic Director's legal guardian	- Greater psychological and rehabilitative attention - Possibility of voluntary admission of the patient to OPs
- Law no. 833 of 1978 (that incorporated the Law no. 180 of 1978)	- Establishment of the SSN - Closure of OPs - Psychiatric wards in General Hospitals - Community model of care - Mental health care as a health service practice - Involuntary hospitalization as an exclusively health care act authorized by a magistrate	- Patient's right to self-determination for treatment - Patient's right to freely consent to treatment - Other civil rights to patient - Rehabilitation goals

Table 17.2 Main innovative laws on forensic psychiatric care in Italy

Italian forensic mental health care laws	System structure	Patients' condition
Italian Security Hospital		
- 1876 Aversa is the first Italian "manicomio criminale"	- Section for "maniacs"	- Internment in Security Hospital as a security measure (Art. 203 Italian Penal Code) for NGRI offenders
- A second one in Montelupo Fiorentino in 1886		- About 200 patients for each OPG
- A third in Reggio Emilia (1892)		
- A fourth in Naples (1922)		
- A fifth in Barcellona Pozzo di Gozzo in 1925		
- Finally, one in Castiglione delle Stiviere in 1939		
- In 1975 the "manicomi criminali" were called "Ospedali Psichiatrici Giudiziari" (OPGs)		
- Constitutional Court Sentence on July 18, 2003, no. 253	- Admission to a different security measure (*libertà vigilata*)	- 1,457 men and 95 women in all OPGs at 2010
- Decree of the Italian Prime Minister of April 1st, 2008, implemented the prior Decree Law (Number 230) on June 22, 1999	- The responsibility of treating OPGs' patients and the mentally ill prisoners were transferred from Department of Justice to Department of Health	- Max 20 patients for each REMS
- Decree Law December 20, 2011, no. 211	- Transfer of the OPGs' patients to the REMS in each Italian region	–
- Law no. 81, May 30, 2014	- OPG closure	- At 2023, there are 32 REMS in Italy

OPGs to one based on REMS in each region, from an asylum model of forensic treatment to a rehabilitative model of care. As a result, the discrepancy between general psychiatry treatment and forensic psychiatry treatment, created almost 40 years ago by Law 833 of 1978, was resolved. This means that also the "dangerous" offenders found NGRI would be treated by the same community treatment model entrusted to the public DSM for general psychiatric public services.

REMS are mental health community facilities with 20 beds operated broadly to the standard of "medium security" in other European states. Commitment to a REMS facility is designed as a custodial security measure, which is "extreme and exceptional." Precisely because of the exceptional nature of the security measure in REMS, the total number of beds in the 32 Italian REMS is ~600 beds. In fact, the average length of stay in REMS is just over a year.[4] The use of security measures with a lower level of security such as *"libertà vigilata,"* a sort of probation measure or supervised outpatient treatment, is more frequent. Even patients with schizophrenic disorders are more often on probation than interned in REMS and demonstrate good functional adaptation to the current community treatment and rehabilitation model. The use of rehabilitation, psychotherapy, and family support activities are common practices in the forensic treatment model of our country and allow for continuous and effective management even of patients with severe mental illnesses. A more problematic and less effective management concerns REMS patients affected by severe personality disorders, who represent approximately one-third of all REMS patients.[4] In recent years, in fact, the need has emerged to provide for a reduced number of patients a higher level of security than that of REMS. During the validation of new assessment tools for the Italian population, this need was quantified in ~5–9% of all NGRI patients who committed crimes socially dangerous.[5]

The Law number 81 of 2014 has also raised criticism not only among psychiatrists who find themselves having to once again manage the dangerousness of their patients, a matter no longer within their competence after Law number 883 of 78, but also in the judicial world.[3, 6]

In fact, in some Italian regions, especially those that make little use of recidivism risk assessment tools[7, 8] waiting lists of patients have been created before they enter REMS. How and where to manage patients during the waiting period is a problem raised above all by jurists. Before 2015, in fact, the placement of the NGRI patient in an OPG occurred without any waiting, immediately after the judge's order (Art. 222 Italian penal code) or even at the request of the prosecutor in a provisional and temporary form (Art. 206 Italian penal code). Further, this naturally allowed for a more immediate and less problematic management of the NGRI mentally ill offender at risk of criminal recidivism by the judicial authority.

The Law number 81, 2014, limits the maximum duration of internment in REMS to the maximum time of imprisonment had the offender been found guilty of the crime and was sentenced. The security measure is applied only for those NGRI patients who are considered socially dangerous, that is, at risk of criminal recidivism. The assessment of social dangerousness must be renewed periodically (every 6 months) and confirmed by the judge.

Concept of social dangerousness is still in the Italian Penal Code (Art. 203) and the judge is the only one who decides whether or not to apply security measures, REMS, or others less severe security measures. Both REMS internment and other security measures are mandatory, decided by the judge; however, the NGRI patient retains the right to consent (and refuse) to treatment.[9]

The exceptional nature of the REMS security measure derives from the intention of the Italian legislature to balance two different principles of equal dignity. On the one hand, there is the principle of patient consent, which consists in the voluntary nature of the medical treatment already recognized for non-forensic patients by Law number 833 of 1978 and now also for forensic patients who committed crimes by Law number 81 of 2014. On the other hand, there is the need to contain patients who have committed crimes with restrictive measures because of their recognized social dangerousness, because they are at a risk of criminal recidivism. By balancing the two requirements, the legislature intended to give REMS measure the character of "last resort," but at the same time with a rehabilitative aim (Tables 17.1 and 17.2).

Conclusion

From this review and analysis of Italy's transformation mental health services for forensic patients requiring security measures, we cannot draw comparisons between the civil mental health systems in Italy and other countries such as the United States. Deinstitutionalization without development of adequately robust community mental health services is an often cited factor in the relentless increase in mentally ill persons entering US jails and prisons.[10] However, the Italian model does demonstrate that, with a robust community system in place, deinstitutionalization is possible without increases in criminalization.

Furthermore, Italy's transition to an informed consent model for involuntary treatment, and away from a dangerousness model, appears to have effectively reduced the need for involuntary treatment. The change in involuntary treatment standard in the context of community treatment has also provided for improved dignity and strengthened therapeutic relationships between psychiatrists and people living with schizophrenia.[11] Policy makers visiting Italy for seeing its model mental health systems should take these factors into consideration.

References

1. World Medical Association. (2013). World Medical Association Declaration of Helsinki: ethical principles for medical research involving human subjects. *Jama*, **310**(20), 2191–2194.

2. Carabellese, F., & Felthous, A. R. (2016). Closing Italian forensic psychiatry hospitals in favor of treating insanity acquittees in the community. *Behav Sci Law*, **34**(2–3), 444–459.

3. Carabellese, F., Parente, L., & Kennedy, H. G. (2024). Reform of forensic mental health services in Italy: stigma and blaming the messenger: Hermenoia. *Int J Offend Ther Compar Criminol*. **68**(15), 1505–1524.

4. Catanesi, R, Mandarelli, G., Ferracuti, S., Valerio, A., & Carabellese, F. (2019). The new Italian residential forensic psychiatry system (REMS). A one year population study. *Rassegna Italiana di Criminologia*, special issue.

5. Parente, L., Carabellese, F., Felthous, A., et al. (2024). Italian Evaluation and Excellence in REMS (ITAL-EE-REMS): appropriate placement of forensic patients in REMS forensic facilities. *Int J Mental Health Syst*. **18**, 33.

6. Mandarelli, G., Coluccia, A., Urbano, M. T., Carabellese, F., & Carabellese, F. (2019). Current issues, penitentiary treatment problems and prospect after law 81/2014. *Rassegna Italiana di Criminologia*. **13**(4): 316–326.

7. Carabellese, F. (2017). Closing OPG: socially dangerous mentally ill offenders' diagnostic tools. From forensic-psychiatric evaluation to the treatment. *Rass Ital Criminol*. **11**, 173–181.

8. Kennedy, H. G., Carabellese, F., & Carabellese, F. (2021). Evaluation and management of violent risk for forensic patients: is it a necessary practice in Italy? *J Psychopathol*, **27**(1), 11–18.

9. Carabellese, F., Parente, L., La Tegola, D., et al. (2022). Il DUNDRUM ToolKit, versione italiana e il suo potenziale utilizzo nel modello trattamentale forense italiano. *Rass Ital Criminol*, **4**, 271–282.

10. Torrey, E.F., Kennard, A.D., Eslinger, D., Lamb, R., Pavle, J. More Mentally Ill Persons Are in Jails and Prisons Than Hospitals: A Survey of the States. Arlington, VA: Treatment Advocacy Center. 2010:1–8.

11. McLaughlin, P., Brady, P., Carabellese, F., et al. (2023). Excellence in forensic psychiatry services: international survey of qualities and correlates. *BJPsych Open*, **9**(6), e193.

Liberty or Life
Mental Health Care in Australia

Kirsty MacDonald and Andrew Ellis

Introduction

The indigenous inhabitants of the Australian continent arrived approximately 65,000 years ago. Treatment for schizophrenia prior to European arrival is not well known by current professionals. The Commonwealth of Australia, a parliamentary democracy, was established in 1901. The Commonwealth is a federation of six states and two territories that were originally colonies of Britain. Australia has a population of 26.8 million people, 30% of whom are born overseas. Indigenous Australians make up 3.8% of the population. Schizophrenia is a complex disorder of brain functioning, which the World Health Organization describes as a "disturbance involving the most basic functions that give the normal person a feeling of individuality, uniqueness and self-direction."[1] Schizophrenia affects up to 1% of the population[2] and is among the top 10 disorders in the global burden of disease and disability.[3] Australian surveys show similar prevalence results to international studies.[4]

Treatment of schizophrenia includes staging of the disorder, psychological interventions (such as Cognitive Behavioral Therapy), addressing co-morbid conditions such as substance use and interpersonal deficits, psychoeducation, and antipsychotic medications.[5] Treatment guidelines detail the management of acute and chronic psychotic symptoms, as well as ongoing evaluation of efficacy, adherence, and addressing co-morbid issues.[5] Indigenous Australians show higher rates of schizophrenia, which may be explained by higher rates of substance use[6] disorders, although other elements such as poverty, racism, and inequitable access to health care also play a role.[6]

Overview of legislation

In Australia, individual states have their own Mental Health Acts to guide decision-making around involuntary treatment and admission. Each piece of legislation falls under the jurisdiction of the State or Territory government. Mental Health Acts guide admission of all civil involuntary admissions, based on current (and future) mental state and risk of harm to self or others.[7] Currently, variations between the definition of mental illnesses and disorders and differing criteria for involuntary treatment are found within the Acts.[8]

Table 18.1 details current legislation for the states and territories in Australia for involuntary commitment and treatment.[8]

All states and territories include a similar definition of "mental illness"; however, only the Australian Capital Territory (ACT) and New South Wales (NSW) have a definition for "mental disorder." Other differences include a "continuing condition" in NSW, which includes potential deterioration or likely deterioration in their care. South Australia (SA) requires a person to have impaired decision-making capacity. As mentioned by Tosson et al.,[9] "Criteria for mental health treatment is too diversely defined in each jurisdiction. While the criteria adhere to the ethical principles of beneficence and non-maleficence, they vary widely in implementation, which may result in differing treatments between States and Territories."

Mental Health Acts are also used to determine acute treatment in inpatient settings and involuntary longer-term treatment in the community, under the provision of compulsory Community Treatment Orders (CTOs). Research of the reporting process of involuntary treatment both in hospitals and in the community is different among jurisdictions and uses differing data (incidents of treatment versus number of individuals affected).[10] There are clear differences regarding the reporting of involuntary treatment across states and territories within Australia and this should be rectified in order to inform current and future practice. Australia is signatory to the Convention on the Rights of Persons with Disabilities (CRPD) and the Optional Protocol to the Convention against Torture and other Cruel, Inhuman or Degrading Treatment or Punishment (OPCAT). The Australian Government interprets the CRPD as allowing for "compulsory assistance or treatment of persons, including measures taken for the treatment of mental disability, where such treatment is necessary, as a last resort and subject to safeguards." Although signatory to OPCAT, Australia has refused entry to international regulatory observers to review facilities where persons are detained (prisons, psychiatric hospitals, and locked community homes).[11]

There are forensic provisions for diversion of persons with mental illness charged with criminal offenses into health systems, with each state administering services in varying fashion.[12] This includes persons who meet legal criteria for not having criminal responsibility for their acts, not being capable of performing trial tasks, or for prisoners who require involuntary treatment of their condition. Lower order offences may be dealt with summarily by diversion to mental health treatment.[13] These provisions are not consistently applied across the country,[14] and persons who may be eligible for diversion can remain in prison settings which is not recommended or effective.

Services for people with schizophrenia

One of the unique health-care differences within Australia is the split between Commonwealth and state funding for health services. The Commonwealth government oversees the broad delivery of health care and funds Medicare (a universal safety net for outpatient care), whereas the individual states and territories are responsible for their hospital care and budget. This impacts the treatment of a chronic and complex illness like schizophrenia, which requires coordinated inpatient and outpatient services for integrated management.

The National Mental Health Service Planning Framework (NMHSPF)[15] is one model that the Commonwealth government has introduced which assists with providing services for their local community. The broad principles are (i) mental health promotion, (ii) mental illness prevention, (iii) primary and specialized clinical ambulatory mental health services, (iv) specialized mental health community support services, (v) specialized bed-based mental health-care services, and (vi) medications and procedures.

Different jurisdictions within Australia broadly offer models of care that include inpatient treatment, community care, and outreach treatment. The specific needs of

an individual should guide treatment.[5] Typically, patients needing acute admissions (due to symptoms and risk) might be treated in an inpatient ward. After some time, they might transition into community care. Some will be managed with community treatment orders (CTOs), as per local legislation and policies.

From a treatment perspective, there has been criticism that the legislative requirements requiring patients to be a danger to others or themselves delay treatment and lead to worsened outcomes.[16] This is because delays in treatment ultimately lead to a longer duration of untreated psychosis, which might be linked to both suicide[17–19] and violence risk[20,21] as well as worsen the prognosis of the illness itself.[22,23] The ethical issues of autonomy and beneficence are raised in this setting, which are keenly monitored in both medical and legislative frameworks.

The current system of having patients present to their local emergency departments for assessment also places pressure on the departments themselves. Poor access to community care flows into increased pressure being placed on emergency departments when dealing with acute presentations of mentally unwell individuals. Poor planning, coordination, and accountability mechanisms need to be addressed to improve equitable access for people who present with mental health concerns to their local hospital. As highlighted by emergency clinicians, the mental health system is "highly fragmented, with unclear roles and responsibilities".[24]

Effectiveness of treatment

Funding for mental health conditions across the Commonwealth and state/territories varies. Additionally, funding addresses both high- and low-prevalence disorders, as well as preventive strategies.[25] It is difficult to find the overall money spent on treatment of schizophrenia within the Australian context. The term "mental health" encompasses many disorders, as well as prevention strategies. This may lead to legislative and service reforms that reflect advocacy from groups representing high-prevalence conditions and neglect the special concerns faced by persons with schizophrenia and their families.

Treatment of mental health conditions should always be individualized and catered to the individual. Individuals suffering from more common disorders such as anxiety and depression tend to have greater insight and adherence to treatment than people suffering from schizophrenia. Management plans that

Table 18.1 Current legislation for the states and territories in Australia for involuntary commitment and treatment

	ACT Mental Health Act 2015s58,66 101	NSW Mental Health Act 2007ss12,14,68	NT Mental Health and Related Services Act 1998s14	QLD Mental Health Act 2016ss3, 12	SA Mental Health Act 2009s21	TAS Mental Health Act 2013ss6, 40	VIC Mental Health and Wellbeing Act 2022s89, 142, 143	WA Mental Health Act 2014s25
Mental illness	The person has a mental illness cr mental disorder.	The person is suffering from mental illness and, owing to that illness, there are reasonable grounds for believing that the care, treatment, and control of the person is necessary:	The person has a mental illness and as a result of the mental illness, without treatment the person is likely to:	The person has a mental illness; because of the person's illness, the absence of involuntary treatment, or the absence of continued involuntary treatment, is likely to result in:	The person has a mental illness and because of the mental illness, the person requires treatment for:	The person has, or appears to have, a mental illness and without treatment, the mental illness will, or is likely to, seriously harm:	The person has a mental illness; and because the person appears to have a mental illness, the person appears to need immediate treatment to prevent:	The person has a mental illness for which the person is in need of treatment and because of the mental illness, there is:
Harm	Is doing, or is likey to do, serious harm to themselves or someone else.	For the person's own protection from serious harm or the protection of others from serious harm.	Cause serious harm to himself or herself or to someone else	Imminent serious harm to the person or others or	The person's own protection from harm (whether physical or mental and including harm involved in the continuation/deterioration of the person's condition) or to protect others from harm and	The safety of the person or others or	Serious harm to the person or to another person	A significant risk to the safety of the person or another, or a significant risk of serious harm to the person or to another or
Need for care	Is suffering, or is likely to suffer, serious mental or physical deterioration.	N/A	Suffer serious mental or physical deterioration and	The person suffering serious mental or physical deterioration.	The person has impaired decision-making capacity relating to appropriate treatment of the person's mental illness.	The person's health and	Serious deterioration in the person's mental or physical health	A significant risk to the health of the person and
Psychiatric treatment	Treatment/care/support is likely to reduce the harm or deterioration (or its	N/A	The person requires treatment that is	N/A	N/A	The treatment will be appropriate and effective in terms of the outcomes	If the person is made subject to a temporary treatment order	Treatment in the community cannot reasonably be

Table 18.1 (cont.)

	ACT Mental Health Act 2015s58,66 101	NSW Mental Health Act 2007ss12,14,68	NT Mental Health and Related Services Act 1998s14	QLD Mental Health Act 2016ss3, 12	SA Mental Health Act 2009s21	TAS Mental Health Act 2013ss6, 40	VIC Mental Health and Wellbeing Act 2022s89, 142, 143	WA Mental Health Act 2014s25
	likelihood) or result in an improvement in the person's condition.		available at an approved treatment facility and			referred to in section 6(1) [see additional criteria] and	or treatment order, the immediate treatment will be provided to them; and	provided to the person and
No less restrictive alternative	The treatment, care, or support cannot be adequately provided in another way that would involve less restriction of the freedom of choice and movement.	No other care of a less restrictive kind that is consistent with safe and effective care, is appropriate and reasonably available to the person.	There is no less restrictive means of ensuring that the person receives the treatment and	The main objects of the Act are to be achieved in a way that is the least restrictive of the rights and liberties of a person who has a mental illness.	There is no less restrictive means than an inpatient treatment order (ITO) to ensure appropriate treatment of the person's illness.	The treatment cannot be adequately given except under a treatment order.	There are no less restrictive means reasonably available to enable the person to receive the immediate treatment.	The person cannot be adequately provided with treatment in a way that would involve less restriction.
Additional criteria	The above criteria must be satisfied before a mental health order can be made for a person with decision-making capacity (DMC) who refuses treatment, care, or support; the harm or deterioration must be so serious that it outweighs the right to refuse. If a person lacks DMC and refuses treatment, care, or support, the only criteria that apply is the existence of a mental disorder or illness.	In considering whether a person is a mentally ill person, the continuing condition of the person, including any likely deterioration in the person's condition, and the likely effect of any such deterioration, are to be taken into account.	The person is not capable of giving informed consent to the treatment or has unreasonably refused to consent to the treatment.	The person does not have consent to be treated for the illness.	In considering whether there is no less restrictive means than an ITO of ensuring appropriate treatment, consideration must be given, amongst other things, to the prospects of the person receiving all necessary treatment on a voluntary basis or in compliance with a community treatment order.	(i) The person does not have DMC (ii) the treatment will: prevent/ remedy mental illness; or manage/ alleviate it where possible; or reduce the risks that persons with mental illness may pose to themselves or others; or monitor and evaluate the person's mental state.	(i) the person does not have the capacity to give informed consent.	(i) The person does not demonstrate the capacity to make a treatment decision about the provision of treatment; (ii) decisions regarding ICT must be made with reference to guidelines published by the Chief Psychiatrist.

address higher prevalent conditions might not adequately meet the treatment needs of people suffering from schizophrenia.

Treatment measures such as CTOs are often used to manage complex clients with schizophrenia in the community. However, CTOs should not be purely used to gain access to services, nor are they effective when services are non-existent or inadequate.[26] Research also highlights that people with culturally and linguistically diverse backgrounds – including Indigenous Australians – are more likely to be placed on compulsory community treatment.[27]

Small studies that have evaluated the experience of people suffering from schizophrenia highlight universal goals – including having a stable place to live, remaining independent, and keeping physically healthy. Additionally, having autonomy and being able to collaborate with their treating team was very important.[28]

Conclusion

Long-term management of complex conditions such as schizophrenia requires individualized and highly specialized care. Current models of care and associated funding arrangements by both Commonwealth and state/territory governments do not adequately address the needs of this vulnerable community. Specialized models of care for people with severe mental illnesses would ensure that breakdowns in treatment provision were minimized and crisis presentations were not the mainstay of obtaining care within the public health system. Schizophrenia is often a forgotten disorder, where the lack of advocacy leads to poorer outcomes – for both the individual and our society.

Overall, the legislative regimes and health systems provided for persons with schizophrenia show confusion, perhaps reflecting the disorganization and lack of insight characteristic of the condition itself. It has been long noted that people without schizophrenia find the condition difficult to understand.[29] On the one hand, legislation for compulsory treatment of mental disorders in general places schizophrenia as no different from other forms of mental disorder and distress and thereby makes compulsory hospitalization difficult to achieve, placing greater weight on autonomy and personal choice around treatments. On the other, hurdles to achieve diversion from justice systems are also high. When involuntary treatment or imprisonment does occur, international scrutiny of practice is then reduced. Services developed around

these seemingly divergent objectives can then fail to develop and provide services relevant to the minority of mental health patients with the arguably more severe condition of schizophrenia. The end result is high rates of persons with schizophrenia in prisons,[30] high and increasing rates of homelessness,[31] and mortality.[32]

References

1. World Health Organization. *The ICD-10 classification of mental and behavioural disorders: Clinical descriptions and diagnostic guidelines.* Vol. **1**. World Health Organization; 1992.

2. Simeone JC, Ward AJ, Rotella P, Collins J, Windisch R. An evaluation of variation in published estimates of schizophrenia prevalence from 1990 2013: A systematic literature review. *BMC Psychiatry.* 2015;15:Article 193. doi:10.1186/s12888-015-0578-7

3. Mathers CD, Loncar D. Projections of global mortality and burden of disease from 2002 to 2030. *PLoS Med.* 2006;3(11):Article e442. doi:10.1371/journal.pmed.0030442

4. Jablensky A, McGrath J, Herrman H, et al. Psychotic disorders in urban areas: an overview of the Study on Low Prevalence Disorders. *Aust N Z J Psychiatry.* 2000;34(2):221–236. doi:10.1080/j.1440-1614.2000.00728.x

5. Castle DJ, Galletly CA, Dark F, et al. The 2016 Royal Australian and New Zealand College of Psychiatrists guidelines for the management of schizophrenia and related disorders. *Med J Aust.* 2017;**206**(11):501–505. doi:10.1177/0004867416641195

6. Ogilvie JM, Tzoumakis S, Allard T, et al. Prevalence of psychiatric disorders for Indigenous Australians: a population-based birth cohort study. *Epidemiol Psychiatric Sci.* 2021;30:Article e21. doi:10.1017/S204579602100010X

7. Kirkby KC, Henderson S. Australia's mental health legislation. *Int Psychiatry.* 2013;**10**(2):38–40. doi:10.1192/S174936760000374X

8. Royal Australian and New Zealand College of Psychiatrists. Royal Australian and New Zealand College of Psychiatrists clinical practice guidelines for the treatment of schizophrenia and related disorders. *Aust N Z J Psychiatry.* 2005;39(1/2):1. doi:10.1080/j.1440-1614.2005.01516.x

9. Tosson D, Lam D, Raeburn T. Why Australia should move towards nationally consistent mental health legislation? *Aust Psychiatry.* 2022;30(6):743–745. doi:10.1177/10398562221116290

10. Clugston B, Young A, Heffernan EB. A comparison of the reported use of involuntary treatment orders

within Australian jurisdictions. *Aust Psychiatry.* 2018;**26**(5):482–485. doi:10.1177/1039856218789787

11. Ouliaris C, Gill N, Castan M, Sundram S. OPCAT: How an international treaty regarding torture is relevant to the Australian mental health system. *Aust N Z J Psychiatry.* 2024;**58**(5):387–392. doi:10.1177/ 00048674231221419

12. Ellis A. Forensic psychiatry and mental health in Australia: an overview. *CNS Spectrums.* 2020;**25** (2):119–121. doi:10.1017/S1092852919001299

13. Davidson F, Heffernan E, Greenberg D, Butler T, Burgess P. A critical review of mental health court liaison services in Australia: A first national survey. *Psychiatry, Psychol Law.* 2016;**23**(6):908–921. doi:10.1080/13218719.2016. 1155509

14. Carroll A, Ellis A, Aboud A, Scott R, Pillai K. No involuntary treatment of mental illness in Australian and New Zealand prisons. *J Forensic Psychiatry Psychol.* 2021;**32**(1):1–28. doi:10.1080/ 14789949.2020.1817524

15. Diminic S, Gossip K, Page I, Comben C. *Introduction to the National Mental Health Service planning framework–Commissioned by the Australian Government Department of Health and Aged Care* (Version AUS V4.3). The University of Queensland; 2023. www.aihw.gov.au/getmedia/976 cb3dd-18f1-4870-8cfb-9406a16dc844/introduction-to-the-national-mental-health-service-planning -framework-v4-3.pdf.aspx

16. Large MM, Nielssen O, Ryan CJ, Hayes R. Mental health laws that require dangerousness for involuntary admission may delay the initial treatment of schizophrenia. *Soc Psychiatry Psychiatr Epidemiol.* 2008;**43**(3):251–256. doi:10.1007/s00127-007-0287-8

17. Altamura AC, Bassetti R, Bignotti S, Pioli R, Mundo E. Clinical variables related to suicide attempts in schizophrenic patients: a retrospective study. *Schizophr Res.* 2003;**60**(1):47–55. doi:10.1016/s0920-9964(02)00164-0

18. Clarke M, Whitty P, Browne S, et al. Suicidality in first episode psychosis. *Schizophrenia Res.* 2006;**86**(1–3):221–225. doi:10.1016/j.schres.2006.05.026

19. Melle I, Johannesen JO, Friis S, et al. Early detection of the first episode of schizophrenia and suicidal behavior. *Am J Psychiatry.* 2006;**163**(5):800–804. doi:10.1176/ajp.2006.163.5.800

20. Milton J, Amin S, Singh SP, et al. Aggressive incidents in first-episode psychosis. *Br J Psychiatry.* 2001;**178** (5):433–440. doi:10.1192/bjp.178.5.433

21. Verma S, Poon LY, Subramaniam M, Chong SA. Aggression in Asian patients with first-episode psychosis. *Int J Social Psychiatry.* 2005;**51**(4):365–371. doi:10.1177/0020764005060852

22. Marshall M, Lewis S, Lockwood A, et al. Association between duration of untreated psychosis and outcome in cohorts of first-episode patients: a systematic review. *Arch General Psychiatry.* 2005;**62**(9):975–983. doi:10.1001/archpsyc.62.9.975

23. Perkins DO, Gu H, Boteva K, Lieberman JA. Relationship between duration of untreated psychosis and outcome in first-episode schizophrenia: A critical review and meta-analysis. *Am J Psychiatry.* 2005;**162** (10):1785–1804. doi:10.1176/appi.ajp.162.10.1785

24. Duggan M, Harris B, Chislett WK, Calder R. *Nowhere else to go: why Australia's health system results in people with mental illness getting 'stuck' in emergency departments.* Victoria University; 2020. https://vuir.vu .edu.au/41956/1/nowhere-else-to-go-people-mental-il lness-stuck-emergency-departments-report-mitchell-i nstitute.pdf

25. Australian Institute of Health and Welfare. *Australia's mental health system;* 2023, October. www .aihw.gov.au/mental-health/overview/australias-men tal-health-services#national-developments

26. Light EM, Robertson MD, Boyce P, et al. How shortcomings in the mental health system affect the use of involuntary community treatment orders. *Aust Health Rev.* 2016;**41**(3):351–356. doi:10.1071/AH16074

27. Kisely S, Moss K, Boyd M, Siskind D. Efficacy of compulsory community treatment and use in minority ethnic populations: A statewide cohort study. *Aust N Z J Psychiatry.* 2020;**54**(1):76–88. doi:10.1177/ 0004867419877690

28. Fifer S, Keen B, Newton R, Puig A, McGeachie M. Understanding the treatment preferences of people living with schizophrenia in Australia; A patient value mapping study. *Patient Preference Adherence.* 2022;**16**:1687–1701. doi:10.2147/ppa.s366522

29. Rümke HC. Das Kernsymptom der schizophrenie und das 'Praecox Gefuhl'. *Z. Gesamte Neurol. Psychiatry* 1942;**102**:168–169.

30. Browne CC, Korobanova D, Yee N, et al. The prevalence of self-reported mental illness among those imprisoned in New South Wales across three health surveys, from 2001 to 2015. *Aust N Z J Psychiatry.* 2023;**57**(4):550–561. doi:10.1177/00048674221104411

31. Buhrich N, Hodder T, Teesson M. Schizophrenia among homeless people in inner-Sydney: Current prevalence and historical trends. *J Mental Health.* 2003;**12**(1):51–57. doi:10.1080/ 09638230021000058292

32. Lawrence D, Hancock KJ, Kisely S. The gap in life expectancy from preventable physical illness in psychiatric patients in Western Australia: retrospective analysis of population based registers. *BMJ.* 2013;**346**: f2539. doi:10.1136/bmj.f2539

Liberty or Life
The Aotearoa New Zealand Perspective

Justin Barry-Walsh

Introduction: Homelessness, prisons, and mental illness

Homelessness is a major problem in Aotearoa New Zealand. According to the OECD report on homelessness, New Zealand's rate of 2.17% of the population is the highest of any of the countries included in the survey.[1] This can be partly explained by the broad definition of homelessness used in New Zealand (New Zealand includes those in emergency accommodation, homeless shelters, nonconventional accommodation such as mobile homes, those temporarily staying with family or friends, and those living in dilapidated buildings such as those without power and/or water) but does not fully account for the high rate in New Zealand. There are differences between ethnicities and Maori are overrepresented in the homeless population.[2] A recent study in Auckland, New Zealand's biggest city, identified that nearly 43% of all those living rough (meaning living in streets or public spaces without a shelter that can be defined as living quarters) in Auckland were Indigenous.[3] Maori make up about 17% of the total New Zealand population. The latest homelessness data is based on the 2018 Census and trends over time are not clear. Official figures between 2013 and 2019 would suggest that the rate of homelessness in New Zealand only increased by 2%.[1]

The drivers of homelessness are similar to other countries. They include increasing problems with housing affordability and lack of available social housing.[2] There is little information about the proportion of people with mental illness who are homeless. A survey in 2001 identified that 70% of all people with mental health problems receiving treatment within the public system had issues with homelessness or housing and 4% were recognized as homeless.[4] Anecdotal and media reports would indicate mentally ill people struggle to be discharged from hospital because of a lack of available housing and impose an increased burden on those working with the homeless.[5] Whether in New Zealand the rates of psychosis amongst homeless are elevated is unknown, but clinical experience and research from overseas would suggest that probably around 15 to 20% of the homeless have a psychotic illness,[6] and it is thought this rate will be higher amongst those who are living rough.

New Zealand has by international comparison a high rate of incarceration. In 2018 there were 201/100,000 population people in prison. There was growth in the prison population of 70% between 1997 and 2011 despite a decrease in the number of people being charged with criminal offenses. As of 31 March 2024, the prison population stood at 9,508 of which 6.5% were women. This represents a rate of 179/100,000. This rate is currently creeping up but had dropped in 2018 due to the changes in policy introduced by the previous government. Of further concern is the rise in the percentage of the prison population on remand. Between 2012 and 2020 the remand population increased by nearly 50%. Indigenous people are grossly over-represented in the prison population, in March 2024 52.4% identified as Maori.[7]

It is well established there are high rates of serious mental illness in the New Zealand prison population. A thorough survey in 1999 identified that 6% of prisoners at that time had schizophrenia or related psychotic illness.[8] In 2015 using a similar methodology 12% of people in prison were reporting psychotic symptoms.[9]

Services

Skipworth et al. examined whether the shift in models of care for people with mental illness was impacting the number of mentally ill people being incarcerated.[10] This study explored whether the risk of imprisonment following discharge from the mental health unit had increased over recent years. It is important to note that there has been a marked decline in the number of inpatient beds available for the treatment of mental illness in New Zealand. In the last 20 years, there was a decline from around 50 per hundred thousand to 28 per hundred thousand.[10] The average length of stay had fallen to 18 days and occupancy is often well over hundred percent. This is consistent with trends seen overseas.[10] Skipworth et al. found an increase in the number of people seen in prison services within 28 days of discharge from .6 to .9% of all discharges between 2012 and 2019. Maori were overrepresented as were Pacific peoples. They identified those released from inpatient units where homelessness and lack of meaningful employment were issues were more likely to find themselves incarcerated. This was noted by them to be congruent with the recognized increase in homelessness and social deprivation that occurred in New Zealand over that time.

The provision of care for people with serious mental illnesses in prisons in New Zealand is the responsibility of regional forensic psychiatric services. There are five regional services in New Zealand.[11] These services were developed in the early 1990s following a scathing review following several high-profile incidents in the community and prison.[12] The model of care developed was influenced by the medium secure care model in the United Kingdom.

The Mental Health (Compulsory Assessment and Treatment) Act 1992[13] allows for the transfer of acutely unwell prisoners to secure hospitals for treatment and this is a major function of the regional inpatient units. However, they are also responsible for the treatment and rehabilitation of mentally disordered offenders coming through the Courts. The combination of necessarily long-term treatment of mentally disordered offenders found unfit to stand trial or not guilty by reason of insanity, in conjunction with the lack of proportionate growth in acute inpatient beds in forensic services to match the growth in prison population, has led to increasing pressure on forensic inpatient units. This is reflected in the rate of transfer from prison to hospital. In 2001, when the forensic services were relatively new and well resourced, 2.31% of the overall prison population was transferred to the forensic units. By 2008 there had been a fall to 1.4%, and by 2015 these transfers were down to 0.67%.[14] Consistent with this the ratio of prison muster to forensic inpatient beds was 28.11 in 2013. By 2019 this had risen to 39.47.[7]

This parlous state of affairs for the treatment of mental illness, including psychosis, in prison has been pointed out. In 2020 the directors of the forensic psychiatric services wrote a critical article in which they highlighted the ways in which the treatment of mental illness in prisons was failing, including failing to meet the standards required of New Zealand, as a signatory to international human rights agreements.[15] This issue has recently been subject to media attention.[16] The lack of appropriately trained forensic psychiatrists has also been noted.[17] Of relevance, the Australian and New Zealand College of Psychiatrists are opposed to the use of involuntary treatment in prison, with good reason.[18] In New Zealand, there is no scope for involuntary treatment of mental illness within prison.[14]

Compulsory treatment in New Zealand

Compulsory treatment in New Zealand is permitted under the aegis of the Mental Health (Compulsory Assessment and Treatment) Act 1992.[13] This act defines mental disorders and allows for a person to be detained and treated without consent if they are mentally disordered. Mentally disordered is defined as "*an abnormal state of mind (whether of a continuous or an intermittent nature), characterized by delusions, or by disorders of mood or perception, volition or cognition, of such a degree that it- (a) poses a serious danger to the health and safety of that person or others; or (b) seriously diminishes the capacity of that person to take care of himself or herself.*" People are initially assessed in a two-step process facilitated by what is known as a Duly Authorized Officer and, with an assessment by a doctor and a further assessment by a psychiatrist, may then be subject to compulsory assessment and treatment for 5 days, usually as an inpatient though occasionally this is done in the community. Within those 5 days, a decision has to be made as to whether they should be subject to further compulsory assessment and treatment for a period of 14 days after which time an application can be made to the Family Court for a compulsory treatment order. These orders can either be as an inpatient or for treatment in the community.[19] Initially, orders can be made for a maximum of 6 months. A person made subject to compulsory treatment has the right to appeal both to a family court judge and subsequently to a tribunal. Repeat orders can be made for a further 6 months and, after recent reform, for a maximum of 1 year.

Several aspects of the definition of mental disorder merit further examination. The intent of the term mental disorder is deliberately to avoid reliance on diagnostic criteria.[20] There are specific exclusions that include substance abuse, intellectual disability, offending behavior, sexual preference, or political, religious, or cultural beliefs.

For practical purposes, the terms delusion and disorder of mood and perception are relatively straightforward. However, cognition and volition have both been recognized as being more difficult to conceptualize and define, noting the lack of a generally accepted psychiatric meaning. It is thought for the most part, these criteria are utilized for identifiable serious mental illnesses such as psychosis or mood disorder.[20] Personality disorders are neither specifically included nor excluded from the Mental Health Act.

Serious danger is generally understood to reflect the risk an individual may be violent toward others or alternatively to be at risk to themselves primarily through deliberate self-harm and attempted suicide. However, the concept can extend to other harms, such as the psychological harm caused by stalking behavior arising out of mental disorders.[19]

Of relevance to the issue of homelessness, seriously diminished capacity to care for oneself is "*not limited to the basic necessities of survival . . . It also includes "the multiplicity of other needs such as achieving financial security, maintaining proper social relationships, maintaining stable accommodation . . .* "[19] On this basis, an individual who suffers from schizophrenia, and as a result of the combination of impairments arising from that has become homeless, may meet the criteria for mental disorder within the meaning of the Act. A case-by-case approach is recognized as being important in analyzing whether they meet the criteria.

The current Act in New Zealand, therefore, allows for the use of compulsory treatment in situations where, as a result of psychotic illness, there is serious impairment in a person's capacity to care for themselves including rendering them homeless. Two questions arise from this. The first is how effective is this as an approach to the treatment of such individuals and the second is how often and what services may be available to assist such an individual?

Unsurprisingly, there is little limited information with regard to these questions. The issue as to whether compulsory treatment in the community is effective and ethical has been subject to debate. Beaglehole, Newton-Howes, and Frampton in 2021 commented on the intrusiveness of compulsory treatment orders, which in New Zealand means, for the most part, individuals are placed on depot antipsychotic medication and are subject to considerable intrusion as treating clinicians are able to enter premises and administer medication.[21] If they refuse, they may be admitted to the hospital for the injection. The authors note a cultural aspect to this issue. In New Zealand there are higher rates of mental illness in Maori compared to non-Maori[22] and Maori are more likely to be subject to compulsory inpatient and community treatment orders.[23] There is also variation in the frequency of the use of compulsory treatment orders between jurisdictions in New Zealand.[23] Encouragingly, Beaglehole et al. found evidence that, for people with psychotic disorders, the use of compulsory treatment orders in the community both reduced the number of admissions they had by a factor of 18% and reduced their length of stay in hospital by about 3 days.[21] This was utilizing a cohort design, and this made these findings more impressive as it may be the study design limited the ability to identify treatment effects for this group, as people who are more seriously unwell are more likely to be subject to compulsory treatment.

Although there is variability between services within New Zealand, often regions have assertive treatment teams to deal with those people with mental illness who are homeless and/or lacking in family support. These services often work with other agencies both publicly funded and NGOs who provide support and often accommodation for such individuals.

Reform of the Mental Health Act

In 2018 the government commissioned a review of mental health and addiction in New Zealand known as He Ara Oranga or the Government Enquiry into Mental Health and Addiction.[24] This wide-ranging review was released in November 2018 after extensive community engagement. It identified major failings in the current mental health services. It recommended a shift from "big psychiatry" to "big community" which was conceptualized as being a more holistic, recovery-based, culturally sensitive approach to dealing with people suffering from distress (rather than mental illness) and targeting around 20% of the population instead of the 3% that had been targeted previously in the development of mental health services. It noted "*People called for repeal and replacement of the mental health (Compulsory Assessment and Treatment) Act 1992 … And an end to seclusion and restraint … The Mental Health Act embeds archaic and risk-averse attitudes that cause clinicians to opt too readily for coercion and control."*

He Ara Oranga when released was not without controversy. It was noted the language within He Ara Oranga had a lineage that dated back to the reforms from the mid-20th century onwards, and that saw the deinstitutionalization and closure of psychiatric hospitals which have subsequently led to low numbers of hospital inpatient psychiatric beds in the English-speaking world. It was observed that ironically New Zealand already had "small psychiatry" by international standards. As a result, concerns have been raised about whether reform to mental health services and the Mental Health Act as recommended will improve the mental health of New Zealanders.[25]

The government on 6 May 2019 decided to repeal the Act. A high-level discussion document was released in 2021[26] and cabinet papers released in August 2023[27] provided clues as to the form the new Act is likely to take. It will focus on recovery, advanced directives, the inclusion of family and cultural bodies, and incorporate concepts from Te Tiriti O Waitangi (The Treaty of Waitangi, a foundational document signed in 1840 between representatives of the British Crown and some Maori iwi (tribes.)) It explicitly intends to reduce and ultimately end seclusion and reduce restraint. The intention is to minimize compulsion. There is an emphasis within the materials released thus far on the preservation of autonomy. It is apparent that there will be a shift to a three-limb test for mental disorder—an abnormal state of mind, serious danger or diminished capacity to care, and a requirement for incapacity. The details of this remain unclear, but an update from the Ministry of Health in April 2024, in the context of a round of consultation with stakeholders, confirms the direction the Act will take as part of an overhaul of services.[28] It is planned to emphasize the preservation of autonomy with supported decision-making, greater incorporation of cultural and family input, reduction in restrictive practices, and strengthened rights.

The move away from the use of language such as mental illness to well-being and distress highlights a key issue. The reforms and approaches outlined within He Ara Oranga and followed in the plans to repeal the Act may work well for individuals in

distress where medicalization of their distress is unhelpful or harmful. However, there is a real possibility that such an approach will not meet the needs of individuals with recognizable serious mental illnesses and associated problems with aggression and violence.[10] Based on what is known at this stage it seems likely that it will be harder to use compulsory treatment, both due to the added requirement for impairment of capacity and because of the expressed intent and changes described above.

A fixated threat perspective

Half of my time is spent working at the Fixated Threat Assessment Centre New Zealand (FTACNZ.) This is based on the United Kingdom (UKFTAC) and Australian models and sees police and mental health staff working together to deal with individuals who correspond or approach in concerning and threatening ways with Members of Parliament. The cornerstone of this service is research that identifies these people are commonly fixated and with high rates of serious mental illness.[29] Since its inception, initially as a small consultative group, and since July 2019 as a full-time service, FTACNZ has dealt with over 700 referrals. Half of those referred are readily identified as suffering from a psychotic illness with another 10% suffering from a mood disorder, usually bipolar affective disorder. Often, these individuals have either fallen out of treatment or have never been engaged in treatment. As senior clinical staff from UKFTAC have reflected, working in these services provides an opportunity to observe and reflect on the vicissitudes and effectiveness of services for those with serious mental illnesses, usually psychosis.[30] I find myself in a similar position in New Zealand. Commonly those referred have serious psychotic illnesses. Often their communications are chaotic, they may be petitioning or pleading for help with delusion-based persecution.

At times they are threatening, and their behavior can be both concerning and bizarre to recipients including staff of electorate offices scattered around the country and those who work at Parliament in Wellington. Usually, the distress these people are experiencing is palpable in their communication.

Commonly these individuals are itinerant and therefore homeless. Frequently, they are disorganized in their social circumstances, strongly motivated by their beliefs, and may travel from various parts of the country to Wellington where they may present at embassies and parliament before vanishing into the streets again. Sometimes they live in cars. These people pose several practical and ethical problems. Often, while their behaviors may be disorganized and bizarre, and they appear to be homeless, we lack sufficient information to be satisfied they meet the legal threshold for compulsory treatment. Further, the logistics of accessing such treatment becomes complex. They may present after hours, in which case it may fall to the police to firstly recognize they are mentally ill and secondly that their detention is justified (if they have committed a criminal offense they can be arrested, and if they are mentally ill in public, under section 109 of the Mental Health (Compulsory Assessment and Treatment) Act 1992,[13] they can be held by the police pending assessment.) A further obstacle to treatment is whether police can elicit an appropriate response from mental health services.

Sometimes, these logistical problems are resolved when the person commits a usually relatively minor offense, often understandable in the context of their illness, and then is forced to attend court where they may be assessed, through the Court Liaison arm of Forensic Mental Health Services. Often, however, we may be aware of individuals who we believe are seriously mentally ill, and likely seriously impaired in their capacity to care for themselves, as well as distressed and causing harm to themselves and those around them yet we are unable to locate them or arrange for them to have assessment and provision of treatment they may need. Often, as psychosis and behavior ebb and flow, the individual may cease to communicate. However, occasionally and tragically, they may engage in low-base rate but high-harm events. In this regard, the recent stabbing and death of six individuals at the Bondi Junction shopping center[31] forces us to consider how we should approach such individuals and whether there is a better way of dealing with the chaos and distress caused by their illness. It would be rare for such individuals to act in such an appallingly violent and tragic manner, yet equally, their combination of distress, psychosis, and poor engagement socially and with mental health services surely merits a more robust, targeted, and compassionate approach.

Conclusions

Existing Mental Health Act legislation in New Zealand does allow for compulsory treatment of people with schizophrenia who, as a result of their illness, are seriously incapacitated in their ability to care for themselves, with a potential outcome of homelessness. Throughout the country, there are services geared toward treating these individuals, although the extent to which they can meet their needs and their effectiveness overall is unclear. Services within prisons have degraded since their inception in the early 1990s because of the increase in demand and the lack of provision of further inpatient beds and services to meet the demand. Similarly, adult mental health services increasingly struggle as the number of beds available to admit seriously mentally ill individuals has decreased. Reform of the current Mental Health Act is likely to be in the direction of emphasizing autonomy, minimizing the use of compulsory treatment, and likely making it more difficult to coercively treat homeless individuals with psychosis. The FTAC perspective allows for a qualitative, meta-position that illustrates the complexities of dealing with homeless people with schizophrenia, endurance of suffering for these people, and the harm they can cause others.

References

1. Database OAH. *HC3.1. Homeless Population.* OECD-Social Policy Division Directorate of Employment, Labour and Social Affairs; 2021.

2. Te Tūāpapa Kura Kāinga – Ministry of Housing and Urban Development. *Homelessness Outlook Indicators of Homelessness.* 2024. Accessed July 01, 2024. www .hud.govt.nz/stats-and-insights/homelessness-out look/homelessness-indicators#tabset

3. Williams A. *Rates of Homeless Māori in Auckland Should Be a Wake-Up Call, Experts Say.* 2019. Accessed July 01, 2024. www.rnz.co.nz/news/te-manu-korihi/3 90553/rates-of-homeless-maori-in-auckland-should-b e-a-wake-up-call-experts-say#:~:text=Experts%20on% 20homelessness%20say%20figures,call%20to%20fix%2 0the%20problem.&text=The%20first%20city%2Dwide %20census,proportion%20living%20in% 20temporary %20accommodation

4. Peace RKS. Mental health and housing research: housing needs and sustainable independent living. *Soc. Policy J N Zeal.* 2001;**17**:101–123.

5. Almeida R. Homeless Missing Out on Vital Psychiatric Care—Researcher. 2024. Accessed July 01, 2024. www .rnz.co.nz/news/national/505899/homeless-missing-o ut-on-vital-psychiatric-care-researcher

6. Ayano G, Tesfaw G, Shumet S. The prevalence of schizophrenia and other psychotic disorders among homeless people: a systematic review and meta-analysis. *BMC Psychiatry* 2019;**19**(1):370.

7. Ara Poutama Aoteatroa Department of Corrections. Prison Facts and Statistics—March 2024. 2024. Accessed July 01, 2024. www.corrections.govt.nz/reso urces/statistics/quarterly_prison_statistics/prison_fact s_and_statistics_-_march_2024

8. Brinded, PM, Simpson AI, Laidlaw TM, Fairley N, Malcolm F. Prevalence of psychiatric disorders in New Zealand prisons: a national study. *Aust N Z J Psychiatry* 2001;**35**(2):166–173.

9. Indig DG, Wilhelm CK. Comorbid Substance Use Disorders and Mental Health Disorders among New Zealand Prisoners; 2016.

10. Skipworth, J, Garrett N, Pillai K, Tapsell R, McKenna B. Imprisonment following discharge from mental health units: A developing trend in New Zealand. *Front Psychiatry* 2023;**14**:1038803.

11. McKenna BSL. Models of Care in Forensic Mental Health Services: A Review of the International and National Literature; 2021.

12. Mason KR, Bennett H. The Committee of Inquiry into Procedures used in Certain Psychiatric Hospitals in Relation to Admission. Discharge or Release on Leave of Certain Classes of Patients; 1988.

13. Parliamentary Counsel Office. *Mental Health Compulsory Assessment and Treatment Act 1992*. New Zealand Parliament; 2023.

14. Carroll A, Ellis A, Aboud A, Scott R, Pillai K. No involuntary treatment of mental illness in Australian and New Zealand prisons. *J Forensic Psychiatry Psychol*. 2020;**32**(1):1–28.

15. Monasterio KE-P, Norris S, Short J, et al. Mentally ill people in our prisons are suffering human rights violations. *N Zeal Med J*. 2020;**133**:9–13.

16. Arnold N. Mentally Ill and Behind Bars: The Poor Guy Shouldn't Be in Jail. 2022. Accessed July 01, 2024. www .rnz.co.nz/news/in-depth/469434/mentally-ill-and-behi nd-bars-the-poor-guy-shouldn-t-be-in-jail

17. Blackwell F. Shortage of Forensic Psychiatrists, In-Patient Beds Could Impact Prisoners. 2023. Accessed July 01, 2024. www.rnz.co.nz/news/national/490928/s hortage-of-forensic-psychiatrists-in-patient-beds-coul d-impact-prisoners

18. Royal Australian and New Zealand College of Psychiatrists. Position Statement: Involuntary Mental Health Treatment in Custody; 2017.

19. Ministry of Health. Guidelines to the Mental Health (Compulsory Assessment and Treatment) Act 1992; 2022.

20. Brookbanks WSS. *Psychiatry and the Law*. First ed. Lexis Nexis; 2007.

21. Beaglehole B, Newton-Howes G, Frampton C. Compulsory Community Treatment Orders in New Zealand and the provision of care: An examination of national databases and predictors of outcome. *Lancet Reg Health West Pac*. 2021;**17**:100275.

22. Wells JO-B, Scott M, McGee K, Baxter M, Kokaua J. Prevalence, interference with life and severity of 12 month DSM-IV disorders in Te Rau Hinengaro: The New Zealand Mental Health Survey. *Aust N Zeal J Psychiatry*. 2006;**40**:845–854.

23. Ministry of Health. Office of the Director of Mental Health and Addictions Services Regulatory Report 1 July 2021 to 30 June 2022. 2023.

24. Paterson RD, Disley M, Rangihuna B, Tiatia-Seath D, Tualamali'i J. He Ara Oranga: Report of the Government Inquiry onto Mental Health and Addiction. 2018.

25. Allison S, Bastiampillai T, Castle D, Mulder R, Beaglehole B. The He Ara Oranga report: what's wrong with 'Big Psychiatry' in New Zealand? *Aust N Z J Psychiatry*. 2019;**53**(8):724–726.

26. Ministry of Health. *Transforming Our Mental Health Law: A Public Discussion Document*. Ministry of Health New Zealand; 2021.

27. Ministry of Health. *Cabinet Material and Briefings: Transforming Mental Health Law: Second Tranche of Policy Decisions*. Ministry of Health New Zealand; 2023.

28. Ministry of Health. *Repeal and Replacement of the Mental Health Act: Summary of What We Heard During the Regional hui Held in March and April 2024*. Ministry of Health New Zealand; 2024.

29. Barry-Walsh J, James DV, Mullen PE. Fixated Threat Assessment Centers: preventing harm and facilitating care in public figure threat cases and those thought to be at risk of lone-actor grievance-fueled violence. *CNS Spectr*. 2020;**25**(5):630–637.

30. Wilson S, Farnham F, Taylor A, Taylor R. Reflections on working in public-figure threat management. *Med Sci Law*. 2019;**59**(4):275–281.

31. Turnbull T. Sydney Stabbing: Bondi Attack on Women Devastates Australia. 2024. Accessed July 01, 2024. www.bbc.com/news/world-australia-68852486

Autonomy and Compulsory Care in the Netherlands

Esther Nauta and Gerben Meynen

Introduction[1]

In the Netherlands, compulsory care of patients with mental disorders such as schizophrenia is regulated by the Law on Compulsory Mental Healthcare[2] (*Wet verplichte geestelijke gezondheidszorg*, or Wvggz). This law replaces its predecessor, the Law on Special Admissions to Psychiatric Hospitals (*Wet bijzondere opnemingen in psychiatrische ziekenhuizen*, or Bopz). The legislative process for this new law took over a decade to conclude. Discussions in parliament, with clinicians, and in civil society focused on the complexity of the relevant legal procedures and on the autonomy and legal position of the patients. In this chapter, we discuss the Wvggz, its background, and the central procedures for the judicial authorization of compulsory care. We also discuss which forms of compulsory care the Wvggz allows – as the Wvggz provides options for compulsory care in mental health clinics, but also at home and in community settings. While the Wvggz is a complex law with many elements, in this chapter we focus on the various ways in which the Wvggz is purportedly aimed at *enhancing autonomy* of patients with severe mental illness. In conclusion, we show how Dutch regulations aimed at enhancing autonomy also create more complexity and bureaucracy.

Background to the law on compulsory mental health care

As of 2020, the Wvggz has replaced the 1994 Bopz.[3] Under the regime of the Bopz, all compulsory care for mental health patients had to take place in psychiatric hospitals. As such, the Bopz was a hospitalization regime. This was considered to be unsustainable, and parliamentary efforts to implement more modern legislation started as early as 2008. The focus of the new regulations was that compulsory psychiatry no longer had to involve the forced hospitalization of the patient in all cases. Under the new system, other forms of compulsory care, such as administering forced medication to the individual at home, would also become possible. Rather than a hospitalization regime, the new legal framework would provide a regime for (coercive) care more broadly.

Moreover, the new legislation, through a distinction between two separate laws, was intended to ensure the provision of treatment that is better tailored to the specific patient group.

During the legislative process, much emphasis was placed on the legal position or protection of the patient. Through new kinds of procedures and more communication with patients and their relatives, the new legal framework was supposed to enhance patient autonomy, which we discuss in more detail later in this chapter.

During the lengthy legislative process, strong criticism was repeatedly voiced regarding the proposals for this new legislation. Practitioners and lawyers alike warned that these laws would cause implementation issues (including a lot of bureaucracy) and allow for excessive intrusion into the patient's personal privacy. Nevertheless, the new legislation entered into force in January 2020. Since then, the Wvggz has been amended multiple times. It has been called a "bureaucratic monster," but it is also considered to be valuable.[4]

A central goal of the introduction of this new legal regime was to reduce coercive care.[5] However, analysis of the data gathered to date shows that such a reduction in coercive measures has not yet taken place.

The Wvggz and the authorization for compulsory care

Procedure

As many politicians, clinicians, and lawyers have noted, the Wvggz is very complex and difficult to comprehend even for lawyers and seasoned practitioners.[6] There are basically two procedures. The first procedure is for very urgent situations in which immediate action needs to be taken. Here, it is not a judge but the mayor who authorizes (temporary) compulsory care. In the second, regular procedure, it is the judge who gives such an authorization (*zorgmachtiging*). Although compulsory care for the interest of the patient and/or interest of society is substantively, of course, a matter of public law, in the Netherlands it is the civil judge who decides whether such an authorization might be given. To make matters more unusual, it is the "civil" public prosecutor who petitions the civil judge for such an authorization.

The Wvggz requires a complicated and elaborate preparation of a petition for an authorization for the compulsory care of mental health patients.[7] As soon as the public prosecutor starts with the preparation of such a petition, they appoint a medical director (*geneesheer-directeur*). The medical director is a psychiatrist affiliated with a mental health care institution, who is responsible for the legal procedures regarding compulsory care. The medical director then appoints an independent psychiatrist who must see the patient and draft a medical statement about the mental health of the individual involved. The psychiatrist has access to relevant information, such as police and judicial data. The medical statement must mention which symptoms the individual exhibits, the (preliminary) diagnosis of the mental disorder, the relationship between the disorder and the behavior leading to the risk of serious harm, and, specifically, what forms of compulsory care are needed to reduce the risk of harm. Several types of disorders are distinguished in the form. The form, for example, includes neurobiological developmental disorders (such as autism), schizophrenia spectrum disorders and other psychotic disorders, and bipolar mood disorders. A study of compulsory admissions in Amsterdam during 15 years under the old legal regime of the Bopz showed that 32.0% of these patients were diagnosed with schizophrenia, and 30.5% with other psychotic illnesses.[8] We expect that under the new law, in principle, the percentages of psychotic illness in general and schizophrenia in particular are likely to be similar, because there have not been drastic changes in the number of people receiving compulsory care.[9]

In addition to a psychiatrist, the medical director also appoints a care manager (*zorgverantwoordelijke*). This care manager establishes a proposal for a care plan, which outlines the compulsory treatment that the patient should receive. After the medical director has determined that the proposed care plan meets the legal requirements of the Wvggz, they pass on their findings and the proposal for a care plan to the public prosecutor. In the petition, the public prosecutor substantiates which forms of compulsory care should be included in the care authorization. Unlike the regime of the Bopz, which only provided for compulsory hospitalization, the Wvggz allows for outpatient care as well. This could include administering medication and supervising the patient in their home or in community care. The forms of compulsory care that can be included in the authorization are listed in the Wvggz. Examples are administering fluids, food, and medication. Notably, patients have the possibility to write their own plan (*plan van aanpak*) in order to avoid compulsory care. If the patient makes use of this possibility, the independent psychiatrist has to take this alternative plan into account and to evaluate its feasibility. Based on the petition and the accompanying information, eventually the judge decides on the authorization for compulsory care. The decision-making framework for the judge is discussed in the next subsection.

Criteria

When deciding whether to authorize compulsory care, the Wvggz stipulates that the judge tests three central criteria. First, the patient must suffer from a *mental disorder*. Second, there must be a *risk of harm* either to the person themselves, to other people, or to both. This risk has to be a result of the mental disorder. Third, the proposed forms of compulsory care have to be *proportionate*. This means that there are no other options to reduce the risk of harm and no options for voluntary treatment (necessity), that it is reasonably expected that the compulsory care will be effective (suitability), and that the giving of compulsory care is proportionate considering the goal of preventing harm (proportionality). The Wvggz explicitly states that compulsory care has to be a *last resort*.

Compulsory care and autonomy

The Wvggz regime has a few components that are meant to enhance the autonomy of the patient.

Some of these were newly introduced with the Wvggz, while others existed under the previous regime of the Bopz as well. First, the possibility of home and community treatment – rather that hospitalization in all cases – is meant to allow for more proportionate and less intrusive forms of compulsory care. This possibility is new and was a core aspiration of the Wvggz.

Second, the Wvggz includes the possibility for self-binding directives (SBDs). Through a SBD, a patient can give advance consent to specific forms of mental health care during a mental health crisis.[10] The Netherlands is one of the very few jurisdictions in the world with provisions for SBDs for mental health patients.[11] SBDs are aimed at enhancing patient autonomy by giving them the opportunity to decide for themselves what kind of compulsory health care they consider to be beneficial in certain scenarios.

Third, the wishes and opinions of a patient have to be respected (*wilsbekwaam verzet*), unless they are incompetent, their life is in immediate danger, or they pose a serious risk to others. In this way, patients can be (co)decision-makers about their own treatment.

Furthermore, the Wvggz stipulates what should be the *purpose* of the compulsory care, and the relevant purposes need to be specified in the proposal for the care plan. In this regard, the Wvggz explicitly mentions restoring the mental health of the person concerned in such a way that they *regain their autonomy as much as possible.*

So, interestingly, while coercive measures are usually considered to be detrimental to the autonomy of the patient, in the regime of the Wvggz coercive measures are (at least in some cases) considered to be aimed at restoring autonomy. The assumption seems to be that a severe mental illness may compromise a person's autonomy, and, consequently, by restoring the person's mental health, autonomy may be restored (on autonomy and coercive measures, see Prinsen and van Delden[12]). This may also be relevant for people who are not competent to decide about treatment of a physical illness due to their mental disorder. In such cases, the coercive measure can be aimed at restoring competency so that the patient can make a competent decision about the treatment of their physical illness.[13]

The new legal regime has in practice resulted in an increase in bureaucracy and paperwork. For example, Van Melle et al. write that "obtaining legal authorization for providing compulsory care based on an SBD remains subject to highly complex and lengthy formal procedures."[14] Barkhof and Niele write: "[T]he law is too complex, and the administrative burden is enormous. The information obligation includes too many letters to the patient, which frustrates both the patient and the care provider, is at the expense of contact and is very expensive."[15] They conclude: "While the Legislature intended to improve the legal position with the introduction of the Wvggz … this was not achieved properly in the implementation." It is our impression that their view about the new law is shared by many. Still, the core ideas behind the law are laudable, and the inclusion of the restoration of autonomy as a goal can be considered valuable.

Conclusions

In 2020, a new legal regime on compulsory care in mental health came into effect in the Netherlands. One of its core aims was to strengthen the position of the patient. Notably, the law also explicitly recognizes that coercive measures may be taken not only for the purpose of preventing harm, but also to restore a patient's autonomy. This is interesting, as coercive measures usually would be conceived of as diminishing a patient's autonomous choice, while here they are meant to increase a patient's ability to make autonomous decisions about their future treatment and their lives in general. We feel that this is a valuable idea. Still, the law has become an administrative burden. Following its requirements takes a lot of time – time that then cannot be spent providing actual care and real contact and support to the patient. In a way, this illustrates that it can be challenging to translate valuable ideas into effective laws, especially in a field as complex as mental health care.

References

1. This paper is partly based on Nauta EE. *Vrijheid, veiligheid en evenredigheid: terbeschikkingstelling in rechtsvergelijkend en grondrechtelijk perspectief*, 1st edition. Den Haag: Boom Juridisch, 2025.

2. See also Scholten M, van Melle L, Widdershoven G. Self-binding directives under the new Dutch law on compulsory mental health care: An analysis of the legal framework and a proposal for reform. *Int J Law Psychiatry.* 2021;76:101699. doi:10.1016/j.ijlp.2021.101699.

3. The Bopz had been split into two mental regimes: one for patients with mental disorders (Wvggz) and one for

patients with mental disabilities or psychogeriatric disorders (Wzd).

4. Ten Houte de Lange, S. Onwerkbaar maar niet onbruikbaar. *Zorgvisie.* 2020;**50**:34–36. doi:10.1007/s41187-020-0951-0.

5. Noorthoorn EO, Gemsa S, Broer J, et al. Trends in gedwongen opnames en zorg in de periode 2003–2023 in Nederland. *Tijdschr Psychiatr.* 2024;**66**(8):483–488.

6. See also Barkhof E, Niele MM. Wetten voor verplichte ggz in Nederland, een verbetering? [Laws for mandatory mental health care in the Netherlands]. *Tijdschr Psychiatr.* 2024;**66**(8): 465–469.

7. See Nauta EE. *Vrijheid, veiligheid en evenredigheid: terbeschikkingstelling in rechtsvergelijkend en grondrechtelijk perspectief,* 1st edition. Den Haag: Boom Juridisch, 2025.

8. Nusselder KJ, Zoeteman J, Buis B, et al. Trends in acute opnames in Amsterdam; 15 jaar acute psychiatrie in een steeds vollere stad [Trends in emergency admissions in Amsterdam. Fifteen years of emergency psychiatry in an increasingly crowded city]. *Tijdschr Psychiatr.* 2020;**62**(7):530–540.

9. Noorthoorn EO, Gemsa S, Broer J, et al. Trends in gedwongen opnames en zorg in de periode 2003–2023 in Nederland. *Tijdschr Psychiatr.* 2024;**66**(8):483–488.

10. See Scholten M, van Melle L, Widdershoven G. Self-binding directives under the new Dutch law on compulsory mental health care: An analysis of the legal framework and a proposal for reform. *Int J Law Psychiatry.* 2021;**76**:101699. doi:10.1016/j.ijlp.2021.101699.

11. Van Melle L, van der Ham L, Voskes Y, Widdershoven G, Scholten M. Opportunities and challenges of self-binding directives: An interview study with mental health service users and professionals in the Netherlands. *BMC Med Ethics.* 2023;**24**(1):38.

12. Prinsen EJD, van Delden JJM. Can we justify eliminating coercive measurements in psychiatry? *J Med Ethics,* 2009;**35**:69–73.

13. Plomp E, Legemaate J. *Verdiepingsonderzoek Uitvoering Wvggz: goede voorbeelden uit de praktijk.* Den Haag: ZonMw, 2024, p. 325.

14. Van Melle L, van der Ham L, Voskes Y, Widdershoven G, Scholten M. Opportunities and challenges of self-binding directives: An interview study with mental health service users and professionals in the Netherlands. *BMC Med Ethics.* 2023;**24**(1):38.

15. Barkhof E, Niele MM. Wetten voor verplichte ggz in Nederland, een verbetering? [Laws for mandatory mental health care in the Netherlands]. *Tijdschr Psychiatr.* 2024;**66**(8):465–469.

Canadian Mental Health Laws
A Review of Involuntary Admission and Treatment Pending Appeal

Lyndal C. Petit, Karen Shin, Nicole Fielding, Mathieu Dufour, and John Gray

Introduction

Canada provides publicly funded health care that is governed regionally by its 10 provinces and three territories. Mental health legislation differs across the country, but most jurisdictions follow similar principles. Instead of being considered a strict legal issue requiring court authorization as in the USA, most Canadian jurisdictions regard involuntary admissions as medical matters that are authorized by physicians, subject to specific criteria set out in the relevant mental health legislation. In all jurisdictions, involuntary admission may be authorized when a person has a mental disorder that poses a risk of harm to self or others. Jurisdictions vary with respect to their definition of a mental disorder, the probability, timing, and nature of harm required for an involuntary admission, deterioration and physical impairment clauses, treatment requirements or clauses, and whether a finding of incapacity is required for the involuntary admission. A number of jurisdictions specify the person must not be suitable as a voluntary patient. In interpreting involuntary admission criteria, one must look at all elements of the criteria and legislation as a whole.

Mental disorder definition

Ontario's Mental Health Act (MHA) contains the broadest definition of a mental disorder, specifying it is "any disease or disability of the mind."[1] In Quebec, the courts can order a temporary confinement if they have "serious reasons to believe that a person is a danger to himself or others owing to his mental state."[2]

All other Canadian jurisdictions have more narrow mental disorder definitions. In British Columbia, a person with a mental disorder "means a person who has a disorder of the mind that requires treatment and seriously impairs the person's ability (a) to react appropriately to the person's environment, or (b) to

associate with others."[3] To meet British Columbia's mental disorder definition, treatment for the disorder must not just be advisable; it must be required. Although differences exist, the remaining jurisdictions define a mental disorder or serious mental illness using similar language. As an example, in the Northwest Territories, a "'mental disorder' means a substantial disorder of thought, mood, perception, orientation or memory that grossly impairs judgement, behaviour, capacity to recognize reality or ability to meet the ordinary demands of life."[4] A number of jurisdictions add that treatment[5] or psychiatric treatment[6–8] is advisable or that the disorder is amenable to treatment,[9] and three have exclusions either related to intellectual disability[10,11] or acquired or congenital irreversible brain injury.[12]

A narrow mental disorder definition helps prevent legislative criteria from being applied over-broadly and focuses involuntary admission to those who require it due to serious mental illness.

Harm timing and probability

All jurisdictions permit involuntary admission when a mental disorder, serious mental illness, or mental state is causing a risk of harm, if all other necessary criteria are met.

Most jurisdictions require the harm risk be likely (Table 21.1), demonstrated on the standard of a balance of probabilities. "Likely" means a probable risk – one that is more likely than not (i.e., one that is greater than 50% on a balance of probabilities). Using this standard excludes involuntary admission for harms of lower likelihood.

Probability estimates have limitations. They are imprecise and have been wrong. A "likely" requirement doesn't adapt to when a <51% risk may warrant involuntary admission, such as for extreme

Table 21.1 Harm probability requirements

Likely to cause	Has caused OR likely to cause	Is threatening or attempting to cause serious harm to self or has recently done so OR has recently caused serious harm to self OR is seriously harming or threatening serious harm to another or has recently done so	The court must have serious reasons to believe that the person is dangerous and that the person's confinement is necessary	Requires care, supervision, and control in or through a designated facility for the protection of the person or the patient or the protection of others
Alberta, Manitoba, Saskatchewan, Ontario, New Brunswick[a], Newfoundland and Labrador, Yukon, Northwest Territories, Nunavut	Prince Edward Island	Nova Scotia	Quebec	British Columbia

[a] New Brunswick: The person's recent behavior must demonstrate that, due to the serious mental illness, the person is likely to cause serious harm.[11]

harm concerns, as with the risk for a bombing or mass shooting. Practically, the acceptable risk varies with the severity of anticipated harm. "Likely" has been interpreted to have a temporal limit. The anticipated harm must be likely to "occur within some reasonably proximate time."[13]

Some jurisdictions do not specify a required likelihood of harm for involuntary admission. Nova Scotia's MHA makes no mention of "likely" harm. Rather, the person "is threatening or attempting to cause serious harm to himself or herself or has recently done so, has recently caused serious harm to himself or herself," or alternatively "is seriously harming or is threatening serious harm towards another person or has recently done so."[6] New Brunswick requires that the likely serious harm or deterioration risk be demonstrated in the person's recent behavior.[11]

Focusing on current or recent harmful behavior, at the exclusion of prior serious harm, removes an important risk factor in harm analysis, particularly when the prior serious harm is likely to be repeated given the patient's presentation.[14]

Prince Edward Island considers prior harm and likely risk of harm by requiring that, because of the mental disorder, the person "has caused or is likely to cause harm to the person or others."[7] In Quebec, the civil code makes no mention of "likely" risk of harm,

and it does not specify a restriction to recent harmful behavior. Rather, the court assesses the person with input from two psychiatric examinations completed by physicians, and it can order confinement if it "has serious reasons to believe that the person is dangerous and that the person's confinement is necessary."[2] However, a decision from the Quebec Court of Appeal specified there must be a significant danger or a high potential for danger. It does not have to be imminent, but must be – if not probable – at least clearly possible in the present or relatively near future, which would justify immediate custody.[15] In British Columbia, a person with a mental disorder can be involuntarily admitted when the person requires it for their or another person's protection.[3] Protection includes the "notion of harm."[16] The harm risk analysis can include the patient's current presentation and prior harm due to mental illness.

Type of harm

Exclusive bodily harm criteria is not a Canadian Charter requirement, and the vast majority of Canadian jurisdictions recognize non-bodily harms as well as bodily harms as grounds for involuntary admission when other criteria are met. When legislation doesn't specify a required harm severity, the presumption is that the harm must be serious enough to require involuntary admission.[14] Non-bodily harms have been interpreted to include vocational, financial, social, or family life serious harms.[16] Recognizing non-bodily harms for involuntary admission allows individuals to access health care when they need it to prevent the serious social harms of no treatment.

Ontario and Yukon specify that there must be a likely risk for serious bodily harm to self or others.[1,17] The Quebec courts interpret "dangerous" to mean physical danger.[18,19] "Danger" is defined in a specific (i.e., personalized) and precise manner by the Quebec Court of Appeal, including that the risk of its realization must be high, without its materialization necessarily being imminent.[20]

Bodily harm is not defined by Ontario and Yukon's mental health legislation. In Canada's Criminal Code, "bodily harm" means "any hurt or injury to a person that interferes with the health or comfort of the person and that is more than merely transient or trifling in nature."[21] Someone who behaves aggressively because of psychiatric symptoms may incur criminal charges without reaching the threshold of warranting involuntary psychiatric care.

Restricting involuntary admission to only bodily harm risks or physical danger excludes individuals who need involuntary admission to address the non-bodily harms and nonphysical dangers of untreated serious mental illness such as scholastic attrition, unemployment, vocational loss, eviction, strained relationships, estrangement, marital separation, loss of child custody, homelessness, isolation, and/or incarceration. Such harms result in detrimental and pervasive consequences that are very difficult to recover from. Families can become burned out trying to compensate for the untreated illnesses' dire effects while trying not to lose their family member to a marginalized life in shelters or on the streets.[22] Without access to involuntary admission, care is either never accessed or is delayed until the person causes serious bodily harm or physical danger or becomes a likely risk for it.

The majority of Canadian jurisdictions allow for a more comprehensive understanding of harm that can be incurred against oneself or others and do not include the wording of "bodily harm." In British Columbia, the criterion of protection includes the social, family, work, or financial life of the patient.[23] Alberta's wording protects individuals from suffering negative effects due to their mental illness.[12] These broader

Table 21.2 Type of harm required

Harm/serious harm/for protection	Bodily harm/ serious bodily harm/dangerous
British Columbia (protection), Alberta (harm to others or suffer negative effects), Manitoba (serious harm), Saskatchewan (harm), New Brunswick (serious harm), Nova Scotia (serious harm), Prince Edward Island (harm), Newfoundland and Labrador (harm), Northwest Territories (serious harm), Nunavut (serious harm)	Ontario (serious bodily harm), Yukon (serious bodily harm), Quebec (dangerous)

definitions in turn promote equitable care access and allow for involuntary admission to address non-bodily harms when other criteria are met (Table 21.2).

Serious physical impairment or substantial mental or physical deterioration

Several jurisdictions allow for involuntary admission to address a likely risk of serious physical impairment, which has been interpreted as the unintentional and serious harm that will likely come to the person because of the risky activities they engage in due to the mental disorder.[24] Examples can include disorganized behaviors due to psychosis that would likely cause a fight or cause a person to walk into traffic and result in serious physical impairment.

Most jurisdictions allow for involuntary admission to address a likely risk for substantial mental or physical deterioration when other criteria are met (Table 21.3).[1,4,5,7–12] These deterioration clauses mean that the mental or physical symptoms or illness will likely get worse unless the person is admitted and treated for the mental disorder. They allow involuntary admission to occur before serious harm.[25]

In New Brunswick, the likely risk for substantial mental or physical deterioration must be in the context of recently demonstrated behavior.[11] Nova Scotia requires that the deterioration or impairment be expected with certainty. Its clause specifies that the person "will suffer serious physical impairment or serious mental deterioration, or both."[6]

Table 21.3 Deterioration and impairment clauses

Substantial or serious mental or physical deterioration	Substantial or serious physical or mental impairment	None
Likely	*Likely physical or mental impairment*	Quebec
Alberta	Yukon[e]	
Manitoba	Prince Edward Island	
New Brunswick[a]	*Likely physical impairment*	
Newfoundland and Labrador	Alberta	
Nunavut	Newfoundland and Labrador	
Northwest Territories	Northwest Territories	
Prince Edward Island	Nunavut	
Saskatchewan	Ontario	
Ontario[b]	*Other*	
Other	Nova Scotia[d]	
British Columbia[c]		
Nova Scotia[d]		

[a] New Brunswick: The person's recent behavior must demonstrate that, due to the serious mental illness, the person is likely to suffer substantial mental or physical deterioration.[11]

[b] Ontario: The patient must have a past response to treatment and be incapable regarding treatment in a psychiatric facility, and substitute decision-maker consent must be obtained.[1]

[c] British Columbia: "requires care, supervision and control in or through a designated facility to prevent the person's or patient's substantial mental or physical deterioration or for the protection of the person or patient or the protection of others."[3]

[d] Nova Scotia: "will suffer serious physical impairment or serious mental deterioration, or both."[6]

[e] Yukon: "the person's impending serious mental or physical impairment."[17]

A likely risk of substantial mental or physical deterioration may be defended when a person is re-presenting with early symptoms of a prior illness or based on the patient's presentation and the physician's knowledge of the illness's course.[25] Deterioration clauses have limitations as they may not apply if the course of illness is unclear or if the patient appears to be at the peak of the deterioration.

In Ontario, the likely risk of substantial mental or physical deterioration can only be relied on to support meeting the criteria for an involuntary admission if the person is currently incapable with respect to psychiatric treatment, substitute decision-maker consent for treatment has been obtained, and the person has demonstrated clinical improvement with prior treatment for the same or a similar mental disorder.[1]

Requiring a past response to treatment can place a person who is mentally or physically deteriorating due to mental illness and who lacks a past response to treatment into a "chicken and egg" situation: They cannot be admitted involuntarily for treatment because they have no past response to treatment, but they do not have a history of response to treatment because they cannot be admitted under involuntary admission criteria.[22]

Requiring a past response to treatment as part of meeting the criteria for an involuntary admission due to a likely risk of substantial deterioration becomes discriminatory because such patients cannot access involuntary admission when needed to address substantial mental or physical deterioration.[22] Even more confoundingly, patients who have made prior expressed capable wishes to receive treatment under these circumstances would not be able to access involuntary hospitalization and psychiatric care unless there is a past response to treatment.

Incapacity

Some jurisdictions require that the person be incapable with respect to treatment or care and supervision for involuntary admission to occur (Table 21.4).

Saskatchewan and Newfoundland and Labrador require enhanced criteria for determining capacity such that people assessed as capable for making treatment decisions are fully aware of the consequences of their decisions.[5,8] For example, Newfoundland and Labrador's legislation says that, as a result of the mental disorder, the person "is unable to fully appreciate the nature and consequences of the mental disorder or to make an informed decision regarding his or her need for treatment or care and supervision."[8] Nova Scotia does not specify "fully" in its criteria. It elaborates in detail

Table 21.4 Jurisdictions that require a finding of incapacity for involuntary admission

Incapacity required	Incapacity not required
Saskatchewan (lack of enhanced capacity)	British Columbia
Newfoundland and Labrador (lack of enhanced capacity)	Alberta
	Manitoba
Nova Scotia[a]	New Brunswick
Ontario[b]	Prince Edward Island
	Ontario[b]
	Quebec
	Yukon
	Northwest Territories
	Nunavut

[a] Nova Scotia: Patients must be incapable of making admission and treatment decisions. Capacity may be with or without support.[6]

[b] Ontario requires that the person be found incapable of consent to treatment in a psychiatric facility and a past response to treatment to allow involuntary admission for a likely risk of substantial mental or physical deterioration when other criteria are met.[1]

what one must be able to understand and appreciate with respect to treatment and specifies capacity may be with or without support.[6]

In practice, the level of capacity required to consent to a treatment depends on the seriousness and complexity of the issue.[14] Minor interventions may require a casual understanding or appreciation to accept treatment. For example, taking a painkiller for a headache might not require detailed discussions of risks and benefits. However, when the consequences of refusing treatment are severe, such as with inpatient psychiatric treatment for serious mental illness to prevent serious harms, a high threshold for being capable of making a decision about treatment ensures informed decisions are made with full awareness of the risks and benefits of the decision. This means that people with low or partial capacity may still access treatment for their illnesses when they don't fully appreciate the likely risks of serious harm, physical impairment, or substantial mental or physical deterioration from no treatment.

In Ontario, an individual can be involuntarily admitted when, due to a mental disorder, they are at likely risk of serious bodily harm to self or others or of serious physical impairment unless they remain in the custody of a psychiatric facility. Incapacity to consent to treatment in a psychiatric facility is required for involuntary admission when it is to address a likely risk of substantial mental or physical deterioration.[1] In Ontario, a person is considered capable of consenting to a particular form of treatment if they "are able to understand the information that is relevant to making a decision about the treatment" and are "able to appreciate the reasonably foreseeable consequences of a decision or lack of decision."[26]

The Supreme Court of Canada held that, in determining capacity to make decisions regarding treatment in Ontario, the patient does not need to agree with the diagnosis or view the condition in negative terms. The patient "must be able to recognize the possibility that he is affected by that condition," and that "if the patient's condition results in him being unable to recognize that he is affected by its manifestations, he will be unable to apply the relevant information to his circumstances, and unable to appreciate the consequences of his decision."[27] A lower threshold for being deemed capable means a person may refuse treatment without fully understanding or fully appreciating the consequences of their decision. The Supreme Court also noted that capacity can fluctuate.[27]

Need for treatment

Most jurisdictions specify a treatment component in their involuntary admission requirements.

Some Canadian jurisdictions have a purpose written in their legislation and include the provision of treatment as a main objective.[7,8,11] Specifying treatment as the purpose helps with Act interpretation. The purpose frames whether the intent of involuntary admission is to treat the mental disorder in order to improve the person's condition and stop the harm caused by the serious mental illness – including, if required, to provide the treatment involuntarily. Alternatively, the purpose of the involuntary admission would be harm prevention through confinement, and treatment would only be given if it is voluntarily accepted.[14]

Including "need for treatment" in involuntary admission requirements ensures that if the disorder does not need treatment, the person cannot be involuntarily admitted. When a mental disorder is defined as requiring treatment, a person who does not need treatment will not meet the mental disorder definition and will not be eligible for an involuntary admission.[14]

Alberta departed from "dangerousness" criteria in 2010 and adopted "harm"-based criteria but did not initially address the role of treatment in its involuntary admission criteria. In *JH vs Alberta Health Services*, Justice Eidsvik described Alberta's involuntary admission criteria as overbroad because "it denies the rights of many individuals who are being detained under the auspices of the MHA when they cannot benefit from treatment."[28] In 2020, Alberta's new MHA included the provision that individuals must have "the potential to benefit from treatment for the mental disorder" to meet involuntary admission criteria.[12]

Justice Eidsvik wrote: "There are several decisions that looked at whether this move to 'harm' based criteria would render the criteria unconstitutional but, in my view, because of the combination of this part of the criteria with other parts, such as the need for treatment, the legislation in Manitoba, British Columbia and Ontario survived the Charter challenges . . ."[28]

In British Columbia's MHA, need for treatment is explicit within the definition of a person with a mental disorder whereby the disorder must require treatment.[3] In Prince Edward Island, involuntary admission criteria state that "the person requires care and treatment in a psychiatric facility."[7] Similarly, Manitoba and Nova Scotia have need for treatment in their involuntary admission requirements, and Saskatchewan and Newfoundland and Labrador include that the person is "in need of treatment or care and supervision that can be provided only" in a mental health center or psychiatric unit.[5,6,8,10] Ontario and New Brunswick's legislation specifies that the attending physician must release the patient if they are of the opinion that the patient doesn't need the "treatment provided in a psychiatric facility."[1,11]

Some jurisdictions do not specify a need for treatment as part of the involuntary admission criteria. Alberta requires that the person has "the potential to benefit from treatment for the mental disorder."[12] Nunavut's criteria don't include treatment requirements, but its mental disorder definition states that it must be "amenable to treatment."[9] Legislation in a number of jurisdictions requires that a treatment plan be prepared for the patient.[6,12,17]

Pairing the need for treatment with other involuntary admission criteria helps keep legislation from being overbroad, narrows involuntary admissions to being available for those individuals with treatable conditions, focuses the purpose of the admission on treatment, and prevents the detaining of people with conditions that are not susceptible to psychiatric treatment. It focuses the admission purpose on treatment and improvement rather than a possibly indefinite detention used to prevent community physical danger, which does not make sense for hospital functioning and may be contrary to the Canadian Charter.[14]

Treatment during an involuntary admission: When incapable of consenting to treatment

A person may appeal a psychiatrist's finding of incapacity for consent to treatment. In some jurisdictions, treatment cannot begin until the appeal is decided by a panel or, when appealed further, by the courts. Delays incurred by a court review can last months or years, resulting in prolonged detainment without treatment.

First-line treatment decision-making in the context of a finding of incapacity for consent to treatment depends on the jurisdiction. Some jurisdictions require the decision-maker to follow prior expressed capable directives, instructions, or wishes of an incapable individual for whom the treatment is proposed.[9,10,26,29,30]

When applying prior capable directives, instructions, or wishes, some jurisdictions specify that these must apply to the current circumstances and must not be impossible. Such safeguards are helpful but have limitations. They require extrapolation of prior wishes as they apply to the current circumstances, which may be difficult to determine. Prior expressed capable wishes may not have been properly informed. Determining capacity retrospectively may be inaccurate, especially so if the determination of prior capable wishes was done by a substitute decision-maker who does not have capacity assessment training.[14]

Adverse outcomes have occurred. This can occur when an incapable person's prior expressed capable wish was for no treatment regardless of the negative consequences.

Solomon et al.[31] describe an example of this with the case of Edwin Sevels. Mr. Sevels was diagnosed with schizophrenia or schizoaffective disorder and had a history of repeated confinement in a high-secure psychiatric facility. He was subsequently detained on a warrant of remand and, after his criminal charges were dropped, was held involuntarily under Ontario's MHA due to his symptoms and associated violent behavior.[31]

He was incapable with respect to treatment, but because he had previously rejected it when apparently capable, his relative refused to consent on his behalf. The Court believed medications would significantly improve his condition and aggression, and that they would stop further mental deterioration. It believed that detaining a person suffering from mental illness for an extended period without the treatment needed for release could not have been the Canadian Charter's intent. However, it voiced that it had to adhere to the *Fleming vs Reid* decision that indicated that it was against the Canadian Charter to medicate a patient without consideration for their prior capable wish for no treatment.[31]

Mr. Sevels remained detained and untreated. He deteriorated, then assaulted and seriously harmed another person. The official guardian changed their decision and provided consent for treatment. After 65 months of involuntary detainment, Mr. Sevels was treated. He improved quickly, was removed from involuntary seclusion, continued to make gains, was eventually transferred to rehabilitation, and was subsequently discharged on a community treatment order, which required ongoing antipsychotic treatment.[31]

When first-line decision-making consists of prior expressed capable directives, instructions, or wishes, some jurisdictions have safeguards that prevent indefinite involuntary admissions without treatment. In Prince Edward Island, a panel can order treatment without consent according to the patient's best interests.[7] While the wording differs among jurisdictions, some include a clause that prior expressed wishes not be followed if they would endanger the physical or mental health or safety of the patient or another person.[4,6,10] Without safeguards regarding prior expressed capable directives, instructions, or wishes, indefinite involuntary admission without treatment can occur.

The remaining jurisdictions follow other first-line approaches in the setting of incapacity for treatment. In Alberta, decision-making is in accordance with best interests.[12] In Newfoundland and Labrador, the attending may, "taking into account the best interests of the involuntary patient, perform or prescribe diagnostic procedures that he or she considers necessary to determine the existence or nature of a mental disorder, and administer or prescribe medication or other treatment relating to the mental disorder without the consent of the involuntary patient during the period of detention."[8] In doing so, the attending will consult with the patient and their representative and consider their views.[8]

In New Brunswick, decision-making is in accordance with best interests and additional criteria.[11] In Saskatchewan, the attending physician may "administer or prescribe any medication or other treatment that is consistent with good medical practice and that he or she considers necessary to treat the mental disorder to a patient who is detained pursuant to

section 24 or 24.1 without that patient's consent."[5] The attending must also, "to the extent that it is feasible given the patient's medical condition," consult with the patient and consider the patient's views.[5] In Quebec, decision-making follows "the sole interest of that person, complying, as far as possible, with any wishes the latter may have expressed," and the decision-maker "shall ensure that the care is beneficial notwithstanding the gravity and permanence of certain of its effects, that it is advisable in the circumstances and that the risks incurred are not disproportionate to the anticipated benefit."[2] However, if the patient categorically refuses to receive care and if the situation is not an emergency or a hygienic care issue, treatment must not be given until the courts authorize it.[2] In British Columbia, the facility director authorizes safe and effective psychiatric treatment that is appropriate to the patient's mental condition.[3]

Treatment during an involuntary admission: When capacity is present

Prolonged involuntary admission can also occur when a detained individual who is capable of making their own decisions about treatment refuses the treatment that is needed to improve the person's condition for a safe discharge.

Solomon et al.[31] describe this outcome in Scott Starson's case. Mr. Starson had bipolar affective disorder and psychosis. He was initially deemed unfit to stand trial for uttering death threats, and the Court ordered detainment and treatment under the Criminal Code's fitness provisions. He subsequently improved, was fit to stand trial, and was found not criminally responsible for the charges. The Criminal Review Board determined the detention's duration and conditions. As with involuntary admissions under Ontario's MHA, treatment decisions were determined by Ontario's Health Care Consent Act. He was detained, refused medications, and was found to be incapable of consenting to treatment. He contested the psychiatrist's incapacity finding, and eventually the issue went to the Supreme Court of Canada. Most of the justices determined that he was capable using Ontario's Health Care Consent Act's incapacity definition. A minority of the justices viewed that he was incapable, that his ability to understand and appreciate were impaired, and that he neared full denial of the mental disorder. He had ongoing delusions such as that he communicated with aliens and that he was at the forefront of building a starship.[31]

Mr. Starson was found capable by the Supreme Court, but the Criminal Review Board declined his release because they determined that he was too much of a public threat. He refused treatment and remained detained and untreated. Over the next ~20 months, he mentally and physically deteriorated to the point at which he was in danger of impending renal failure and possibly of dying. His psychiatrist deemed him incapable with respect to treatment again. The finding was upheld by the Consent and Capacity Board (CCB), who acknowledged that capacity can change with time. His substitute decision-maker consented to treatment based on best interests, presumably because she believed his prior wishes did not apply to the current circumstances. He significantly improved with antipsychotic treatment, to the point at which, over the next couple of years, the Criminal Review Board approved short passes outside of hospital and eventually allowed him to live in an approved setting contingent on a minimum of monthly follow-up by his treatment team.[31]

Of the jurisdictions that allow capable people to be involuntarily admitted, some have provisions to avoid the indefinite detainment of a capable person refusing the treatment required for a safe discharge. Some allow a panel to order treatment without consent if the treatment is in accordance with the person's best interests and, depending on the jurisdiction, additional criteria.[4,7,11,12]

In British Columbia, the definition of a person with a mental disorder includes that it is a disorder of the mind that requires treatment. "Treatment" is defined as "safe and effective psychiatric treatment and includes any procedure necessarily related to the provision of psychiatric treatment."[3] If a person does not meet the mental disorder definition or the involuntary admission criteria's need for protection or deterioration clauses, they cannot be involuntarily admitted. They can be voluntarily discharged. Accordingly, if they do meet the mental disorder definition and the involuntary admission criteria and they refuse the safe and effective treatment required for the mental disorder, they are determined to be incapable regarding treatment, and the hospital director authorizes treatment according to what is safe, effective, and appropriate to the person's medical condition.[3,23]

Best interests

Controversy exists regarding whether best interests should be applied in treatment decision-making and whether following best interests is contrary to the Canadian Charter because of the *Reid vs Fleming* decision that prior capable wishes had to be respected before applying best interests. However, during a Canadian Charter challenge in 1999, the Ontario Court of Appeal asserted that it did not find the best interest standard to be unconstitutional, and it noted that it was a broadly accepted standard for decision-making.[14] Alberta requires the substitute decision-maker to decide according to best interests, and a review board can overrule a treatment refusal if it determines that the treatment is in the person's best interests.[12]

Although some differences exist across Canada, best interests, as they are described by jurisdictional legislation, generally include regard for whether the condition will likely be improved by the treatment, what will likely happen to the condition if treatment is not provided (i.e., whether the condition will likely deteriorate or likely improve without treatment), whether the anticipated benefits from treatment outweigh the risks of harm, and whether the treatment meeting those requirements also constitutes the least restrictive and least intrusive treatment option.

Best interests may explicitly consider current wishes and/or prior capable wishes, as well as prior capable values and beliefs.[4,8,9,26,29,30] If not explicitly stated in legislation, it can be argued that considering patient wishes is an implicit requirement.[14] Treatment decisions according to best interests help to prevent indefinite detention because the treatment must be the least restrictive and least intrusive applicable treatment. They automatically apply to the current circumstances. They weigh the anticipated benefits and harms, and this would consider any potential harms linked to the administration of involuntary treatment such as any possible harms linked to the involuntary admission itself. The benefit of the involuntary admission and treatment must outweigh the anticipated harms.

Appealing incapacity for treatment in Canada and treatment pending appeal

In British Columbia, Newfoundland and Labrador, Nova Scotia, and Saskatchewan, meeting involuntary admission criteria will result in an individual being eligible for treatment.

In Newfoundland and Labrador, Nova Scotia, and Saskatchewan, involuntary admission requires a finding of incapacity for treatment.[5,6,8] If a person disagrees with the involuntary admission, they may seek review of the involuntary admission to a tribunal authorized to review the decision. The panel may uphold the involuntary admission, which would include the incapacity status and allow for involuntary admission and treatment or rescind the involuntary status and the person can be voluntarily discharged without treatment.

In British Columbia, before an involuntary patient is treated, they must be assessed for capacity by the treating physician. If found to understand the treatment and its consequences (i.e., capable), the patient can consent to their own treatment if they agree with it. If found incapable because they do not appreciate the treatment, including their need for treatment, they are found to be incapable. The director of the psychiatric unit, on the advice of the treating physician, then consents or can refuse. There is no appeal to the review board on a finding of incapacity as such, but a patient could argue that treatment is not required or that they are competent and therefore suitable as a voluntary patient. Treatment continues during the review panel process.[3,23]

In the remaining jurisdictions, except for Quebec, people who are involuntarily admitted may seek a legal review of the involuntary admission status and/or the incapacity finding from an administrative tribunal or reviewing body. In Quebec, involuntary hospitalization and an incapacity finding would need to be reviewed by the courts.[2]

If a party is dissatisfied with a review board's or court's decision, they may seek an appeal to a reviewing court and even up to the Supreme Court of Canada. Appeals addressed through the courts can take months or years to be resolved as a result of various factors. However, when a review board confirms an incapacity finding regarding a proposed treatment, most jurisdictions allow for treatment to commence during the appeal process. A minority of jurisdictions do not allow treatment to start or to be significantly modified until the court makes a decision on the appeal, which can unfortunately result in prolonged involuntary admissions without treatment. Because of the severity of symptoms of patients requiring involuntary admission, which can center around risks of bodily harm or dangerousness, sometimes physical restraints or seclusion are unfortunately required due to violent untreated illness.

Many Canadian jurisdictions – Alberta, New Brunswick, Nova Scotia, Northwest Territories, and Prince Edward Island – permit treatment pending appeal, meaning that the involuntarily hospitalized person can be compelled to receive treatment for the mental disorder while they appeal the incapacity determination to the court system.[4,6,7,11,12] Jurisdictions that do not allow treatment to start until the issue is resolved in court include Ontario, Manitoba, Nunavut, and the Yukon.[9,10,17,26] There is no mandated time frame for an appeal to be heard by the courts. Typically, the waiting period is several months, but it can take up to a year. A study in Ontario showed an average initial treatment delay of 253 days for patients who appealed a panel's decision.[32] In Quebec, when there is a request to review a finding of incapacity in the courts, an application for treatment pending a potential appeal can be made concurrently, so even if there is a subsequent appeal, treatment can commence in the interim.[2,33–35]

Most appeals delay treatment and do not reach the courts. For example, in Ontario, the most populous jurisdiction in Canada, its CCB's 2022–2023 Annual Report reveals that since the data recorded in 2012, the majority of appeal outcomes were identified as withdrawn, abandoned, or unknown.[36] The minority of appeals actually reach the courts, and, when they do, the courts overturn only a small minority of the review board's original decisions. Appeals can rely on arguing that the board made errors in facts, law, or both,[37] but the majority of appeals are dismissed after careful court review. In communication with Ontario's CCB, from 2018 to 2023, there were 346 appeals regarding treatment incapacity. Over this period, only four appeals were allowed by the courts and overturned the review board's decision; there were two additional cases remitted back to the CCB for new hearings (CCB, email communication, June 12, 2023). While it is impossible to track the whereabouts of all such patients and the trails of all appeals, these data collected by the CCB are the best available. When considering the small number of successful appeals, there are enormous harms caused by delays in treatment – or potentially no treatment – if patients are discharged from hospital prior to the appeal reaching the court.

Delaying treatment until a court decision takes into consideration individual rights for autonomy, self-determination, and bodily integrity. However, in clinical practice, delayed treatment in this manner is at the expense of the rights to liberty and freedom and the best interests of vulnerable populations. It denies the provision of wellness and health, and protection from harm. The finding of incapacity is generally upheld by the courts, and so it can also be argued that disallowing treatment pending appeal systematically delays treatment to the personal detriment of patients through prolonged hospital detention and the risk of worsening illness prognosis. One can contend that delaying treatment while awaiting an appeal infringes on a person's right to autonomy and self-determination should the person's prior capable expressed wishes or values regarding treatment be prevented because the person makes impaired decision-making and directions while they are unwell. Bodily integrity is also at risk given any potential self-inflicted bodily harm or agitation driven by untreated illness.

For patients, hospital treatment delays contribute to prolonged suffering, loss of liberty, and poorer prognosis when involuntary admission remains necessary. Patients and their families may endure extended disruption of family life. Delays in discharge can increase socioeconomic disruption for patients, not to mention the risk of worsening illness and poorer prognosis.[38,39] A higher level of psychosis can be a predictor of violence in an inpatient setting,[40,41] increasing the risk of restraint use and seclusion, which can place patients at greater risk of physical injury.

The risk of patient violence also poses a threat to hospital staff and co-patients. Antipsychotic medication can lower patient hostility, potentially mediating aggressive behavior[42]; thus, treatment delays create a barrier to increasing the safety of the hospital setting. Jurisdictions that permit treatment pending appeal address these adverse outcomes, striking a balance that allows individuals to receive treatment while they appeal a panel's decision about an incapacity finding to the court.

Canadian mental health legislation, the Canadian Charter of Human Rights and Freedoms, and the Canada Health Act

Canadian mental health legislation must consider the interests both of society and of individuals with mental illness and consider a person's right to liberty, autonomy, protection from harm, procedural fairness, and equality.[43] It must consider one's right to wellness. It must adhere to the Canadian Charter of Human Rights and Freedoms and to the Canada Health Act.

During an involuntary admission, a person loses their liberty, and potentially their autonomy to decide their treatment.[43]

Liberty, autonomy, and procedural fairness

When a person's liberty is restricted, Section 7 of the Canadian Charter states that it must occur in "accordance with the principles of fundamental justice,"[44] meaning the law must follow fair legal principles that are generally agreed upon by society and must consider a balance of individual and society interests.[14]

In alignment with the principles of fundamental justice, Canadian MHAs have procedural safeguards in place for involuntary admission and treatment. The Canadian Psychiatric Association's (CPA) position paper on "Principles Underlying Mental Health Legislation" states: "Procedural safeguards should generally include, but not be limited to, provision of rights information, the right to retain counsel, the right to an independent review of committal, or a finding of incapacity, and appropriate review by the courts. Safeguards might also include such things as a requirement to provide a second opinion on a plan of treatment, if requested."[43] Following the principles of fundamental justice has kept the liberty loss from involuntary admissions adherent to Section 7 of the Canadian Charter.[43]

With respect to the individual's interests, the CPA describes that the loss of liberty from an involuntary admission should benefit the person and that the associated treatment should be financed by the government, follow best medical practices, and be the least intrusive and the "least restrictive alternative treatment that is appropriate."[43]

Liberty loss must not be arbitrary. In alignment with Section 9 of the Canadian Charter,[44] involuntary admissions must comply with specific criteria that ensure that the law is not overbroad and that the detainment is not arbitrary.[14]

Legislation has similar considerations for the loss of autonomy that occurs when a person loses capacity to consent to treatment. The CPA's position includes that treatment should be the least restrictive alternative that is appropriate, that it should have procedural safeguards in place, that patients should have an active role in the formulation and integration of their treatment, and, when appropriate, that close support(s) should be involved.[43]

It can be argued that involuntary admission and treatment can restore a person's right to freedom of thought unplagued by the irrationality of psychosis, restore a person's freedom when they have required involuntary admission to address serious harms,[14] and restore their autonomy to make treatment decisions regarding mental and medical illness.

Equality and health care accessibility

Health care should be accessible to all residents. The Canada Health Act identifies that the primary objective of Canadian health care policy is "to protect, promote and restore the physical and mental well-being of residents of Canada and to facilitate reasonable access to health services without financial or other barriers."[45] Section 12(1) of the Act asserts that a province's health care insurance plan "must provide for insured health services on uniform terms and conditions and on a basis that does not impede or preclude, either directly or indirectly whether by charges made to insured persons or otherwise, reasonable access to those services by insured persons."[45]

People with severe mental illness who refuse treatment because they do not realize they are ill and because they are incapable with respect to treatment do not have reasonable access to health care when they need it and are discriminated against for their health status. The CPA asserts that "all citizens have the right to access publicly funded treatment," and that "access to psychiatric treatment should not be denied to a person simply because that person does not have the capacity to recognize his or her illness."[43]

Section 12 of the Canadian Charter says: "Everyone has the right not to be subjected to any cruel and unusual treatment or punishment."[44] It can be argued that detaining people with schizophrenia for long periods without the treatment they need to be safely released violates Section 12.[14] When a person is involuntarily admitted because of the serious harm from the mental disorder, treatment can restore their liberty.

Access to health care should be consistent across Canada and respect Section 15 of the Canadian Charter, which ensures equality rights.[44] Critics have argued that Section 15 is violated by involuntary admission, because they frame involuntary patients as the same as voluntary medical patients but not treated the same. They are involuntarily admitted and treated and therefore discriminated against because they do not consent, violating Section 15. The opposing argument is that they are not the same. Medical patients must consent to admission, or the substitute decision-maker must consent on their behalf. Involuntary psychiatric patients are not asked to consent to admission; indeed, by definition they refuse admission. When a medical patient refuses treatment, they can walk out of the hospital at any time. In contrast, the untreated involuntary patient is detained until they meet the discharge criteria without treatment, which may result in an indefinite detainment when the serious mental illness requires treatment for the person to be safe for discharge. Should the untreated mental illness cause violent behaviors during the detainment, the person can end up physically and chemically restrained to ensure their and other co-patients' safety.

Section 15 also says that it "does not preclude any law, program or activity that has as its object the amelioration of conditions of disadvantaged individuals or groups including those that are disadvantaged because of race, national or ethnic origin, colour, religion, sex, age or mental or physical disability."[44] This means that programs aimed at reducing apparent discrimination are not contrary to Section 15. Involuntary treatment is what restores a person to having the same privileges and rights as a voluntary patient.

Individuals have the right to equal protection and equal benefit from the law without discrimination based on mental disability. It is arguable that the jurisdictions that restrict involuntary admission to bodily harm or physical danger criteria breach Section 15.[14] Such jurisdictions deny individuals with mental illness causing serious non-bodily harms or mental or physical deterioration the protections and health rights they would obtain in most other Canadian jurisdictions.

Conclusion

Mental health legislation across Canadian jurisdictions has overlapping principles with respect to involuntary admission and access to treatment. Legislation must consider the individual's interests and the interests of society, as well as a person's right to liberty, autonomy, procedural fairness, wellness, protection from harm, and equality.

Most jurisdictions allow for involuntary admission to address non-bodily harms or mental or physical deterioration due to a mental disorder when other criteria are met. Legislation that limits involuntary admission to when there is concern for physical danger or bodily harm forces people to suffer the serious non-bodily harms and mental or physical deterioration of untreated mental illness. Individuals with serious mental illness who refuse involuntary admission and treatment because of anosognosia – a common symptom of psychosis that impairs awareness of one's own mental condition – are discriminated against in those jurisdictions. Access to involuntary admission and treatment when it is needed should not be restricted to bodily harm or physical danger. Individuals with mental illness should have equal access to care and treatment. Safeguards should be in place to ensure involuntary admission is accompanied by appropriate treatment and that prolonged detention without treatment does not become a common deleterious outcome for people with severe, but treatable, conditions.

When the purpose of involuntary admission is to provide needed treatment that cannot be provided voluntarily, the concept of stopping treatment, which leads to increased detention and suffering, might be questioned. As Solomon et al.[31] described regarding Ontario's MHA, "In attempting to protect autonomy, the Ontario law has imperilled the physical and mental health of involuntary psychiatric patients and exposed them to indeterminate detention. In our view, a better balance needs to be struck among the competing interests of these patients. In striking this balance, consideration must be given to the impact that the law has on the lives of those it seeks to protect. As our study indicates, treatment delayed results in liberty denied."

A review of the mental health legislation across Canada's provinces and territories demonstrates how various jurisdictions have grappled with the complex balance between competing rights, principles, and ethical considerations when it comes to involuntary hospitalization, capacity, and treatment decision-making. The nuanced and different approaches played out across the country allow for comparisons and the potential for each jurisdiction to review their system in order to seek improvements. There are opportunities to fine-tune laws to eliminate unintended and significantly harmful consequences and to incorporate new knowledge and societal expectations for timely care. Mental health legislation must consist of living documents and align with best practices and recognized guidelines related to pharmacotherapy, psychosocial treatments, and comprehensive community treatment.

References

1. Mental Health Act [Ontario], RSO 1990, c M.7, https://canlii.ca/t/52kkd, retrieved on January 5, 2025.

2. Civil Code of Québec, CQLR c CCQ-1991, https://canlii.ca/t/56cfw, retrieved on January 5, 2025.

3. Mental Health Act [British Columbia], RSBC 1996, c 288, https://canlii.ca/t/5643r, retrieved on January 5, 2025.

4. Mental Health Act [Northwest Territories], RSNWT 1988, c M-10, https://canlii.ca/t/568qn, retrieved on January 5, 2025.

5. Mental Health Services Act [Saskatchewan], SS 1984–85–86, c M-13.1, https://canlii.ca/t/56b6d, retrieved on January 5, 2025.

6. Involuntary Psychiatric Treatment Act [Nova Scotia], SNS 2005, c 42, https://canlii.ca/t/56bmd, retrieved on 5 January, 2025.

7. Mental Health Act [Prince Edward Island], RSPEI 1988, c M-6.2, https://canlii.ca/t/5664k, retrieved on January 5, 2025.

8. Mental Health Care and Treatment Act [Newfoundland], SNL 2006, c M 9.1, https://canlii.ca/t/52950, retrieved on January 5, 2025.

9. Mental Health Act [Nunavut], SNu 2021, c 19, https://canlii.ca/t/55w0s, retrieved on January 5, 2025.

10. Mental Health Act [Manitoba], CCSM c M110, https://canlii.ca/t/569hs, retrieved on January 5, 2025.

11. Mental Health Act [New Brunswick], RSNB 1973, c M-10, https://canlii.ca/t/566m2, retrieved on January 5, 2025.

12. Mental Health Act [Alberta], RSA 2000, c M-13, https://canlii.ca/t/56flt, retrieved on February 6, 2025.

13. BI (Re), 2022 CanLII 39864 (ON CCB), https://canlii.ca/t/jp7ww, retrieved on July 1, 2024.

14. Gray JE, Shone MA, Liddle PF. *Canadian Mental Health Law and Policy*, 2nd edition. LexisNexis; 2008.

15. A c. Centre hospitalier de St. *Mary*, 2007 QCCA 358 (CanLII), https://canlii.ca/t/1qszr, retrieved on January 27, 2025.

16. McCorkell v. Director of Riverview Hospital, 1993 CanLII 1200 (BC SC), https://canlii.ca/t/1dk2g, retrieved on January 9, 2025.

17. Mental Health Act [Yukon], RSY 2002, c 150, https://canlii.ca/t/525lk, retrieved on January 5, 2025.

18. Centre intégré de santé et de services sociaux des Laurentides c. G.V., 2018 QCCQ 642 (CanLII), https://canlii.ca/t/hqgb3, retrieved on January 30, 2025.

19. Centre intégré de santé et de services sociaux de la Montérégie-Centre c. J.A., 2017 QCCQ 1137 (CanLII),

https://canlii.ca/t/h2m4d, retrieved on January 30, 2025.

20. J.M. c. Hôpital Jean-Talon du Centre intégré universitaire de santé et de services sociaux (CIUSSS) du Nord-de-l'Île-de-Montréal, 2018 QCCA 378 (CanLII), https://canlii.ca/t/hqznz, retrieved on February 8, 2025.

21. Criminal Code, RSC 1985, c C-46, https://canlii.ca/t/56crs, retrieved on January 26, 2025.

22. Ho A, Petit L, Pirzada K, Shin K. Ontario's mental health laws must change to protect our most vulnerable patients. *Healthy Debate*. 2022. https://healthydebate.ca/2022/07/topic/ontario-mental-health-laws/, retrieved on January 30, 2025.

23. British Columbia Ministry of Health. *Guide to the Mental Health Act*, 2005 edition. British Columbia Ministry of Health; 2005.

24. M.T. *(Re)*, 2004 CanLII 56536 (ON CCB), https://canlii.ca/t/1r71l, retrieved on January 16, 2025.

25. Government of Saskatchewan. *A Guide to the Mental Health Service Act. V1.0*. Government of Saskatchewan; 2015.

26. Health Care Consent Act [Ontario], 1996, SO 1996, c 2, Sch A, https://canlii.ca/t/55kk2, retrieved on January 16, 2025.

27. *Starson* v. *Swayze*, 2003 SCC 32 (CanLII), [2003] 1 SCR 722, https://canlii.ca/t/1g6p, retrieved on January 14, 2025.

28. *JH* v. *Alberta Health Services*, 2019 ABQB 540 (CanLII), https://canlii.ca/t/j1hjk, retrieved on January 26, 2025.

29. Care Consent Act [Yukon], SY 2003, c 21, Sch B, https://canlii.ca/t/55lwx, retrieved on January 17, 2025.

30. Consent to Treatment and Health Care Directives Act, RSPEI 1988, c C-17.2, https://canlii.ca/t/5664n, retrieved on February 3, 2025.

31. Solomon R. O'Reilly R, Gray J, Nikolic M. Treatment delayed – Liberty denied. *Can Bar Rev*. 2009;**87**(3):679–719.

32. Kelly M, Dunbar S, Gray JE, O'Reilly R. Treatment delays for involuntary psychiatric patients associated with reviews of treatment capacity. *Can J Psychiatry*. 2002;**47**(2):181–185.

33. C.R. c. *Centre intégré de santé et de services sociaux du Bas-Saint-Laurent*, 2017 QCCA 328 (CanLII), https://canlii.ca/t/h03ld, retrieved on February 8, 2025.

34. Centre hospitalier de l'Université de Montréal c. *K.D.*, 2019 QCCS 7 (CanLII), https://canlii.ca/t/hwvlw, retrieved on February 8, 2025.

35. Centre intégré de santé et de services sociaux du Bas-Saint-Laurent c. M.M., 2016 QCCS 5772 (CanLII), https://canlii.ca/t/gvsx4, retrieved on February 8, 2025.

36. Consent and Capacity Board. Annual Report; 2022–2023. www.ccboard.on.ca/english/publications/documents/CCB%20AR%2022–23%20Final%20-%20with%20FR%20note_FINAL-s.pdf, retrieved on January 30, 2025.

37. *Bennett v. Sutton*, 2023 ONSC 6902 (CanLII), https://canlii.ca/t/k1k4n, retrieved on January 29, 2025.

38. Marshall M, Lewis S, Lockwood A, et al. Association between duration of untreated psychosis and outcome in cohorts of first-episode patients: A systematic review. *Arch Gen Psychiatry*. 2005;**62**(9):975–983.

39. Penttilä M, Jääskeläinen E, Hirvonen N, Isohanni M, Miettunen J. Duration of untreated psychosis as predictor of long-term outcome in schizophrenia: Systematic review and meta-analysis. *Br J Psychiatry*. 2014;**205**(2):88–94.

40. Radisic R, Kolla NJ. Right to appeal, non-treatment, and violence among forensic and civil inpatients awaiting incapacity appeal decisions in Ontario. *Front Psychiatry*. 2019;**10**:752.

41. Steinert T. Prediction of inpatient violence. *Acta Psychiatr Scand Suppl*. 2002;(412):133–141.

42. Volavka J. Violence in schizophrenia and bipolar disorder. *Psychiatr Danub*. 2013;**25**(1):24–33.

43. O'Reilly R, Chaimowitz G, Brunet A, Looper K, Beck P. Principles underlying mental health legislation. *Can J Psychiatry*. 2010;**55**(10):1–5.

44. The Constitution Act, 1982, Schedule B to the Canada Act 1982 (UK), 1982, c 11, https://canlii.ca/t/ldsx, retrieved on January 14, 2025.

45. Canada Health Act, RSC 1985, c C-6, https://canlii.ca/t/532qv, retrieved on January 26, 2025.

Chapter 22

The Current Situation of Treatment for Patients Suffering from Schizophrenia in the Austrian Forensic System

Alexander Dvorak, Patrick Swoboda, and Thomas Stompe

Introduction

Treatment of patients suffering from schizophrenia in Austria

Treatment of patients with schizophrenia in the healthcare system is generally voluntary. This applies both to outpatient care provided by specialists in private practice, hospital outpatient clinics, or social psychiatric outpatient clinics and to inpatient care in hospitals. However, there is an exceptional situation in which the patient's freedom of will is restricted by law. This is the case when acute danger to self or others caused by the disorder is present. With the involvement of the district court, the patient advocate, a possible adult representative, and an external expert, the patient's freedom of movement can be restricted for a certain period of time to enable treatment. The acceptance of psychopharmacological therapy remains the patient's decision in this situation, with the exception of explicit authorization by the court. Treatment under the consideration of proportionality, meaning that coercion is only applied in the case of an acute risk of severe bodily harm, is therefore possible for the majority of patients with schizophrenia.

However, this does not mean that patients are able to connect to the care network in all cases. Some patients fail because the contact threshold is still too high. In order to reduce this, outreach care has been integrated into the existing services in many cases. These multi-professional teams often manage to establish contact with the patients and thus create a willingness to undergo treatment in order to counteract the long-term consequences, including complete social isolation and disintegration.

Increase in patients with schizophrenia in the forensic system

As in many other European countries, the number of mentally ill patients in prison is increasing. In Austria, the number of inmates placed in forensic institutions has doubled in the last 20 years. This is due to both the rising number of admissions and the fact that releases have not kept pace with this increase. As far as admissions are concerned, there is a trend among people with schizophrenia, to name just one example, toward a shift in offense severity toward comparatively less serious offenses. During care in an inpatient forensic psychiatric setting, delays can occur due to limited therapeutic resources. Finally, in many cases, the search for a suitable outpatient aftercare facility once again proves to be a bottleneck. In order to take this development into account, an amendment to the law, the Measures Enforcement Adjustment Act, was passed in 2022. The plan was to ease the burden on the Austrian penitentiary system and improve legal certainty for mentally ill offenders who had committed relatively minor offenses such as resistance to state authority or dangerous threats.

Legal situation to date

This legal package regulates the admission of mentally ill or disturbed criminals who are not guilty for reasons of insanity. The prerequisite for this is incapacity according to Section 11 of the Austrian Criminal Code (StGB), defined as follows:

Section 11 StGB: *Any person who, at the time of the offence, is incapable of understanding the injustice of his deeds or of acting in accordance with this understanding because of mental illness, mental disability, a profound disturbance of consciousness, or because of another serious mental disorder equivalent to one of these conditions, is not culpable.*

Preventive detention for mentally ill offenders who are not culpable

If the person is incapable of guilt, it was previously sufficient for him/her to have committed an offense punishable by more than 1 year and a negative criminal prognosis to be committed to detention in accordance with Section 21 (1) StGB.

Around 75% of mentally ill offenders suffer from a schizophrenic disorder, 15% from an intellectual disability, and 10% from an acquired organic brain disorder. Approximately half of them are housed in the three institutions belonging to the justice system (Forensic Therapeutic Centers), the rest in closed forensic wards in regional psychiatric hospitals. The resulting costs are reimbursed to the facilities by the Ministry of Justice.

If, after the arrest, there are sufficient grounds to assume that the requirements of Section 21 (1) StGB are met, the public prosecutor's office must file an application for placement in an institution for mentally disturbed offenders.

If the offender's mental state improves during provisional detention prior to the main hearing to such an extent that no further serious offense is to be feared, the court may refrain from unconditional committal.

Patients provisionally detained are also treated primarily in judicial departments of prisons.

If a person is unconditionally admitted to the preventive measure, the following legal requirements for conditional release apply:

The purpose of placement in an institution for mentally disordered offenders is to prevent those placed there from committing punishable acts under the influence of their mental or emotional abnormality. The placement is intended to improve the condition of the inmates to such an extent that they can no longer be expected to commit punishable acts and to help the inmates to adopt a law-abiding attitude to life that is adapted to the requirements of community life.

Duration of preventive measures associated with deprivation of liberty:

Preventive measures shall be ordered for an indefinite period. They must be enforced for as long as their purpose requires. The court shall decide whether to end the preventive measure. Whether placement in an institution for mentally disturbed offenders is necessary shall be reviewed by the court ex officio at least once a year.

Release from a preventive measure involving deprivation of liberty

Release from a preventive measure involving deprivation of liberty shall be ordered if it can be assumed from the performance and development of the detainee in the institution, his/her person, his/her state of health, his/her previous life, and his/her prospects for an honest future that the dangerousness against which the preventive measure is directed no longer exists (Figure 22.1).

The length of stay in detention thus depends on the reduction of the disease-specific dangerousness that led to the admission offense. In principle, it is not limited in time. Release is always subject to conditions.

The Ministry of Justice is responsible for the financing and logistics of the Austrian penitentiary system. The previous legal regulations led to two problems, which the legislator wanted to solve with the new Act of 2022.

Increase in the prevalence of inmates in correctional facilities

Since 1980, the prevalence of offenders considered not guilty for reasons of insanity has risen continuously. Since 2015, the prevalence of offenders incapacitated for measures doubled to almost 800 inmates between 2014 and 2022 (Figure 22.2).

With only a few exceptions, the number of annual admissions clearly exceeded the number of discharges (Figures 22.3 and 22.4).

Most recently, 220 people were admitted to the penitentiary system in accordance with Section 21 (1) of the Criminal Code, compared to only 120 inmates who were released in the same year. However, the significant increase in admissions to the penitentiary system cannot be explained by a general increase in crime. Between 1980 and 2020, the number of offenders sentenced to unconditional custodial sentences fell by almost half (Figure 22.5), while the incidence of admissions to detention under Section 21 (1) quadrupled.

Provisional detentions of mentally ill offenders who were not ultimately committed to detention, also increased continuously from 2000 to 2020 (Figure 22.6).

Reasons for the increase in forensic patients

If we look at the increase in the number of patients being cared for as part of forensic detention, it is clear that there is no monocausal explanation for this. When

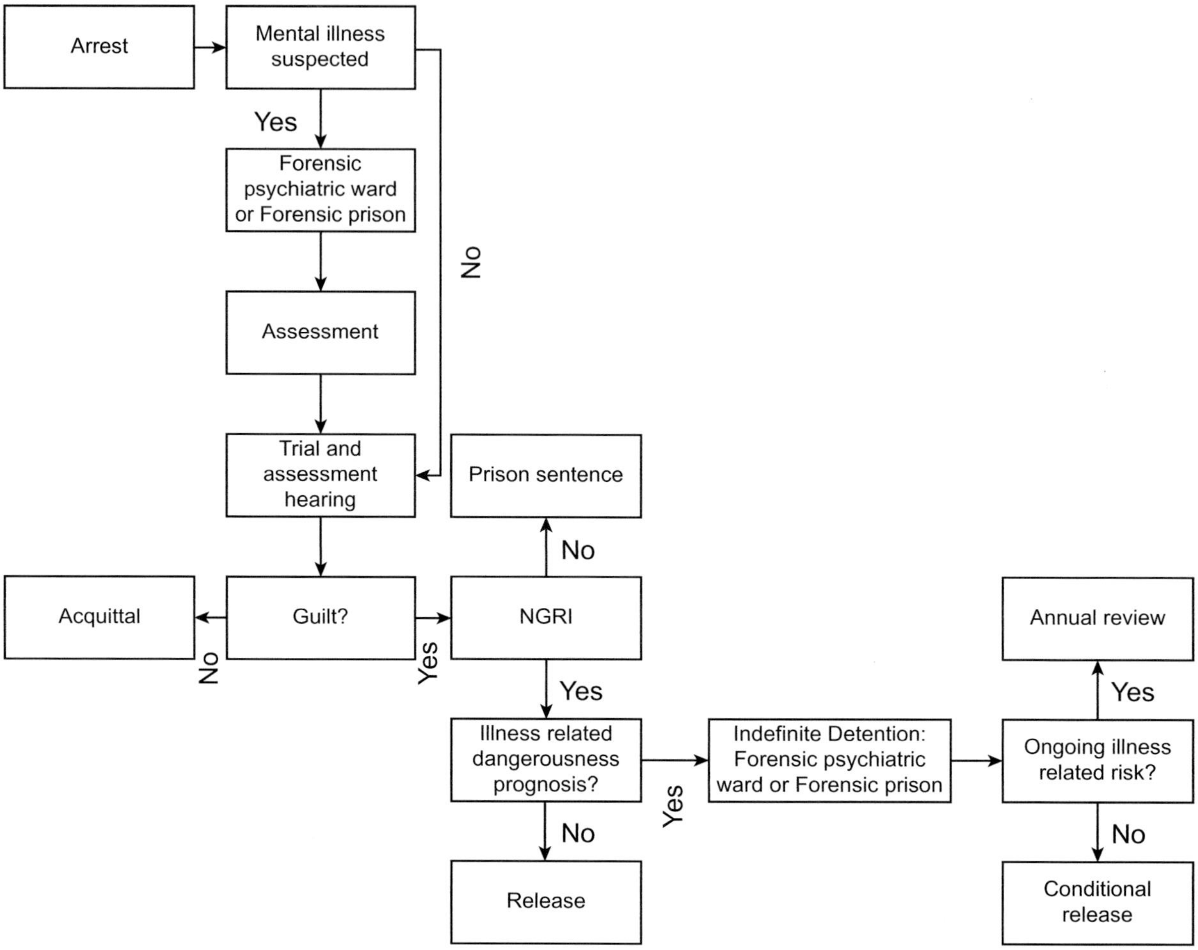

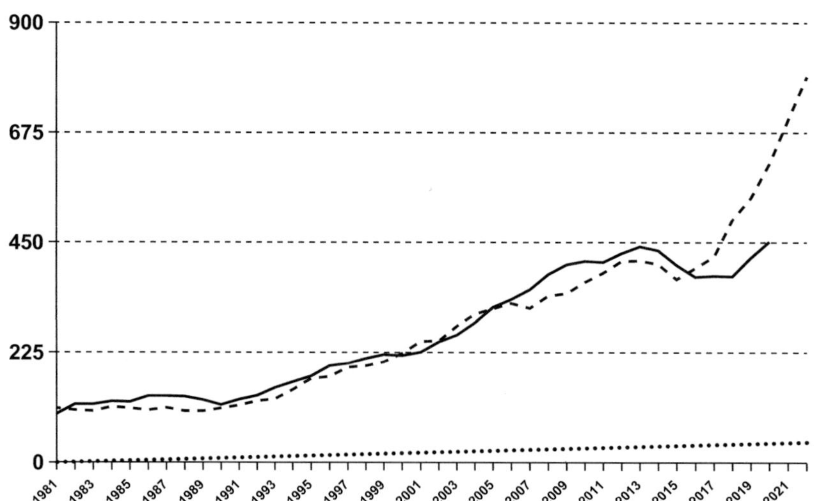

Figure 22.1 Flow chart showing considerations in the release from a preventive measure involving deprivation of liberty.

Figure 22.2 Prevalence from 1981 to 2022 of those placed in detention in accordance with Section 21 (1) (dashed line) and (2) (solid line) StGB.

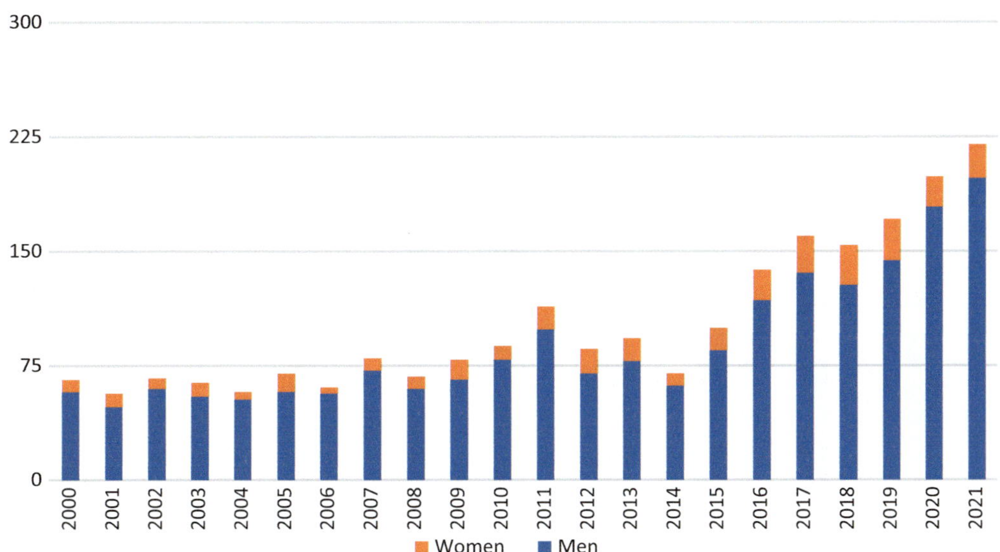

Figure 22.3 Admissions to detention in accordance with Section 21 (1) StGB by year (2000 to 2021), broken down by women and men (according to Ref.[1]).

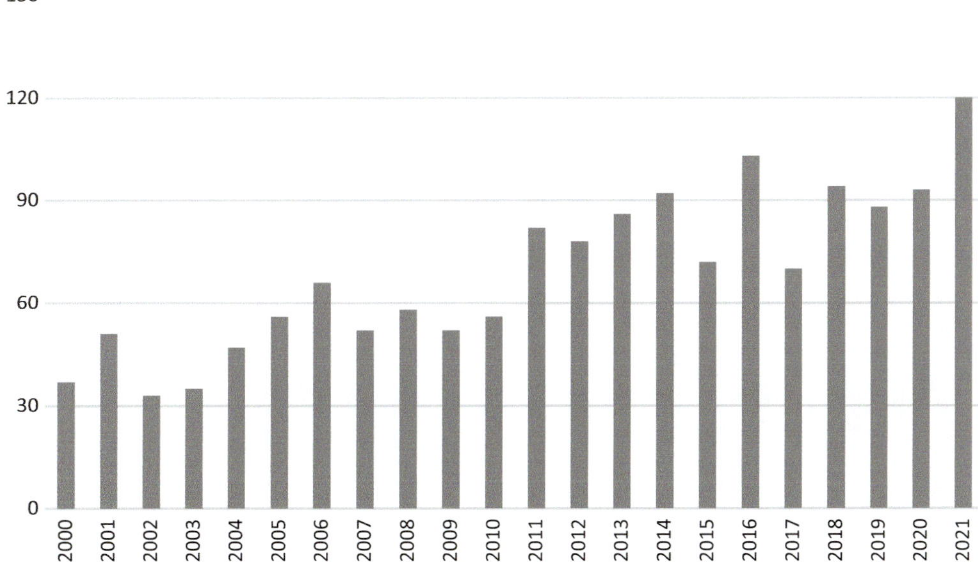

Figure 22.4 Conditional releases from detention under Section 21 (1) of the Criminal Code (according to Ref.[1]) from 2000 to 2021.

attempting to classify these reasons, a distinction can be made between pre-offense and post-offense treatment.

Before the offense, the changed conditions in general psychiatric care come to mind first. Without being able to break down the causes in detail, there was a reduction in available beds without outpatient care being able to compensate for this change. This is linked to a simultaneous reduction in admission times, also in order to have the necessary beds available for crisis interventions. However, this development also meant that the reasons for discharge from inpatient treatment changed. For example, patients who escaped the hospital were not readmitted or were discharged prematurely for disciplinary offenses

173

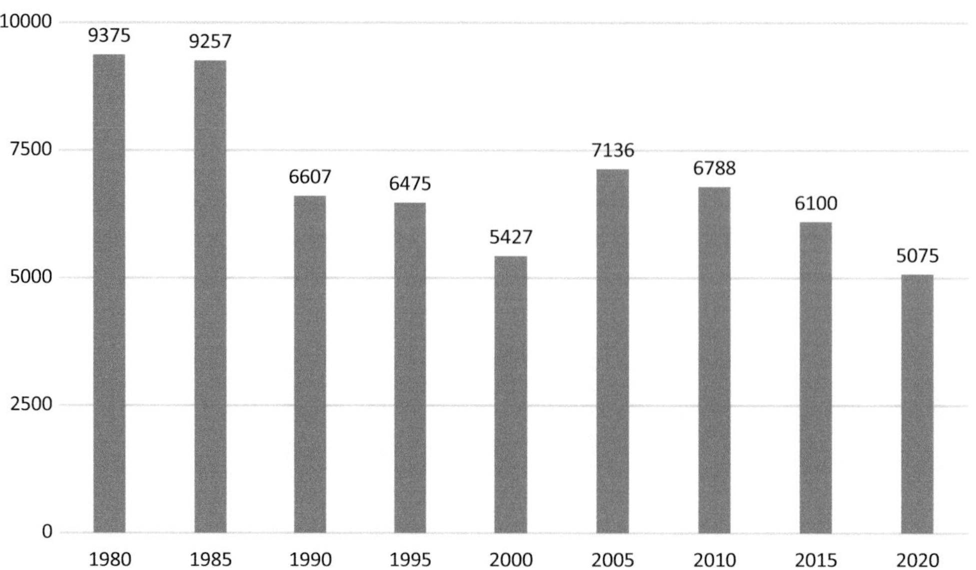

Figure 22.5 Final convictions for unconditional prison sentences 1980–2020 (Statistics Austria 2020 – Crime statistics).

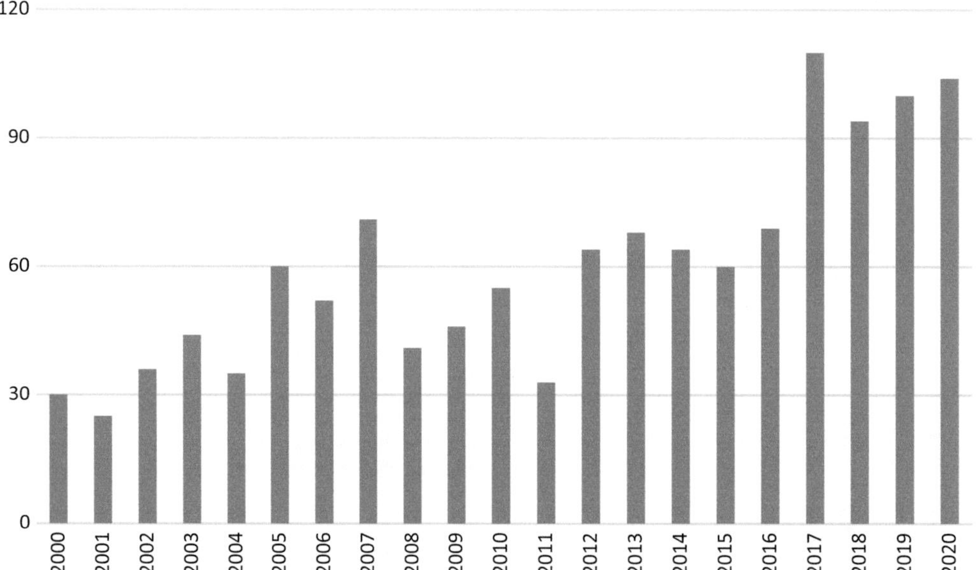

Figure 22.6 Provisional detentions under Section 429 (4) of the Code of Criminal Procedure by year (2000 to 2020), without subsequent committal to detention under Section 21 (1) of the Criminal Code (according to Ref.[1]).

such as illicit substance use or socially inadequate and aggressive behavior toward patients or staff.

In the category of post-offense reasons, at least three points should be mentioned here.

On the one hand, psychiatric experts are consulted by the court, perhaps even in the case of minor suspicions, with the result that patients who would not have been recognized as such in the past are now committed to preventive detention.

More far-reaching, however, are two points that influence the length of time patients spend in detention. The first point is that the personnel resources for treatment have not been able to keep pace with the increase in patients. This can delay the assessment of the relevance of the case and thus the start of treatment and extend the overall duration of treatment. Even if treatment in inpatient detention has been successfully

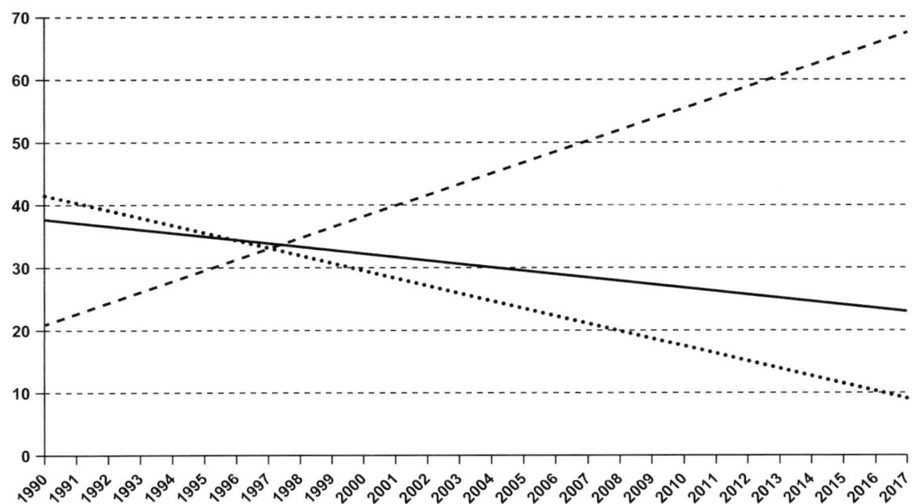

Figure 22.7 Change in the percentage shares of different offense types in the annual incidence of admissions to detention in accordance with Section 21 (1) StGB (1990–2017). Dashed line represents minor offenses such as dangerous threats and resistance to state authority; solid line represents sexual offenses; dotted line represents homicide.

completed, there is still one key point that needs to be clarified before discharge. And this key area is outpatient psychiatric and psychotherapeutic after-care as well as a suitable place to live.

In addition to these reasons, a significant increase in the number of migrants admitted has been particularly noticeable in recent years (Stompe and Keckeis, 2017[3]). In recent years, the proportion of inmates with a migration background has already exceeded the 50% mark.

All in all, multiple factors and participants play a role, which is why the number of patients in forensics continues to increase despite the commitment of treatment providers.

The increase in the prevalence of sane mentally abnormal offenders, which has, however, reached a plateau since 2014, probably has other causes. In the execution of measures in accordance with Section 21 (1), it is mainly personality disordered and/or paraphilic offenders who are treated for offenses against sexual self-determination, primarily child sexual abuse and rape. The increase in prevalence is most likely due to the increasingly critical attitude of the population toward sexual offenses.

Violation of the principle of proportionality

In addition to the question of how to ensure adequate care for mentally ill or disturbed lawbreakers given the sharp rise in incidences of admission and the relatively moderate rise in incidences of discharge, the proportionality of measures involving deprivation of liberty was increasingly discussed in Austria, as in Germany.

The available data show that the increases in the incidence and prevalence of imprisoned and the number of offenders imprisoned, particularly in correctional facilities in accordance with Section 21 (1) of the Criminal Code, are primarily attributable to persons who had committed relatively minor offenses such as dangerous threats or resistance to state authority, that is, offenses that are normally punishable by 1 year's imprisonment (Figure 22.7).

Our research in the Forensic Therapeutic Center in Göllersdorf showed that there is no correlation between the severity of the offense and the length of stay. This result is not entirely surprising, as treatment in the correctional facility is aimed at reducing the disease-specific dangerousness that led to the offense. The severity of the offense is not a criterion. The legislature clearly states that the dangerousness against which the preventive measure is directed should no longer exist and that there should be prospects of a fair future. However, there are no indications that the severity of the offense for which the offender has been committed should be a criterion for the length of stay in preventive detention. Our research revealed that the type of illness also plays no role concerning how long a person is placed in a detention center. The decisive factors were an early age at the time of the first offense and an early onset and extent of the illness. Furthermore, patients with psychopathic personality traits were detained for longer, as they exhibited a higher degree of intramural deviant and aggressive behavior.

From the perspective of the principle of proportionality, the fact is that mentally ill offenders who

Table 22.1 Relationship between the length of stay in detention and the sentencing range provided for in the Criminal Code (StGB)

Offense	Penalty range	Relation to the penalty range		
		under	in the	about
Dangerous threat: § 107(2)	1–3 y	0	28.6%	71.4%
Serious coercion: § 106	6 mo to 5 y	0	63.6%	36.4%
Serious bodily injury: § 84	1–5 y	0	51.3%	48.7%
Murder/attempted murder: § 75	10 y to life	76.7%	23.3%	–
Sexual offenses: §§ 205–207	6 mo to 10 y	0	76.5%	23.5%
Robbery: § 131	6 mo to 5 y	0	42.9%	57.1%
Theft: §§ 127–129	6 mo to 5 y	0	40.0%	60.0%
Arson: § 169	1–10 y	0	62.5%	37.5%
Resistance to state power	6 mo to 5 y	0	100%	0

Table 22.2 Length of stay in penal institutions and detention centers by offense

Offense	Measure § 21/1 ($N = 235$)	Detention ($N = 800$)	p
Dangerous threat	4.2 ± 3.7	1.6 ± 2.9	0.049
Serious coercion	4.5 ± 2.8	2.6 ± 0.9	n.s.
Serious bodily injury	4.9 ± 4.9	2.5 ± 1.3	0.000
Murder/attempted murder	5.8 ± 6.4	11.2 ± 5.5	0.000
Sexual offenses	4.2 ± 5.6	3.9 ± 2.4	n.s.
Robbery	6.9 ± 8.4	4.4 ± 3.1	0.042
Theft	6.5 ± 3.1	2.2 ± 1.3	0.025
Arson	8.0 ± 4.8	5.5 ± 1.3	n.s.
Resistance to state power	2.1 ± 1.2	1.5 ± 2.6	n.s.

have committed less serious offenses, such as resistance to state authority or dangerous threats, are treated for significantly longer in detention than is legally required for healthy offenders (Table 22.1). A comparison of the actual periods of imprisonment of healthy offenders and the stay of mentally ill offenders of unsound mind in detention for minor offenses also showed a clear disadvantage for the patient group, who were admitted for an average of 4–5 years (Table 22.2).

Changes due to the new legislation

In all relevant legal texts, the term "institution for mentally abnormal offenders" has been generally changed to "Forensic Therapeutic Center," which is intended to emphasize the therapeutic nature of this kind of detention. It is expected that this will also make more therapeutic resources available in the future. However, the more important changes concern the modalities of admission to detention and the responsibility for the treatment of persons provisionally admitted to detention.

By increasing the sentencing range to offenses punishable by more than 3 years, the legislature hopes to reduce the burden on the prison system. In addition, the aim is to prevent patients with minor offenses (resistance to state authority, dangerous threats) from remaining in detention for significantly longer than healthy offenders in prison for comparable offenses.

Criminal placement in a forensic therapeutic center

Any person who has committed an offense under the significant influence of a serious and persistent mental disorder and who cannot be punished solely because of being mentally incompetent (Section 11) at the time of the offense due to this disorder shall be placed in a forensic therapeutic center if there is a high probability that he/she will otherwise commit a punishable offense with serious consequences in the foreseeable future under the significant influence of his/her mental disorder. If there is such a fear, a person who, without being mentally incompetent, has committed an act pursuant to subsection (3) under the significant influence of a serious and persistent mental disorder shall also be placed in a forensic therapeutic center. In this case, placement shall be ordered at the same time as the sentence is imposed. Only acts punishable by more than 1 year's imprisonment may give rise to a criminal detention order. If the threatened custodial sentence for this offense does not exceed 3 years, the apprehension under subsection (1) must relate to an offense of bodily harm punishable by more than 2 years' imprisonment or to an offense against sexual integrity and self-determination punishable by more than 1 year's imprisonment. Acts against another person's property that are punishable by a custodial sentence are not considered to be a triggering offense unless they were committed using violence against a person or under threat of a current danger to the victim's life.

Comment

Whereas under the old legislation, mentally ill or disturbed offenders who had committed an offense punishable by at least 1 year's imprisonment could be committed, the de facto sentencing range has now been raised to 3 years. Only if there is a high probability of a repeat offense using bodily force that is punishable by more than 2 years' imprisonment or if there is a high probability of acts against sexual integrity and self-determination that are punishable by more than 1 year's imprisonment will the offender be committed to a detention facility.

On the one hand, the legislature obviously hopes that this will relieve the burden on the facilities by reducing the incidence of admissions, but on the other hand, the principle of proportionality will be upheld. However, the increase in the sentencing range creates a "blind zone." Mentally ill persons who are mentally incompetent and have committed crimes punishable by 1–2 years, in particular patients who have made dangerous threats, have no further legal sanctions or conditions to fear. As an Austrian study has shown,[2] civil law restrictions on liberty under the

Hospitalization Act often fall short, especially in the case of patients who have been admitted due to dangerous threats. This group of people, in particular, was admitted under the Hospitalization Act much more frequently in the run-up to the crime, than, for example, sane patients who have committed a homicide. They frequently discontinued treatment in psychiatric wards, even under conditions of detention, fled the ward and were often no longer able to be readmitted. The Austrian Hospitalization Act recognizes three criteria for hospitalization that must be present at the same time: (a) an acute psychiatric illness or disorder, (b) an associated serious and significant danger to self or others, or (c) the absence of an effective treatment alternative. If only one of these three criteria relevant to placement is not met, the placement must be lifted. As the willingness of mentally ill persons who pose a threat to others to undergo treatment is usually considered to be very low, the Hospitalization Act is likely to fall short of providing adequate treatment under the conditions of general psychiatric care for persons who have been committed to detention for making dangerous threats.

Crisis intervention

According to Section 157 of penal law, instead of revocation, the court shall suspend the provisional suspension of enforcement (Section 157 a) for a maximum period of 3 months and provisionally enforce the criminal placement if it can be assumed that treatment and care in a forensic therapeutic center, a public psychiatric hospital, or a public hospital with a psychiatric ward can improve the condition of the person concerned during this period to such an extent that a continuation of the provisional suspension of enforcement is possible again.

As inpatient detention facilities are generally operating at more than full capacity, it is to be expected that the courts will make frequent use of this option.

Comment

This immediately led to a statement by the Austrian Society for Psychiatry and Psychotherapy (ÖGPP). As the currently valid and available planning principles of the healthcare system (Austrian Healthcare Structure Plan, Regional Healthcare Structure Plans) take into account the care needs of a region, but not the psychiatric care of offenders in terms of the execution of measures, this group of people is neither included in the existing structures nor in the current plans. Experience has shown that a longer planning and implementation phase will be required before the existing structures can be expanded appropriately. As the admission of offenders in the sense of the execution of measures can be imposed on psychiatric hospitals or psychiatric departments of public hospitals, it must be assumed that in this case, the spatial and personnel structures in the general psychiatric departments for other mentally ill persons will not be available to a sufficient extent.

For around 2 decades, the duration of inpatient treatment in psychiatric hospitals and psychiatric departments in general hospitals has mostly been reduced to a few days to a few weeks at most. Under the new law, in addition to 50–70 general psychiatric patients who can be discharged after 2–3 weeks, there would be 2 or 3 patients who would have to be treated for up to 2 years. It is doubtful that adequate treatment for forensic patients can be offered under these conditions.

It is considered extremely problematic to treat forensic patients together with general psychiatric patients. The different length of stay, the different risk prognosis, and the different legal and assessment practices alone must cause tensions between the two patient groups. This results in a considerable additional workload for the staff working in these areas. The shortage of nursing staff that has arisen in recent years is also increasingly noticeable in psychiatric hospital departments. An additional burden caused by the admission of forensic patients to general psychiatric wards is likely to encourage nurses to leave psychiatry.

Forensic psychiatry has developed considerably in recent years and is a highly specialized field within psychiatry with elaborate methods of prognosis and treatment. Forensic psychotherapy and criminal therapy, in particular, require a high level of expertise that is not available in general psychiatry. It would require time-consuming and intensive training for all professional groups working in this field in order to further develop the relevant knowledge, skills, and abilities so that the dangerousness of forensic patients can be correctly assessed and treatment can be provided to the required quality.

The responsibility for securing, detaining, and monitoring patients to be treated in general psychiatric wards as part of provisional placement is completely unclear. Within the existing structures, these requirements go beyond the given framework and

pose a considerable risk potential both for the general psychiatric patients undergoing joint treatment and for the staff.

In recent decades, the former large psychiatric hospitals have largely been replaced by regional psychiatric departments at general hospitals. In addition to psychiatric departments, these general hospitals also have departments for internal medicine, obstetrics, pediatrics, and other medical specialties. As the psychiatric wards at general hospitals are often not locked, but are run openly, this means that their patients can sometimes leave the psychiatric ward without permission. If offenders are also admitted to these psychiatric wards without the staff being appropriately qualified, this also increases the risk for patients in other hospital departments.

Involuntary treatment in the forensic system

Psychopharmacological treatment against the will of the person concerned is only possible in forensic psychiatry to avert a significant and immediate danger to themselves or others if no less severe means appear sufficient and promising for this purpose. The need for such a measure is determined by the attending physician. Authorization to carry out such measures is granted following a written application to the Ministry of Justice. Subsequently, in order to enable an external review, the doctor responsible must send a protocol of the procedure to the authorizing body.

This procedure is modeled on the procedure in general psychiatry in terms of documentation and indication.

Relapse prevention

The treatment of the individual in correctional facilities, with all its difficulties and challenges, aims to reduce the specific danger posed by the illness to such an extent that reintegration into society is possible. This goal is pursued with a high expenditure of resources and always requires an individualized treatment of risk factors, the strengthening of resources, and the development of protective factors. Progress can be assessed in the course of gradual relaxation measures.

The success of this system can ultimately be measured, from a legal perspective, by the recidivism rates. And here, a long-term comparison consistently shows that patients who are released from the measure have a significantly lower reconviction rate than is the case for offenders with the same offenses.

References

1.   Eher R, Domany S, Engel F. Monitoring report 2021 enforcement of measures pursuant to Section 21 (1) StGB; 2022.

2.   Meuschke N. Typological description of the inpatient utilization behavior of mentally abnormal lawbreakers suffering from schizophrenia. Unpublished diploma thesis; 2014.

3.   Stompe T, Keckeis K. Diagnosen, Delikte und Migrationshintergrund. *Clinicum Neuropsy*, 2017.

Interventions for the Unhoused Individual with Schizophrenia
A Civilized Plan

Charles L. Scott

Introduction

Globally, nearly 24 million individuals are afflicted with schizophrenia[1], a severe and frequently disabling disorder vastly overrepresented among the homeless population. Schizophrenia involves a loss of touch with reality, with symptoms characterized by hallucinations, delusions (fixed false beliefs), disorganized speech and behavior, diminished emotional expression, and a loss of motivation.[2] Coupled with the presence of these devastating symptoms, individuals with schizophrenia are often unaware that they have this disease, a phenomena known as "anosognosia."[3]The combination of having a psychotic illness while being unaware of the illness makes interventions for unhoused individuals with schizophrenia particularly challenging. The faces and deteriorating lives of this population are increasingly impossible to ignore. As one walks down the street of a major urban city, seeing a disheveled and often half-naked human screaming in agony at voices that do not exist and running in fear from unfounded foes, society is faced with an obvious moral question: Is this the best we can do for those most in need?

This article provides an overview of individuals with schizophrenia who are unhoused and explores current approaches to managing this severe illness in those who often do not want care or believe they need it. For purposes of this article, the terms "homelessness" and "unhoused" are used interchangeably.

Homelessness definitions

When reviewing the prevalence of homelessness in any community or country, one must first consider the definition of homelessness used to calculate this statistic. In the United States, the Department of Housing and Urban Development (HUD) defines "literally homeless" as an "individual or family who lacks a fixed, regular, and adequate nighttime residence" as exemplified by one of the following 3 categories[4]:

1. The individual resides at night in a private or public place that is not meant for human habitation. This situation is often referred to as unsheltered homelessness or "sleeping rough" and includes living on the street, in a vehicle, or in an abandoned building.
2. The individual lives in some type of temporary shelter, such as an emergency or crisis shelter, transitional housing, or safe haven (SH) program. This category is considered "sheltered homelessness."
3. The individual resides in an institution for 90 days or less and immediately prior to living in the institution experienced either sheltered or unsheltered homelessness. A person who is briefly incarcerated or hospitalized yet did not have a fixed regular nighttime residence prior to institutional placement meets this definition of being homeless.[4]

Some individuals who do not have a fixed regular residence may not be included in the above definition and are referred to as the "hidden homeless." For example, a person who is "couch surfing" and stays with different friends or family because they do not have their own housing is likely not counted in official homelessness statistics.

Homelessness can also be categorized based on the time frame that the individual is unhoused. According to HUD, chronic homelessness involves an individual with a disability (such as a substance use disorder or mental illness) who has lived in a sheltered or unsheltered living environment for at least 12 months or at least four separate occasions during the last 3 years (if the combined occasions are at least 12 months in duration). Transitional homelessness, therefore, involves individuals who do not have housing for less than 12 months. Transitional homelessness is the most common type of homelessness and may result from a major life stressor, such as losing a job, experiencing a change in relationship status, enduring a natural disaster, or having a sudden change in financial circumstances.[4]

Schizophrenia and homelessness

Individuals with a serious mental illness (SMI) are at a substantial risk of facing homelessness when compared to the general population. Of note, men and women in the United States who are diagnosed with a SMI such as schizophrenia have a risk of becoming unhoused that is 10–20 times greater than the general population.[5] US veterans diagnosed with schizophrenia are likewise at increased risk of facing homelessness. In their study of 102,207 veterans, Lin et al. (2022)[6] found that the frequency of homelessness for veterans with schizophrenia was 28.2%, dramatically higher than the frequency of homelessness in a matched cohort of veterans without schizophrenia (7.2%) and even higher when compared to the prevalence of homelessness of 0.2% found in the general population.

Researchers have also studied unhoused individuals to assess the prevalence of schizophrenia or other psychotic disorders in this population. In 2019, Ayano et al.[7] published a systematic review and meta-analysis describing the prevalence of schizophrenia and other psychotic disorders among homeless people. Their review included 31 studies involving 51,295 unhoused individuals. The authors included studies from both developed and developing countries. Developed countries were described as those with a longstanding market economy and strong research traditions. Developed countries included in this study were the United States of America, Canada, Germany, Spain, France, Scotland, the United Kingdom, Japan, and Australia. Developing countries for purposes of this study included China, Ethiopia, Ireland, and Serbia.

The definition of homelessness used for this review was broad, including people sleeping in public places, living in shelters, or marginal accommodations. Most studies included in this meta-analysis utilized the DSM criteria for diagnosing schizophrenia and other psychotic disorders. The authors found the following prevalence of schizophrenia and other psychotic disorders among homeless people: overall, psychosis – 21.21%; schizophrenia – 10.29%; schizophreniform disorder – 2.48%; schizoaffective disorder – 3.53%, and psychotic

disorders not otherwise specified – 9%. Similar results were noted by Gutwinski et al.[8], which noted a 12-month prevalence rate of schizophrenia spectrum disorders of 12.4% from their systematic review and meta-analysis of the published literature on this topic.

Barry et al.[9] conducted a meta-analysis to also assess the current and lifetime prevalence of mental health disorders among people experiencing homelessness age 18 or older. These authors included 85 studies in their final review, which consisted of 48,414 participants (77% male; 22% female). Most studies included in this review were from the United States (n = 36), with studies from Canada (n = 8) and Germany (n = 7) rounding out the top three. Although the definition of homelessness varied among the studies, the majority (n = 71) included individuals who were either living in a shelter or other places not intended for housing, such as the streets. Findings indicated a current prevalence of mental health disorders of 67% and lifetime prevalence of mental health disorders of 77% among people experiencing homelessness. Although substance use disorder had the highest current prevalence of all disorders (44%) in this population, the current prevalence of schizophrenia and psychotic disorders was 21% and the lifetime prevalence was 25%.

The results of these studies are clear. Both current and lifetime prevalence of schizophrenia/psychotic disorders in the homeless are substantially higher than found in the housed general population. To more clearly illustrate, 1 in 5 unhoused individuals living in shelters or on the streets are suffering from a current psychotic disorder and 1 in 4 have a lifetime history of schizophrenia or a psychotic disorder. This finding contrasts dramatically with the estimated prevalence in the general population, which ranges from 0.3% to 0.7%.[2] These numbers become even more alarming when reviewing the prevalence of schizophrenia in transitional shelters (whose goals is to assist unhoused persons with a SMI). Viron et al.[10] found that schizophrenia spectrum disorders were present in 67.6% of this group, far greater than mood disorders present in 35.1% of the sample.

With the high prevalence of psychosis in unhoused individuals, the following question arises: Are those with schizophrenia or other psychotic disorders at risk to move into chronic homelessness, including homeless shelters? Burton et al.[11] examined this question by comparing homeless men with psychosis who lived in central Melbourne over a 12-month period in 2018 with data related to homeless men with psychosis in 2006. These authors found that the mean time spent without shelter for homeless psychotic men in 2018 (149 days) was over double that in 2016 (72 days). Greater than 40% of the 2018 sample were "sleeping rough." The findings raise concern that a significant number of unhoused men with psychosis are becoming increasingly entrenched in homeless settings, which results in worsened continuity of care combined with suboptimal treatment of psychosis.

With research confirming that those with schizophrenia have higher rates of experiencing homelessness in their lifetime and that up to 25% of homeless have a schizophrenia spectrum disorder, is there somehow a link between this severe mental illness and homelessness? Several proposed theories may account for why individuals with schizophrenia are at an increased risk for becoming unhoused when compared to the general population. First, many individuals with schizophrenia, particularly when untreated, experience a gradual deterioration that adversely impacts reality testing, cognition, and functioning. A cascade of negative outcomes results in social withdrawal and difficulty maintaining employment with a loss of income necessary to fund housing. Second, persons with schizophrenia have a high comorbidity of alcohol or other substance use disorder, both additional risk factors related to becoming homeless.[12] Third, with the deinstitutionalization movement that began in the 1960s, the community mental health system did not have the resources to manage a severely mentally ill patient population. Without an appropriate level of intervention, many individuals with schizophrenia failed to receive appropriate medication, monitoring, and follow-up in the community with a subsequent shift of psychiatric inpatient care from hospitals to jails and prisons.[13]

Impact of homelessness on individuals with schizophrenia

Individuals with schizophrenia experience higher rates of co-occurring medical disorders, substance use disorders, other psychiatric disorders, premature mortality,[12,14] and suicide when compared to the general population.[15] For the unhoused person with schizophrenia, these adverse consequences are heightened as they have limited access to medical and mental health treatment. It is no surprise, therefore, that unhoused individuals with schizophrenia face more frequent psychiatric hospital readmission rates, an emotional burden for the individual as well as a financial burden for society. In their retrospective study of 207 patients who had been psychiatrically hospitalized, Lorine et al.[16] evaluated 207 patients who were discharged and followed up at 3 different time periods to examine readmission rates. The time frames were readmission within 15 days (Group 1), readmission within 3–6 months (Group 2), and not being readmitted from at least 12 months (Group 3). Of this sample, 50% had schizophrenia or schizoaffective disorder and 24% of the sample were homeless. The study found that having a diagnosis of schizophrenia or schizoaffective disorder increased the odds of being readmitted within 15 days versus not being readmitted within 12 months by nearly 18 times. For those with a diagnosis of schizophrenia or schizoaffective disorder, being homeless increased their odds of readmission within 15 days versus not being readmitted by nearly 30 times. These results highlight the particular risk that having both a schizophrenia spectrum disorder and being unhoused plays in hospital readmission.

Unhoused individuals with schizophrenia are also at an increased risk of becoming both perpetrators and victims of violence. A diagnosis of schizophrenia in and of itself confers an increased risk of violence toward others when compared to the general population.[17] Untreated schizophrenia is characterized by active psychosis, which typically includes symptoms of paranoia, hallucinations, and false beliefs about others and one's environment. In an analysis of 204 studies examining the relationship between psychopathology and aggression, Douglas et al.[18] found that psychosis was the most important predictor of violent behavior in an individual. Although significant research indicates that unhoused individuals without schizophrenia have higher rates of violence and criminal offending,[19, 20] does the combination of both circumstances heighten the risk of criminal offending further? The answer is yes. Research by Nilsson et al.[21] indicates that individuals with a severe mental illness (e.g., schizophrenia or bipolar disorder) who are unhoused have higher rates of violence than those who are housed.

Unhoused individuals with schizophrenia are at increased risk of being victims of violence in addition to their increased risk of victimizing others. In their study, Roy et al.[22] reviewed 21 studies investigating the relationships of persons experiencing homelessness with serious mental illness (PEHSMI) to violence and victimization. The authors reviewed 15 studies specific to contacts with the criminal justice system and 6 studies specific to the prevalence of victimization. Their analysis indicated that PEHSMI had lifetime arrest rates ranging from 63% to 90%, lifetime conviction rates ranging from 28% to 80%, lifetime incarceration rates ranging from 48% to 67%, and lifetime victimization rates ranging from 74% to 87%.

Interventions for unhoused individuals with schizophrenia

With the goal of implementing the most effective treatment approaches for unhoused individuals with schizophrenia or other psychotic disorders, two competing models have been implemented: Treatment First versus Housing First (HF). The Treatment First model, also known as the "Continuum of Care" model, was the dominant model for managing psychiatric patients who had been discharged into the community during the deinstitutionalization movement of the 1960s and 1970s. This model typically consists of a linear model of care, where individuals with a psychiatric disorder have a stepwise progression of services that help prepare the individual for independent living, a process known as "housing readiness."[23]

Under the Treatment First model, the unhoused individual is typically expected to demonstrate sobriety and readiness to accept mental health treatment while in temporary housing. In the Treatment First model, case managers evaluate whether the person has sufficient life skills to live without onsite supervision.[24] Once the individual is deemed "housing ready," then independent housing is considered. Individuals who refuse to engage in psychiatric treatment, who continue to use substances, have a history of violence or incarceration, or problematic behaviors are not typically placed in independent housing under this model.

In contrast, the HF model emphasizes the importance of first being placed in permanent housing regardless of whether the person is actively psychotic, using alcohol or drugs, agrees to occupational rehabilitation, or accepts recommended treatment interventions. The HF model's origins can be traced to the Consumer Preference Supported Housing (CPSH) model that arose from a private non-profit

social services organization in New York City known as Pathways to Housing, Inc. Under this model, housing is considered a right for all individuals and interventions are client centered. The CPSH model is the precursor for the HF model, and its foundation includes the following tenants[25]:

1. Unhoused individuals with a SMI can successfully live independently in housing of their choice with appropriate supports;
2. The individual chooses their own housing;
3. Housing is rented from a community landlord who does not provide the support services;
4. The individual does not lose their housing when they are in a clinical crisis, such as a substance use relapse or psychotic episode;
5. Services are provided by a community ACT team and available 24 hours a day;
6. The individual selects the type, frequency, and order of services chosen;
7. No form of treatment is required, including sobriety or medication compliance. Instead, the harm reduction model is used to address alcohol and drug abuse.

In their 2004 research examining the longitudinal effects over a 2-year period of a HF program for homeless individuals with severe mental illness, Tsemberis et al.[26] compared 126 participants assigned to the Continuum of Care model to 99 participants assigned the HF model program. Fifty-three percent of those enrolled in the study had a psychotic disorder diagnosis. Although those placed into the HF program were able to maintain their independent housing over the 24-month period, no differences were found in substance use or psychiatric symptoms between HF versus the Continuum of Care participants.

In their systematic review of 72 articles, Aubry et al.[27] examined the effectiveness of permanent supportive housing and income assistance for homeless individuals in high-income countries. According to these researchers, most of the studies on permanent supportive housing they reviewed included individuals with severe mental illness who had been unhoused. The authors concluded that both permanent supportive housing and income assistance significantly improved housing stability at 6 years of follow-up.

However, this systematic review did not provide evidence that unhoused individuals with permanent supportive housing had improvements in their mental health or substance use compared with controls. In other words, HF may increase housing stability but has not been shown to decrease symptoms of SMI. This finding should inform public policy that to decrease the psychiatric disease burden, antipsychotic medications should be combined with HF to improve the mental health outcomes of unhoused individuals with schizophrenia and other forms of active psychosis.

In their subsequent study, Loubiere et al.[28] studied the effects of the HF model among homeless people regarding housing stability, quality of life, healthcare use, mental symptoms, and addiction issues. Researchers examined data from a randomized controlled trial involving homeless or precariously housed adults with severe mental illness from four French cities. A total of 703 participants were selected for this study, and all had a diagnosis of either bipolar disorder (30%) or schizophrenia (70%) according to the Diagnostic and Statistical Manual of Mental Disorders, 4th edition, text revision (DSM-IV-TR). In addition to having a bipolar disorder or schizophrenia disorder diagnosis, participants had to have at least one of the following: (1) two or more psychiatric hospitalizations in the past 5 years; (2) co-occurring alcohol or substance use disorder; or (3) history of arrest or incarceration within the previous 2 years. Participants who could not provide informed consent for the study were excluded.

The study participants were divided into two groups for comparison outcomes: a treatment-as-usual (TAU) group (n = 350) and a HF group (n = 353). For those who were assigned to the TAU group, their housing situations varied, with some individuals living on the streets, with friends or families, or in slums. TAU interventions involved preexisting programs and services for the homeless. These services included outreach teams, day-care facilities, access to emergency shelters and transitional shelters, residential facilities with medical accommodations if needed, and independent housing. In contrast, the HF model involved the provision of independent housing with housing subsidies and assertive community treatment provided by a mobile support team. Both groups were followed over a 48-month period. Both the TAU and HF groups improved in measures of recovery although no statistical difference in recovery outcomes was noted. The HF group compared to the TAU group had a lower use of hospital services. However, no significant differences were found between the two groups related to self-reported

mental symptoms or substance dependence. In fact, HF participants experienced higher alcohol consumption between baseline and 40 months. The findings in this study that HF did not reduce mental health symptoms replicate the results from the Aubry et al.'s[27] meta-analysis described above.

Whether or not a homeless individual with schizophrenia is housed, does compulsory treatment, most often involuntary medication administration, improve outcome? Compulsory community treatment orders (CTOs) are legally mandated orders that require psychiatric treatment for identified individuals with severe mental illness who do not voluntarily accept treatment and are considered a risk of harm to self or others or are unable to care for themselves. Failure to follow requirements in CTOs may result in involuntary psychiatric hospitalization. In some jurisdictions, CTOs require a showing that the individual lacks medical decision-making capacity regarding the use of psychotropic medications.[29] In the 2017 Cochrane review of compulsory community treatment (CCT) for people with mental illness, Kisely and Campbell[30] reviewed three randomized controlled clinical trials of CCT compared with standard care for people with SMI. The authors concluded that their review did not demonstrate that those receiving CCT had differences in improvement in the areas of service use, social functioning, or quality of life compared with those who received voluntary care or brief supervised discharge. However, those receiving CCT were less likely to be victims of violent or nonviolent crime.

CTOs are considered controversial with debated pros and cons of their usage. Suggested benefits of CTOS include earlier treatment intervention that helps prevent mental health deterioration, increased involvement of family and monitoring clinicians, decreased recurrent hospitalizations, decreased interaction with the criminal justice system, and decreased victimization. Concerns regarding the use of CTOs include therapeutic alliance disruption, adverse medication side effects, stigmatization, disproportionate application to people of color or indigenous populations, and a resulting reluctance of the patient to seek future treatment.[31]

Perhaps CTOs are more effective for some individuals than others, depending on the diagnosis. For example, Beaglehole et al.[32] reviewed nearly 15,000 patients in New Zealand who were placed on a CTO over a 10-year period between January 2009 and December 2018. This study examined the number of psychiatric inpatient admissions per year for individuals on CTOs for a range of psychiatric disorders. These researchers found that the use of CTOs for individuals with a psychotic disorder resulted in reduced hospitalization admissions and frequency. In contrast, individuals with dementia, bipolar disorder, major depressive disorder, and personality disorder had more frequent hospital admissions that were also of longer duration. The authors concluded that compulsory treatment for individuals with psychotic disorders appeared effective in reducing psychiatric hospital admissions and, therefore, relevant in decreasing the disease burden of psychosis.

Optimizing interventions for unhoused individuals with schizophrenia

Unhoused individuals with schizophrenia face an array of challenges, not the least of which is survival. With increased mortality and suicide rates, what are common-sense approaches to caring for these persons who may not want and even refuse treatment? First, practitioners and policymakers should be familiar that many persons with schizophrenia suffer from anosognosia, thereby limiting their ability to appreciate their symptoms and robbing their rational capacity to accept or refuse treatment. Research indicates that between 30 and 50% of patients with schizophrenia lack insight as a prevalent feature of their disorder.[33]

When assessing for decisional capacity to accept or refuse treatment, evaluating the individual's insight into their mental illness may assist in determining whether treatment refusal is linked to an unawareness that they are psychotic and could benefit from treatment. A consensus definition for assessing insight includes addressing the following questions[34]:

1. Is the person aware that they have a mental illness?
2. Does the person understand the need for treatment?
3. Is the person aware of the potential adverse social consequence related to their mental disorder?
4. Is the person aware that they have symptoms?
5. Is the individual able to attribute their symptoms to a mental disorder?

One widely used tool to assess insight in clinical trials and epidemiological studies is the Scale to Assess Unawareness in Mental Disorder (SUMD).[35]

An abbreviated and more practical version of the SUMD has been developed to assist clinical evaluators assess a patient's insight into their mental illness. In contrast to the full SUMD, which has 74 items, the abbreviated SUMD has only 9 items which are rated on a severity scale. This abbreviated version rates the following 9 items as related to their mental awareness:

1. mental disorder;
2. consequences of a mental disorder;
3. effects of drugs;
4. hallucinatory experiences;
5. delusional ideas;
6. disorganized thoughts;
7. blunted affect;
8. anhedonia; and
9. lack of sociability.

This abbreviated version has demonstrated that it is a valid instrument for measuring insight in patients with schizophrenia and can accurately assess insight in clinical settings.[36]

Second, when balancing liberty interests in refusing effective medication treatments for schizophrenia versus the treatment benefits, the reality that medications decrease psychotic symptoms and improve outcomes should not be ignored. Large meta-analyses have demonstrated that oral antipsychotics effectively decrease acute psychotic symptoms.[37] Research also indicates that long-acting antipsychotic injectables are efficacious in treating acutely psychotic individuals with schizophrenia spectrum disorders.[38] Because many individuals with schizophrenia have poor medication adherence, the use of a long-acting injectable helps optimize the delivery of an effective medication for often debilitating symptoms. Failure to provide antipsychotic treatment as early as possible has been associated with negative outcomes. In their research studying two longitudinal cohorts of patients with first-episode psychosis, Drake et al.[39] found that a long duration of untreated psychosis (DUP) was associated with a reduced treatment response over time. DUP represents the time between onset of the first threshold psychotic episode and the initiation of treatment. Longer DUP has demonstrated numerous negative outcomes including less likelihood of symptoms going into remission along with a decreased quality of life and level of functioning.[40] When faced with individuals with schizophrenia who refuse treatments that assist in bringing them closer to reality, psychiatrists should be knowledgeable about the negative impact of delaying treatment so that they can meaningfully inform the relevant decision-maker responsible for treatment refusal overrides. As highlighted above, individuals with schizophrenia are at a much greater risk of early death, completed suicides, and becoming unhoused. These adverse consequences of remaining untreated are relevant when considering compulsory medication to maximize positive treatment outcome.

Third, although the HF approach has shown that individuals with a severe mental disorder who are placed into housing have less days homeless, the research has not demonstrated that those with SMI experience actual symptom reduction with HF alone. Although being placed into housing may decrease the stress and trauma of living on the streets, the HF model by itself is not an effective treatment for the psychotic symptoms of schizophrenia. Combining the HF approach with consideration of compulsory anti-psychotic treatment in symptomatic treatment refusers is essential to prevent deterioration and maximize functioning. As noted above, compulsory treatment orders for individuals suffering from psychosis have demonstrated their utility in decreasing hospitalizations for individuals experiencing psychosis.

Fourth, intensive case management and assertive community treatment provide meaningful support and assistance for individuals with schizophrenia. However, for some individuals with schizophrenia, this level of care does not adequately manage their needs or symptoms. Lamb and Weinberger[13] emphasize the need for more 24-hour structured care facilities as part of the community mental health system. This level of community care will assist those individuals whose psychosis is refractory to treatment as well as decrease the risk of diversion into the criminal justice system. Future policymakers and stakeholders should recognize that current long-term care facilities are not the equivalent of the "snake pit" hospitals of the past, whose horrific conditions understandably played a role in deinstitutionalization of the mentally ill. Moving forward, such 24-hour treatment facilities will likely have an important role in the continuum of care for individuals with schizophrenia who are unhoused or at risk for becoming homeless due to their disability.

Summary

Individuals with schizophrenia are at an increased risk of becoming chronically homeless. While attempting to survive on the streets or in a shelter, they face an onslaught of challenges, from being personally victimized, diverted into the criminal justice system, developing serious untreated medical complications, and dying prematurely. Being untreated and actively psychotic represents its own form of psychic torture. What "works best" includes the following key principles:

1. A rational balance of the individual with schizophrenia's liberty interests with restoration of their sanity and dignity through implementation of compulsory treatment orders when indicated.

2. A recognition that the HF approach alone for individuals with active symptoms of schizophrenia does not address the negative long-term medical and societal outcomes of untreated psychosis. More structured interventions with required treatment involvement are necessary as part of the permanent housing approach.

3. The Harm Reduction approach for individuals with schizophrenia and a co-occurring substance use disorder is unlikely to be effective and may actually perpetuate psychosis, particularly with substances such as cannabis, stimulants, and hallucinogens.

Psychiatrists and mental health professionals play a crucial role in educating policymakers, judges, and other stakeholders that effective treatment and medication therapy work. Society does not have to ignore psychotic humans in despair on the street under the guise of respecting them. In the novel "My Several Worlds," Pearl S. Buck may have said it best when she writes "The test of a civilization is in the way that it cares for its helpless members."[41] Moving forward, we should better care for members of our society who need our help. We should pass this basic test of civilization.

References

1. Institute of Health Metrics and Evaluation. Global Health Data Exchange (GHDx). https://vizhub.health data.org/gbd-results/. Accessed August 27, 2024.

2. American Psychiatric Association. *Diagnostic and Statistical Manual of Mental Disorders,* Fifth Edition, Text Revision. Washington, DC, American Psychiatric Association; 2022.

3. Amador X. Denial of anosognosia in schizophrenia. *Schizophrenia Res.* 2023;252:242–253.

4. Category 1: Literally homeless. HUD Exchanged. hudexchange.info. Accessed August 27, 2024.

5. Treatment Advocacy Center. Serious mental illness and homelessness. www.TreatmentAdvocacyCenter.org. 2016. Accessed August 27, 2024.

6. Lin D, Kim H, Wada K, et al. Unemployment, homelessness, and other societal outcomes in patients with schizophrenia: a real-world retrospective cohort study of the United States Veterans Health Administration database. *BMC Psychiatry*. 2022;**22**:458. doi:10.1186/s12888-022-0422-x.

7. Ayano G, Tesfaw G, Shumet S. The prevalence of schizophrenia and other psychotic disorders among homeless people: a systematic review and meta-analysis. *BMC Psychiatry*. 2019;**27**(1):1–14.

8. Gutwinski S, Schreiter S, Deutscher K, Fazel S. The prevalence of mental disorders among homeless people in high-income countries: an updated systematic review and meta-regression analysis. *PLoS Med*. 2021;**18**(8):e1003750. doi:10.1371/journal.pmed.1003750

9. Barry R, Anderson J, Tran L, et al. Prevalence of mental health disorders among individuals experiencing homelessness. *JAMA Psychiatry*. 2024;**81**(7):691–699.

10. Viron M, Bello I, Freudenreich O, Shtasel D. Characteristics of homeless adults with serious mental illness served by a state mental health transitional shelter. *Community Ment Health J*. 2014;**50**:560–565.

11. Burton D, Jones S, Carlisle T, Holmes A. Homeless men with psychosis are spending more time shelter less. *Australas Psychiatry*. 2021;**29**(2):145–148.

12. Olfson M, Gerhard T, Huang C, Crystal S, Stroup TS. Premature mortality among adults with schizophrenia in the United States. *JAMA Psychiatry*. 2015;**72**(12):1172–1181.

13. Lamb HR, Weinberger LE. The shift of psychiatric inpatient care from hospitals to jails and prisons. *J Am Acad Psychiatry Law*. 2005;**33**(4):529–532.

14. Tsai J, Rosenheck RA. Psychiatric comorbidity among adults with schizophrenia: a latent class analysis. *Psychiatry Rex*. 2013;**210**(1):16–20.

15. Palmer BA, Pankratz VS, Bostwick JM. The lifetime risk of suicide in schizophrenia: a reexamination. *Arch Gen Psychiatry*. 2005;**62**(3):247–253.

16. Lorine K, Goenjian H, Kim S, et al. Risk factors associated with psychiatric readmission. *J Nerv Ment Dis*. 2015;**203**:425–430.

17. Wallace C, Mullen P, Burgess P. Criminal offending in schizophrenia over a 25-year period marked by deinstitutionalization and increasing prevalence of comorbid substance use disorders. *Am J Psychiatry*. 2004;**161**:716–727.

18. Douglas K, Guy L, Hart S. Psychosis as a risk factor for violence to others: a meta-analysis. *Psychol Bull*. 2009;**135**:679–706.

19. Gonzales RJ, Jetelina KK, Roberts M, et al. Criminal justice system involvement among homeless adults. *Am J Crim Just*. 2018;**43**:158–166.

20. Snow DA, Anderson L. *Down on Their Luck: A Study of Homeless Street People*. Berkeley: University of California; 1993.

21. Nilsson SF, Laursen TM, Andersen LH, Nordentoft M, Fazel S. Homelessness, psychiatric disorders, and violence in Denmark: a population-based cohort study. *Lancet Public Health*. 2024;**9**:e376–e386.

22. Roy L, Crocker AG, Nicholls TL, Latimer E, Isaak C. Predictors of criminal justice system trajectories of homeless adults living with mental illness. *Int J Law Psychiatry*. 2016;**49**:75–83.

23. Tsemberis SJ, Moran L, Shinn M, Asmussen SM, Shern DL. Consumer preference programs for individuals who are homeless and have psychiatric disabilities: a drop-in center and a supported housing program. *Am J Commun Psychol*. 2003;**32**(3/4):305–317.

24. Dordick GA. Recovering from homelessness: determining the "quality of sobriety" in a transitional housing program. *Qual Sociol*. 2002;**25**:7–32.

25. Tsemberis S, Asmussen S. From streets to homes: the pathways to housing consumer preference supported housing model. *Alcohol Treat Q*. 1999;**17**(1–2):113–131.

26. Tsemberis S, Gulcur L, Nakae BA. Housing first, consumer choice, and harm reduction for homeless individuals with a dual diagnosis. *Am J Public Health*. 2004;**94**:651–656.

27. Aubry T, Bloch G, Brcic V, et al. Effectiveness of permanent supportive housing and income assistance interventions for homeless individuals in high-income countries: a systematic review. *Lancet Public Health*. 2020;**5**(6):342–360.

28. Loubiere S, Lemoine C, Boucekine M, et al. Housing First for homeless people with severe mental illness: extended 4-year follow-up and analysis of recovery and housing stability from the randomized *Un Chez Doi d/ Abord* trial. *Epidemiol Psychiatr Sci*. 2022;**31**.e14. doi:10.1017/S204579602000026.

29. Beaglehole B, Tennant M. Compulsory community treatment orders (CTOs): recent research and future directions. *BJPsych Open*. 2023;**9**,e86. doi:10.1192/bjo.2023.71

30. Kisely SR, Campbell LA. Compulsory community and involuntary outpatient treatment for people with severe mental disorders. *Cochrane Database of Syst*

Rev. 2014;**12**:CD004408. doi:10.1002/14651858
.CD004408.pub4

31. De Waardt DA, van Melle AL, Widdershoven GAM,
et al. Use of compulsory community treatment in
mental health care: an integrative review of
stakeholders' opinions. *Front Psychiatry.* 2022;
13:1011961. doi:10.3389/fpsyt.2022.1011961

32. Beaglehole B, Newton-Howes G, Porter R,
Frampton C. Impact of diagnosis on outcomes for
compulsory treatment orders in New Zealand. *BJPsych
Open.* 2022;**8**:e415. doi:10.1192/bjo.2022.547

33. David AS. Insight and psychosis. *Br J Psychiatry.*
1990;**156**:798–808.

34. Thompson KN, McGarry PD, Harrigan SM. Reduced
awareness of illness in first-episode psychosis. *Compr
Psychiatry.* 2011;**42**(6):498–503.

35. Amador X. Denial of anosognosia in schizophrenia.
Schizophr Res. 2023;**252**:242–253.

36. Michel P, Baumstarck K, Auquier P, et al.
Psychometric properties of the abbreviated version of
the Scale to Assess Unawareness in Mental Disorder in
schizophrenia. *BMC Psychiatry.* 2013;**13**:229.

37. Huhn M, Nikolalopoulou A, Schneider-Thoma J.
Comparative efficacy and tolerability of 32 oral
antipsychotics for the acute treatment of adults with
multi-episode schizophrenia: a systematic review and
network meta-analysis. *Lancet.* 2019;**394**
(10202):939–951.

38. Vita G, Pollini D, Canozzi A, et al. Efficacy and
acceptability of long-acting antipsychotics in acutely ill
individuals with schizophrenia-spectrum disorders:
a systematic review and network meta-analysis.
Psychiatry Res. 2024;**340**:116124. doi:10.1016/j
.psychres.2024.116124

39. Drake RJ, Husai N, Marshall M, et al. Effect of delaying
treatment of first-episode psychosis on symptoms and
social outcomes: a longitudinal analysis and modelling
study. *Lancet Psychiatry.* 2020;**7**:602–610.

40. Frischherz M, Conus P, Golay P. Reduction of DUP in
early intervention programmes: no pain … almost no
gain. *Early Interv Psychiatry.* 2025;**19**(1):e13580.
doi:10.111/eip.13580

41. Buck PS. *My Several Worlds: A Personal Record.* John
Day Company; 1954.

Chapter 24

What Role Did Serious Mental Illness Play in Jackson Pollock's Drip Paintings?

Abstract Expressionism and Possible Links to Serious Mental Illness and to Encrypted Images (Polloglyphs)

Stephen M. Stahl, Debbi Ann Morrissette, Jahon Jabali, and Jon A. Gates

Introduction

Chronic and severe mental illnesses such as bipolar disorder and schizophrenia often have poor outcomes, especially if available treatments are not implemented and housing is not consistent.[1,2] On the other hand, numerous observers have long noted the shared genetic vulnerability of serious mental illness (SMI) disorder with creativity,[3–13] with this observation attributed to Aristotle himself: "no great genius has ever existed without a strain of madness." Many artists, writers, and celebrities are said to have an SMI including Vincent Van Gogh, Edvard Munch, and Jackson Pollock.[11,12] Here, we explore the relationship of Jackson Pollock's disorder both to the manic energy he exhibited while painting his drips and the proposal that he used symbolic images across his lifetime to articulate his unconscious thoughts and conflicts within his art.

Experts have been fascinated with Jackson Pollock (born 1912, died 1956) and the meaning of his famous "drip paintings" ever since he began producing them in the 1940s.[14–19] Winston Churchill used the phrase "a riddle, wrapped in a mystery, inside an enigma" to describe a situation that was difficult to understand. This quote can undoubtedly be applied to the 70+ years of attempting to comprehend the meaning of Jackson Pollock's famous drip paintings. Some of the currently unresolved questions include: Is there more to them than just the representation of the motion and frenetic activity that occurred during the act of painting, often given as the classical explanation of his genre, abstract expressionism[14–19]? Do his drip paintings incorporate images he expressed in earlier work and possibly arising from his troubled and chaotic inner world? If so, are these images accidental, unconscious, or purposeful to tell a story?

Did Jackson Pollock have an SMI and was it linked to his creation of drip paintings?

It is well documented that Pollock began to have mood swings as a child, with symptoms of social anxiety relieved by alcoholic binges from his teen years until his death (see timeline in Figure 24.1A).[14–19] He received psychiatric treatment from age 23 until his death at age 44 (Figure 24.1B), mostly in the form of outpatient psychoanalytic psychotherapy, with several psychiatric hospitalizations and some psychopharmacologic treatments (Figure 24.1A and Figure 24.1B).[19] Most of his treatment was ineffective by psychiatrists trained in Jungian or Freudian psychoanalysis and at times homeopathic practitioners prescribing "healing minerals".[19]

Pollock's first psychoanalyst was Joseph Henderson, who began treating Pollock during his first year in practice and diagnosed Pollock with schizophrenia and alcoholism (Figure 24.1A).[19] Henderson found that Pollock was not very verbal about his problems or drinking habits so they communicated by means of artistic sketches. The 83 sketches on 69 pieces of paper published in Wysuph's book[18] were thought by Henderson to represent Jungian symbolism and illustrate Pollock's psychiatric illness and unconscious conflicts.[18,19] Henderson also took possession of Pollock's sketches as a form of payment while ignoring doctor–patient confidentiality. However, Henderson wrote and lectured extensively on his sessions with Pollock. He also sold these "therapeutic" drawings for his fame and profit once Pollock became prominent.[14,18,19] Likely, these "sessions" with Henderson were not therapeutic for Pollock, as discussing art in a Jungian psychoanalytic setting today would

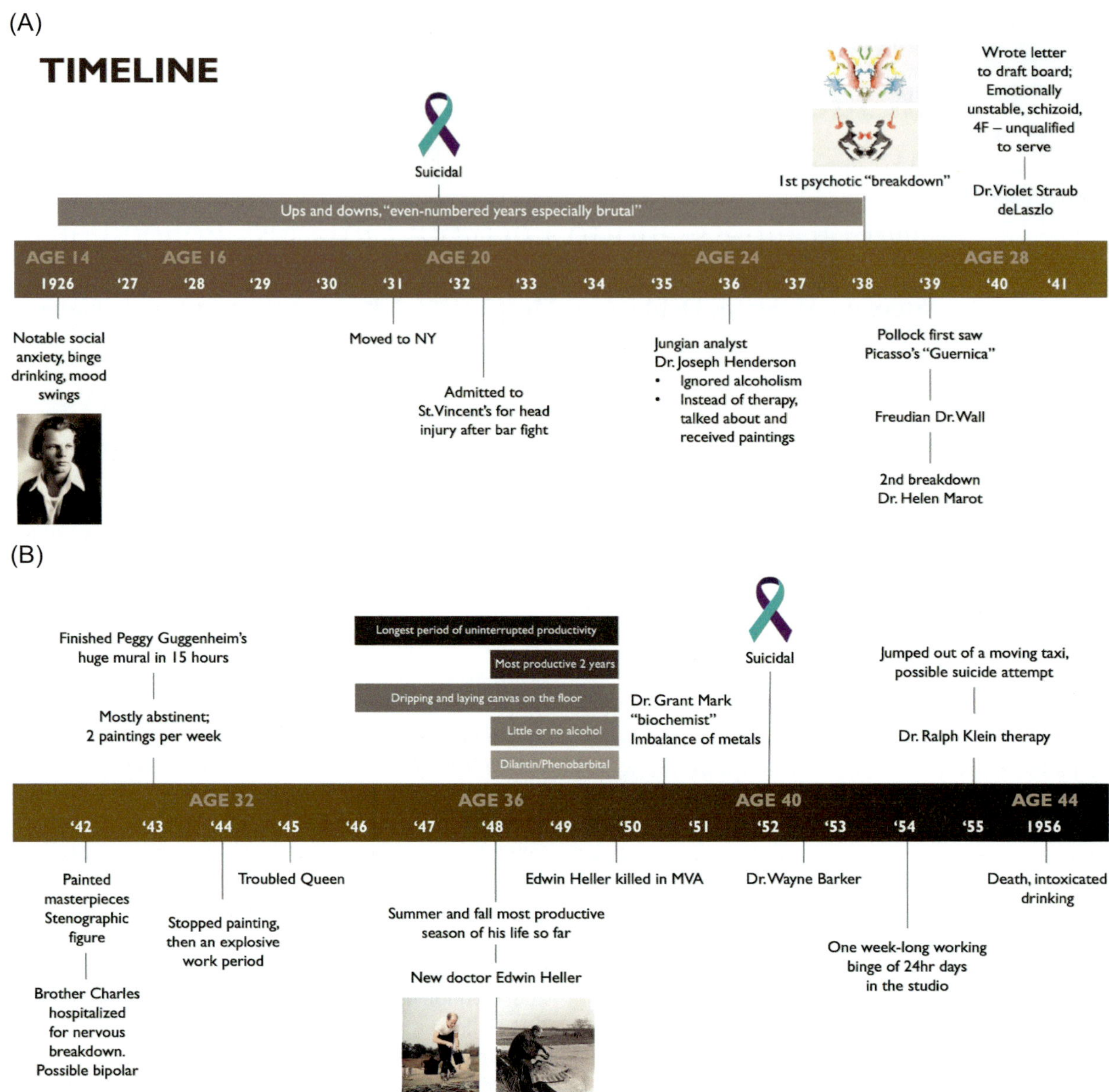

Figure 24.1 (A) Timeline of psychiatric events for Jackson Pollock, ages 14 to 28 (1926–1941). (B) Timeline of psychiatric events for Jackson Pollock, ages 30–44 (1942–1956).

be considered ineffective treatment if not unethical practice for his disorder. In fact, while working with Henderson, Pollock deteriorated. He was psychiatrically hospitalized for the first time at New York Westchester Hospital in 1938 at the age of 26 with his first "breakdown," likely a manic or psychotic episode combined with alcohol intoxication.[19] Without modern mood-stabilizing antipsychotic medications or lithium at the time, Pollock was treated mostly with rest.

Although according to his biographers, Pollock was variably diagnosed by his psychiatrists as "alcoholic psychosis," "schizoid," or "a schizophrenia like disorder characterized by alternating periods of violent agitation and paralysis or withdrawal."[19] In today's world, he would more likely be diagnosed as bipolar. That is, Pollock did not experience the classical paranoid delusions and auditory hallucinations with thought disorder that are now the core diagnostic criteria for schizophrenia.[2] Instead, he experienced very unstable moods with devastating periods of depression alternating with high energy, irritable mania, and hypomania while he self-medicated with huge intakes of alcohol.[19] For example, when Jackson Pollock was living with his brother Sanford and Sanford's wife Arloie, she recalls in Wysuph's book[18] a pattern of mood cycling consistent with bipolar disorder: "Pollock would become unusually quiet and depressed for a few days before going on a "binge." The binge would in turn be followed by a period of solitude and depression. Then, sober, Pollock would begin a period of intense painting and drawing." Pollock's own wife Lee Krasner similarly noted that this very pattern "continued into the late 40s and that during periods of depression, Jackson would become so withdrawn as to be impenetrable."[18]

This cycling of mood that Pollock experienced is typical of bipolar disorder in contrast to periodic episodes of paranoid psychosis with auditory hallucinations which is typical of schizophrenia and which Pollock did not experience. The diagnosis of bipolar disorder is further supported by other comments from Pollock's biography[19] that "more and more the schizophrenic like state described by his psychiatrist was playing itself out in a binary drama of depression and elation." The observation that Jackson's older brother Charles – who exhibited no signs of schizophrenia – was hospitalized in 1942 for a "nervous breakdown" possibly a bipolar episode is also suggestive of a positive family history of bipolar disorder in the Pollock family.[19]

During Pollock's first psychiatric hospitalization, he was tested extensively with Rorschach inkblots, a new way of evaluating psychiatric disorders at the time and adapted from the 1921 publication of inkblots by the Swiss psychiatrist and psychoanalyst Hermann Rorschach.[19] Exposure to Rorschach inkblots would have introduced Pollock to the phenomenon of pareidolia, perceiving specific images out of random or ambiguous visual patterns – which could have very well influenced Pollock's drip technique of camouflaging polloglyphs in his later works. It is now well-known that fractal edges – uneven edges with random patterns – can provoke viewers to see images.[20-23] Rorschach inkblots have fractal edges and are used in psychiatry to provoke the patient to project images onto the inkblots and thereby determine what the patient is thinking to help make a diagnosis.

Pollock's drip paintings also have fractal edges, and the question is whether fractal edges in his drip paintings are an accident of throwing paint, with unintended provoking of images in the observer, or if Pollock recognized that fuzzy edges would provoke images, so he did this on purpose as a component of a technique to consciously or unconsciously create camouflaged images. Art critics generally do not believe Pollock did this on purpose and tend to focus on Pollock's actions during the performance of painting rather than on the images resulting from these actions.[14,19,24,25] If the principal meanings of Pollock's drip paintings are pictorial energy, and a new sense of motion, with the dripped line imparting a sense of constantly changing velocity, then Pollock's bipolar disorder may have been at the heart of how he created this revolutionary new genre in the art world. That is, bipolar mania or hypomania, associated with increased activity, energy or agitation, likely was linked to the creation of Pollock's drip paintings, perhaps nowhere better demonstrated than in Namuth's famous film of Pollock painting where "it is almost impossible to keep track of where Pollock's rapidly launched strokes are landing. The almost inevitable effect is to reinforce the cliché that he is flinging paint at random."[14,19,24]

Pollock's disorder could have also been linked to his embedding images and camouflaging them in his drip paintings. It is well documented that Pollock was afflicted with hallucinatory spells, particularly visual.[19] With his eyes wide open, he would suddenly begin to see whirling images, and Pollock himself realized that for his drip paintings, he had seen those images before he painted them. Bipolar experts have written about altered sensory phenomena experienced in bipolar disorder and even theorized a suprasensory world for some patients with enhanced visual perceptual abilities especially when manic or hypomanic.[25-29] Given that Pollock included images in his pre-drip paintings, and some of these same images occur repeatedly in several of his drip paintings, it is possible that Pollock's bipolar visual perceptions allowed him to develop a unique technique to camouflage images beneath drippings. Pollock himself gave conflicting information on whether his paintings contained images, on the one hand stating, not only "I choose to veil the image"[24] but also "I deny the accident" and "it took a long time to learn how to pour and drip paint like using a giant fountain pen" as though he was painting purposely in the air above the canvas.[19]

About 1947, Jackson Pollock began his drip paintings and his longest period of uninterrupted productivity until about 1950 (Figure 24.1B).[19] During this period, he created his masterpieces, especially during the years between 1948 and 1950, a time when he drank little and was treated with the early mood stabilizers dilantin/phenytoin and phenobarbital.[14,19] These agents are not effective for the treatment of schizophrenia but can improve bipolar disorder, particularly mania.[1,30] Additional evidence is that Pollock had bipolar disorder and not schizophrenia. These observations of improved artistic output and productivity while undergoing effective bipolar disorder treatment support the proposal that serious and disabling mental illness such as bipolar disorder can nevertheless be associated with productive output from creative genius when properly treated. But for the treatment Pollock received during this time, Pollock's greatest masterpieces of abstract expressionism in drip paintings might have never been created. Unfortunately for Pollock and his subsequent productivity, the only psychiatrist who prescribed effective psychiatric treatment for Pollock's bipolar disorder was Edwin Heller, who unfortunately died after just two years of treating Pollock with mood stabilizers.[19] After Heller's death, Pollock stopped his medications, resumed drinking with the return of unstable moods and suicidal ideation, and lost his high productive output for the rest of his life despite seeing others for ineffective treatments and quackery.[19] Pollock eventually crashed his car a few years later after drinking in a possible suicidal act and died at age 44.

Pollock's images in his sketches and paintings prior to his drip paintings

Although Jackson Pollock is most famous for his drip drawings, these occurred late in his career, starting around 1947. Prior to that he produced sketches for his psychoanalyst Henderson in the 1930s as mentioned above, and after that, several nondrip paintings including some "surrealist inflected" paintings and "gestural abstraction" paintings.[19,24]

One example of the earliest sketches of Pollock from the Wysuph book[18] is shown here in Figure 24.2A which we will call "Drunken Ape" (18, plate 76 rotated 180 degrees). This sketch is best observed upside down from the way it is presented in the Wysuph book, a trick Pollock used throughout his career perhaps to better camouflage his images. Figure 24.2A shows a monkey along with a wine bottle and a booze bottle. An outline of these images is

(A)

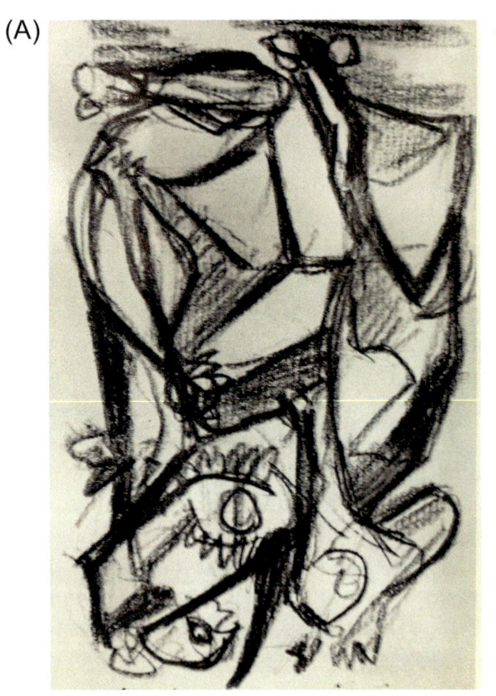

(B)

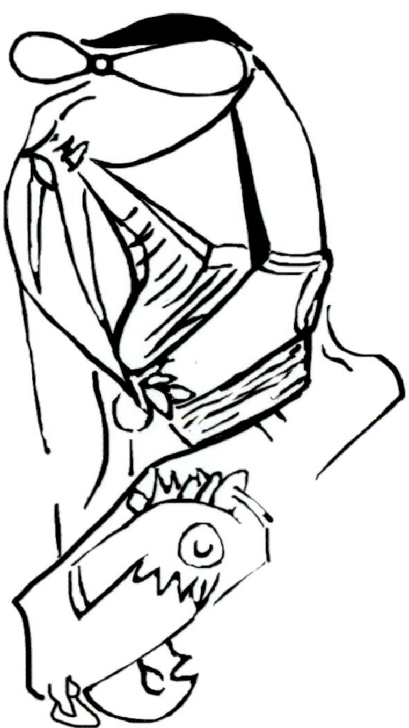

Figure 24.2 "Drunken monkey" untitled sketch from the Wysuph sketchbook utilized by psychiatrist and psychoanalyst Dr. Joseph Henderson to interpret Jungian psychoanalytic conflicts. Plate 76 in reference [18]. (A) Drunken Monkey rotated 180 degrees (upside down). Here, a monkey with glasses can be seen holding a wine bottle with another booze bottle visible. (B) Drunken Monkey with outlines of the embedded images of the monkey, booze and wine bottles, without the background of the original sketch. Compare Figures 24.2A and 24.2B to better visualize the embedded images.

shown in Figure 24.2B and can facilitate recognition of these same images in the original sketch (compared to Figure 24.2A). Monkeys, gorillas, wine bottles, and booze bottles are seen not only in these earliest primitive sketches given to his psychoanalyst in the late 1930s but also throughout Pollock's later abstract paintings and drip paintings (see Figures 24.2–24.5). Pollock was obsessed with drinking and was a very severe alcoholic,[19] which could explain the recurrence of alcohol representations in his work. But what does the monkey represent? Pollock himself? Other sketches from the Wysuph book (18, not illustrated here) include "Highway Robbery," plate 39 showing a shootout of banditos with the driver of a car with

a little boy inside. Another example is "Car Crushed" (18; plate 15) showing what at first glance may look like a Native American sketch, but on closer analysis shows a car running over someone, perhaps Pollock, with paint brushes impaling the tire of the car, possibly to show that painting was literally killing him. Many other sketches contain additional images not only in the Wysuph book but also in subsequent paintings.

For example, not shown here is what we will call "Smoking Monkey" (actually untitled from 1938–41, Art Institute of Chicago) which shows an upside-down monkey in glasses smoking a cigarette. Another example illustrated here in Figure 24.3 is the far more

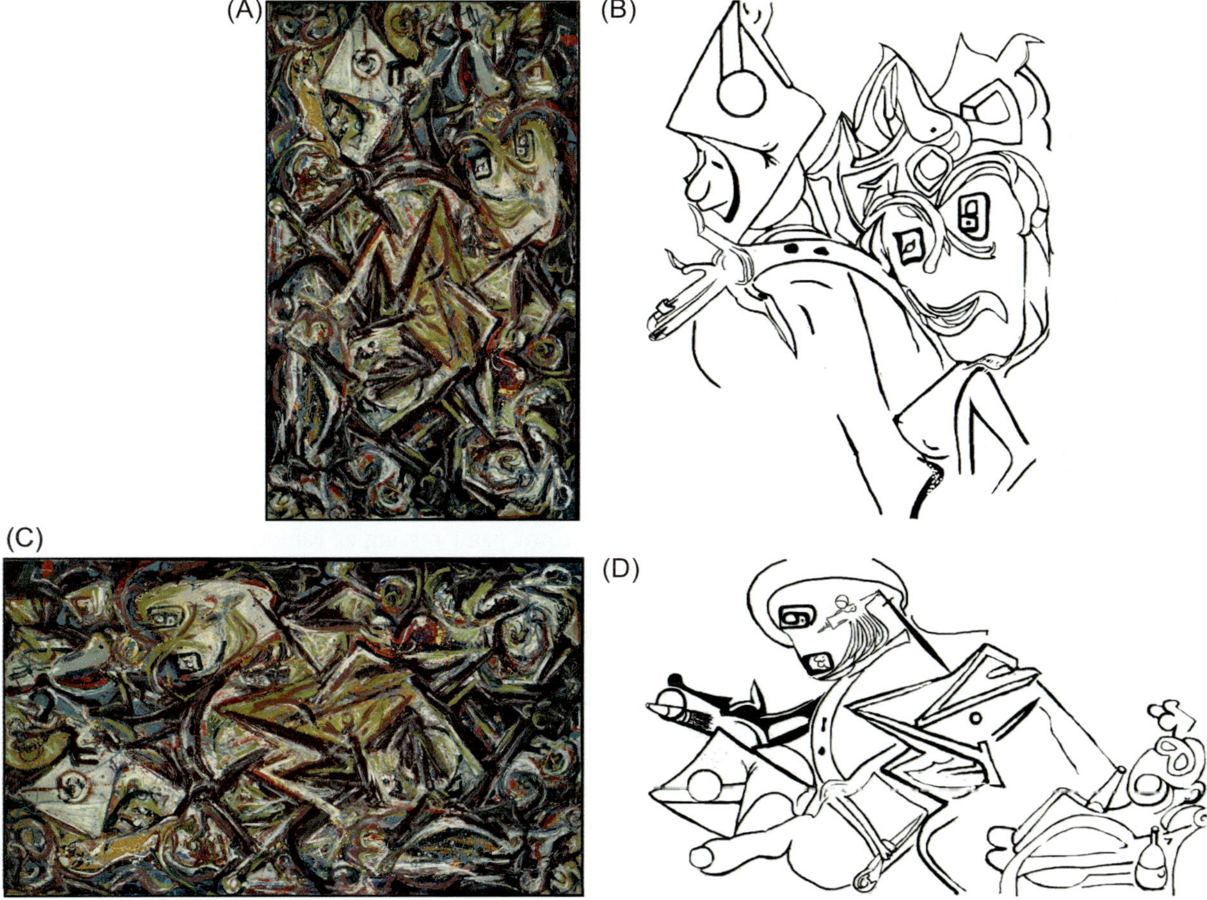

Figure 24.3 Troubled Queen (1945, Museum of Fine Arts, Boston). (A) Troubled Queen upright, original display. Not only a "troubled queen" but also another figure, possibly a soldier, and other images are shown. (B) Troubled Queen. Images of the troubled queen and a soldier in outline without the background of the original painting are shown. Compare Figures 24.3A and 24.3B to better visualize the embedded images. (C) Troubled Queen, rotated 90 degrees counterclockwise. A charging soldier holding a hatchet and a pistol with a bullet in the barrel; a Picasso-esque rooster; a monkey with goggles and wine; and one of the clearest images, the angel of mercy and her sword are shown. (D) Images outlined here without the background of the original painting show soldier, rooster, monkey, and angel of mercy with a sword. Compare Figures 24.3C and 24.3D to better visualize the embedded images.

(A) 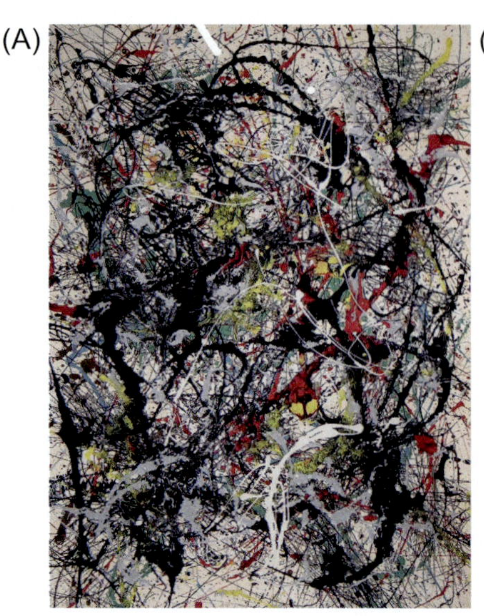

(B) 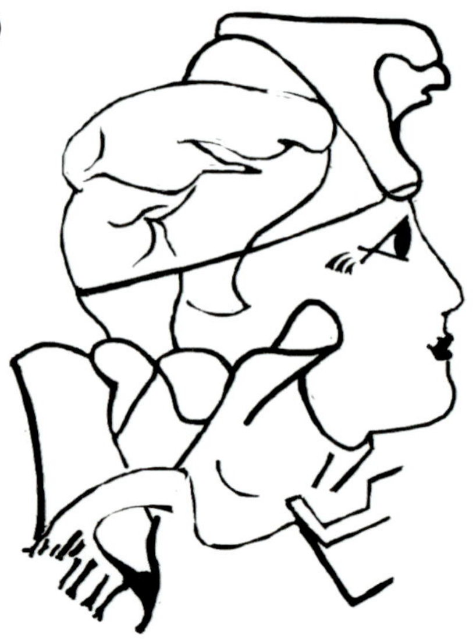

Figure 24.4 "Pretty lady" rotated 90 degrees clockwise (number 34, 1949 Munson-Williams-Proctor Institute Utica NY), one of his drip paintings, which we will call "Pretty Lady." Pollock was rumored to be dedicated to the actress Lauren Bacall and one can see her image in this rotated drip painting (compare Figure 24.4A). Here is a profile of a pretty lady looking to the right. (B) The pretty lady is outlined here without the background of the original painting. Compare Figures 24.4A and 24.4B to better visualize the embedded images.

revealing set of images clearly present in the work titled "Troubled Queen" from 1945 and the Museum of Fine Arts Boston (Figure 24.3). Troubled Queen is considered to be Pollock's masterful transitional work from the regionalist figurative paintings of his early years to the passionate "drip paintings" for which he is best known.[19,24] As stated by Elliot Bostwick Davis et al. (mfashop.com/9020398034), "As Troubled Queen shows, Pollock had begun to work in a very large scale by this time; his paint was dragged over, dripped on, and flung at the canvas. His subject matter was no less highly wrought: emerging from the churning coils and jagged lines of this life-sized canvas are two face-like forms, one a leering mask and the other a one-eyed diamond shape. Their nightmarish presences reflect not only Pollock's agitated psyche but also the years of violence that had torn the world apart through war" (see Figure 24.3A and Figure 24.3B). Thus, Troubled Queen shows convincingly that Pollock included images, which we call polloglyphs, in his painting prior to his "drip paintings," rendering it feasible that he continued to include images in his later classical "drip paintings" using the new technique begun at this time.

Exploiting Pollock's trick to better visualize and uncover many other polloglyphs, Troubled Queen can be rotated 90 degrees counterclockwise (Figure 24.3C) to reveal more images (Figure 24.3D) including a charging soldier holding a hatchet and a pistol with a bullet in the barrel; a Picasso-esque rooster; a monkey with goggles and wine; and one of the clearest images, the angel of mercy and her sword. Troubled Queen was completed in 1945, during World War II, and specifically after 1939, the time when Pollock first saw Picasso's famous Guernica about the Spanish Civil War, which was painted in 1937. Pollock had been excused as unfit to serve in the US army during World War II due to his psychiatric disorder, and one wonders whether the images and timing of Troubled Queen could be telling a story of how Pollock felt about the war and might be his own "Guernica." Pollock was obsessed with Picasso and felt an intense competition with him, always hoping to better that giant with his own work.

Although some of the later polloglyphs shown in later drip paintings and discussed below may be more difficult to see or "decode" from the chaotic layers of thrown paint serving as camouflage (see Figures 24.4 and 24.5), we propose that the images up to this point in Pollock's career are not Rorschach inkblots with fractal edges fooling the eyes and only in the mind of the viewer but represent images purposely put on canvas. Clearly, there is a "troubled queen" in Troubled Queen.

Did Pollock suddenly stop including images in his work and move into abstract expressionism only representing frenetic action painting with no content and the drips only showing the aftermath of movement with fractal edges and false images? Or did he consciously or unconsciously embed polloglyphs as well during his action painting to tell a story?

Art critics state "Once in a while a lifelike image appears in the painting by mistake. But Pollock cheerfully rubs it out because the picture must retain a life of its own".[19,24] Also, "the conscious part of his mind," he says plays no part in the creation of his work. It is

(A) 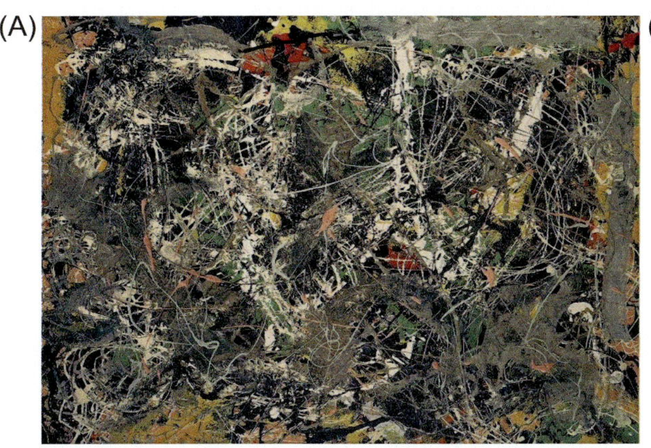 (B) 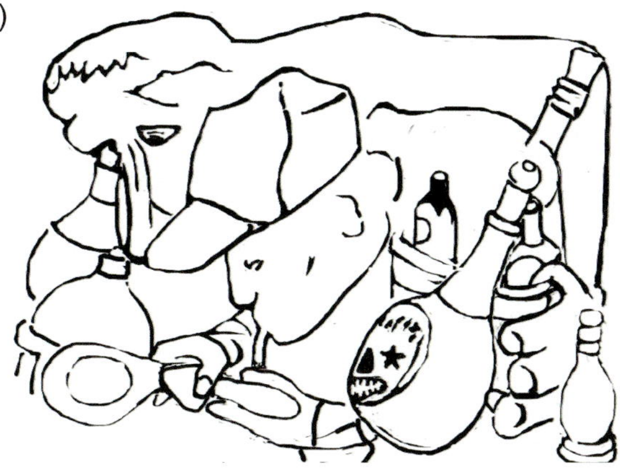

Figure 24.5 (untitled 1949, Foundation Beyeler Reihen/Belel Beyeler Collection, rotated 90 degrees clockwise) which we will call "Monkey on My Back". (A) The original rotated 90 degrees where these images are visible (a smoking Pollock with his signature baseball cap looking at something with a magnifying glass; a monkey (or guerilla) with his arm around Pollock looking on; and also those notorious booze bottles). (B) These images listed in the legend for Figure 24.5A are outlined here without the background of the original painting. Compare Figures 24.5A and 24.5B to better visualize the embedded images.

relegated to the duties of a watchdog; when the unconscious sinfully produces a representational image, the conscience cries alarm and Pollock wrenches himself back to reality and obliterates the offending form".[24] This is why experts not only do not believe there are any images in Pollock's drips, and that any accidental fractal fake images (such as we identify in Figures 24.4 and 24.5) were neither conscious nor unconscious.

Images in Jackson Pollock's drip paintings – polloglyphs. Do these arise purposely from his conscious mind or from his repressed unconscious mind, or are they all in the viewer's mind?

Figure 24.4 shows a 90-degree clockwise rotation of Pollock's painting he numbered #34 (1949 Munson-Williams Proctor Institute Utica NY), one of his drip paintings, which we will call "Pretty Lady." Pollock was rumored to be dedicated to the actress Lauren Bacall and one can see her image in this rotated drip painting (compare Figure 24.4A and Figure 24.4B).

Figure 24.5 (untitled 1949, Foundation Beyeler Reihen/Belel Beyeler Collection, rotated 90 degrees clockwise) which we will call "Monkey on My Back" shows a smoking Pollock with his signature baseball cap looking at something with a magnifying glass, a monkey (or guerilla) with his arm around Pollock looking on, and also those notorious booze bottles (compare Figure 24.5A and Figure 24.5B).

These paintings and several more were presented at a psychiatric congress in November 2023,[26,31,32] and the results of a survey of 48 mental health observers showed that a large majority (75%) felt that Pollock had bipolar disorder, whereas 85% saw images in Pollocks paintings with 58% seeing them in both Troubled Queen and in the drip paintings, and 27% seeing them in Troubled Queen but not in the drip paintings. Finally, 67% thought that images were purposely included by Pollock but disguised, whereas 17% thought the images arose from Pollock's unconscious and even he was not aware of them and another 15% thought that the images were in the viewer's mind not in Pollock's paintings. Only 2% thought there were no images present.[26,31,32]

Discussion

Hamlet: Do you see yonder cloud that's almost in the shape of a camel?

Polonius: By th' mass, and 'tis like a camel indeed.
Hamlet: Methinks it is like a weasel.

Polonius: It is backed like a weasel. Hamlet: Or like a whale?

Polonius: Very like a whale.

This famous dialog from Shakespeare's Hamlet is an example of pareidolia and is used by Hamlet in this case to feign madness on his girlfriend's father Polonius. Perhaps Shakespeare is also using Hamlet to play with the act of perception and ask how can a person ever know what is real? In this case, Polonius cannot be trusted; He is a sycophant, and Hamlet will stab him to death two scenes later. Are polloglyphs present in Jackson Pollock's drip paintings or are they the mad product of viewers' misperceptions? Seeing images in Pollocks drip paintings has been a controversy ever since these paintings were created. So, was Jackson Pollock "Jack the dripper" with paintings "that a dog or cat could have done better," or did Pollock insert polloglyphs – images that are encrypted that tell a story about Pollock's inner being – into his paintings and then disguise them with drippings? On the one hand, some – especially art critics – have emphasized the formal elements of Pollock's work, arguing that no images are present and viewers can find whatever they are looking for because such images are artefacts of the "fractal" fuzzy edges to the drippings and are just fooling the eyes. Thus, maybe Pollock's paintings are just a massive set of new Rorschach inkblots to provoke the viewer to project their own emotions onto the painting, where there is actually nothing at all in the painting from the artist.

On the other hand, seeing an image once in a drip painting could be random; seeing the same image twice in different paintings could be a coincidence; seeing it three or more times, as is the case for booze bottles, monkeys/gorillas, elephants, and more, make those images very unlikely to be random provoked pareidolia (Box 24.1).

Furthermore, from a psychiatric point of view, Pollock had bipolar disorder and painted when he was euthymic or manic and not intoxicated or depressed. He had extensive exposure to Rorschach inkblots during his own psychiatric treatment and had visual images and hallucinations of images, clearly incorporated images into his pre-drip paintings (e.g., see Troubled Queen; Figure 24.3), and he used repeatedly the same images in multiple drip paintings (e.g., booze bottles, images of himself, monkeys, clowns, elephants, and more). The alternate point of view is that Pollock either consciously or unconsciously encrypted images in his drip paintings to tell us a story. His remarkable ability to do this with polloglyphs hiding in plain sight may be part of Pollock's creative genius and could have been enhanced by the endowment of extraordinary visual–spatial skills that have been described in some bipolar patients.[27–30] If so, painting could have been Pollock's way to rapidly unspool his images and to do this onto canvas and thus communicate his personal stories.

In favor of the images being accidental, Pollock himself stated that consciously "I try to stay away from any recognizable image; if it creeps in, I try to do away with it."[19] However, he also admitted "recognizable images are always there in the end."[19] If coming from his deep unconscious creativity and genius, such images may have appeared in spite of himself. Pollock thus may indeed not have been mindful of creating Polloglyphs as he stated "When I am in my painting, I'm not aware of what I am doing."[19] He painted in air, letting gravity make the picture, and dripping became not just another way of obscuring images but also a new way of creating them. Ultimately, we may never know if there are polloglyphs present in Jackson Pollock's famous drip paintings, nor can we know for sure whether they are merely in the mind of the beholder or put there consciously or unconsciously by the artist. In the meantime, it can be enlightening to view Pollock's works and decide for oneself while keeping in mind that chronic and severe mental illnesses such as

---

Box 24.1 Glossary

Abstract expressionism – the representation of free, spontaneous, and personal emotional expression that occurred during the act of painting.

Fractal edges – uneven edges with random patterns which can provoke viewers to see images. Rorschach inkblots have fractal edges and are used in psychiatry to provoke the patient to project images onto the inkblots and thereby determine what the patient is thinking to help make a diagnosis.

Pareidolia – perceiving specific images out of random or ambiguous visual patterns.

Polloglyphs – images arising from Jackson Pollock's conscious or unconscious creativity, and embedded in his paintings, especially his drip paintings, often camouflaged with layers of dripped paint and often to tell a story about something significant in his life.

bipolar disorder can be associated with creativity and genius, with a good outcome, especially with effective treatment.

References

1. Correll CU, Solmi M, Croatto G, et al. Mortality in people with schizophrenia: a systematic review and meta-analysis of relative risk and aggravating or attenuating factors. *World Psychiatry.* 2022;**21**:248–271.

2. Stahl SM. *Stahl's Essential Psychopharmacology,* 5th edition. Cambridge University Press; 2020.

3. Greenwood TA, Creativity and bipolar disorder: a shared genetic vulnerability. *Ann Rev Clin Psychol.* 2020;**16**:239–264.

4. Kyaga S, Lichtenstein P, Boman M, et al. Creativity and mental disorder: family study of 300,000 people with severe mental disorder. *B J Psychiatry.* 2011;**199**:373–379.

5. Biasi B, Dahl MS, Moser P, The role of bipolar disorder and family wealth in choosing creative occupations. *Sci Rep.* 2024;**14**:10703.

6. Johnson SL, Murray G, Fredrickson B, et al. Creativity and bipolar disorder: touched by fire or burning with questions? *Clin Psychol Rev.* 2012;**32**:1–12. doi:10.1016/j.cpr.2011.10.001.

7. Greenwood TA. Positive traits in the bipolar spectrum: the space between madness and genius. *Mol Neuropsychiatry.* 2017;**2**:198–212. doi:10.1159/000452416.

8. Bass M, Nijstad BA, Boot NC, DeDreu CKW. Mad genius revisited: vulnerability to psychopathology, biobehavioral approach- avoidance and creativity. *Psychol Bull.* 2016;**142**:668–692. doi:10.1037/bul0000049.

9. Taylor CL. Creativity and mood disorder: a systematic review and meta-analysis. *Perspect Psychol Sci.* 2017;**12**:104076. doi:10.1177/1745691617 699653.

10. McCraw S, Parker G, Fletcher K, Friend P. Self-reported creativity in bipolar disorder: prevalence, types and associated outcomes in mania versus hypomania. *J Affect Disorders.* 2013;**151**:831–836.

11. Jamison KR. *An Unquiet Mind: A Memoir of Moods and Madness.* Penguin Random House; 1995.

12. Jamison KR. *Touched with Fire: Manic Depressive Illness and the Artistic Temperament.* Simon and Schuster; 1993.

13. Perko M, Stahl SM. *Tesla: His Tremendous and Troubled Life, The Story of Tesla's Genius and Bipolar Disorder.* Prometheus Books/Rowman and Littlefield; 2022.

14. Landau EG. *Jackson Pollock.* Harry N. Abrams Publishers; 1989.

15. Varnedoe K, Karmel P. *Jackson Pollock.* Tate Gallery Publishing, Museum of Modern Art; 1988.

16. Harrison H, ed. *Such Desperate Joy: Imagining Jackson Pollock.* Thunder's Mouth Press/Nation Books; 2000.

17. Friedman BH. *Jackson Pollock: Energy Made Visible.* McGraw-Hill; 1972.

18. Wysuph CL, Jackson P. *Psychoanalytic Drawings.* Horizon Press; 1070.

19. Naifeh S, Smith GW. *Jackson Pollock: An American Story.* Clarkson N. Potter/Publishers; 1989.

20. Abbott A. Fractal secrets of Rorschach's famed ink blots revealed. *Nature.* 2017. doi:10.1038/nature.2017.21473.

21. Taylor R. The facts about Pollock's fractals. 2017. blogs.uoregon.edu/richardtaylor/2017/01/04/the-facts-about-pollocks-fractals/

22. University of Oregon. Fractal edges shown to be key to imagery seen in Rorschach inkblots. 2017. phys.org/news/2017-02-fractal-edges-shown-key-imagery.html

23. Kikon NO. Quasi Jackson Pollock with Rorschach and a hint of Projective test. 2018. medium.com/@mzanokharskikon-/quasi-jackson-pollock-with-rorschach-and-a-hint-of-a-projective-test-1aeea17b7429

24. Karmel P. A sum of destructions. In: Varnedoe K, Karmel, P, eds. *Jackson Pollock.* Tate Gallery Publishing, Museum of Modern Art; 1988: 71–100.

25. Marr D. *Vision: A Computational Investigation into the Human Representation and Processing of Visual Information.* Freeman and Co.; 1982.

26. Parker G, Coroneo MG, Spoelma MJ. Bipolar eyes: windows to the pole? *Aust NZJ Psychiatry.* 2023;**57**:1405–1406. doi:10.1177/00048674231195259.

27. Parker G. The suprasensory world of bipolar II disorder. *Am J Psychiatry.* 2014;**171**:614–615.

28. Parker G, Paterson A, Romano M, Graham R. Altered sensory phenomena experienced in bipolar disorder. *Am J Psychiatry.* 2017;**174**:1146–1150.

29. Parker G, Paterson A, Romano M, Smith, IG. Suprasensory phenomena in those with a bipolar disorder. *Australas Psychiatry.* 2018;**26**: 384–387. doi:10.1177/1039856218 762306.

30. Hesselink Keppel JM, Stahl SM. Phenytoin in bipolar depression: an old chapter, but not yet properly evaluated. *J Mood Disorders Therapy*. 2018;1:24–28.

31. Morrissette DA, Gates, JA, Stahl SM. Pollock's abstract images in paintings prior to his drip paintings. In: *CNS Spectrums, Abstracts of the 19th Annual Neuroscience Education Institute Psychopharmacology Congress*, Colorado Springs, November 8–12; 2023.

32. Gates, JA, Morrissette DA, Stahl SM. Do images in Jackson Pollock's paintings – polloglyphs – arise from his conscious and unconscious or are they all in the viewers' mind? In: *CNS Spectrums, Abstracts of the 19th Annual Neuroscience Education Institute Psychopharmacology Congress*, Colorado Springs, November 8–12; 2023.

The Behavioral Health Care Continuum in the USA

What It Should Look Like and How We Can Pay for It

Elinore F. McCance-Katz

Introduction

The numbers of Americans affected by serious mental illness (SMI), often complicated by substance-use disorders, is rising in the USA. The National Survey on Drug Use and Health (NSDUH) shows marked increases in Americans affected by substance-use and mental disorders. Substance-use disorders rose by 125% over the course of the COVID-19 pandemic.[1,2] There have been increases in the numbers of individuals with mental disorders, and the 2022 NSDUH estimated that 52.9 million Americans met the criteria for a mental illness, and 26% of those have SMI. The numbers with co-occurring mental and substance-use disorders have also increased from 9.5 million in 2019 to 21.5 million in 2022. Of great concern is the finding that in the USA fully one-third of those with SMI get no treatment for their debilitating conditions, impacting quality of life and increasing the likelihood of worsening mental disorders that may be more refractory to symptom-relieving medication when treatment is provided. What follows is a discussion of the current approach to paying for behavioral health care in the USA and future directions to improve clinical services for mental and substance-use disorders, as well as of existing means by which to pay for those enhanced services.

Paying for mental and substance-use disorder care: The current system

Health care insurers reimburse expenses related to the care and treatment of mental disorders. In 2019, USD 106.5 billion was spent on mental health services for 43.9 million (17.3% of the adult population) American adults. Private insurance covered 31.8% of these costs, followed by Medicaid, which paid 25.9%, 19.1% was paid by Medicare and families paid the remaining 14.7%.[3] These estimates do not include costs for children with mental health conditions and

serious emotional disturbance (SED), nor do they include costs for those institutionalized, such as costs related to hospitalization in state hospitals for those with SMI refractory to currently available treatments. Further, these estimates do not include payments for the unique needs of the population of Americans with SMI, including those with psychotic disorders such as schizophrenia, schizoaffective disorder, and bipolar disorder. These individuals need intensive outreach and treatment of mental disorders and co-occurring substance abuse problems because the impairments of their illnesses often prevent them from understanding that they have a mental disorder and that they need care and assistance. Traditional health care insurance fails to adequately compensate for the services necessary to maintain the most seriously mentally ill in treatment, nor does it pay for services that can provide the wraparound support that this vulnerable population requires.

When all costs related to the care and treatment of mental disorders are considered, Medicaid is the largest single payer for these services in the USA. Medicaid is a government program that is a partnership between state governments and the federal government. Its purpose is to provide health insurance coverage to American adults and children who are low income and would not otherwise be able to afford to pay for health care. Increasingly, Medicaid pays for services related to substance-use disorder treatment needs as well.[4] Each state determines the extent of services to be paid for with state tax dollars within the constraints of federal law regarding service coverage. The federal government determines its contribution to these costs using the federal medical assistance percentage (FMAP), which is based on per capita income relative to the national average. It ranges from a low of 50% to a maximum of 83% of the cost of care.[5]

Medicaid is a state program that provides health care services to those with limited income and resources determined by state criteria. Each state develops its own Medicaid plan and makes decisions regarding who qualifies to be a Medicaid beneficiary – the latter being an area of significant shifts with the COVID-19 pandemic and its resolution. States also differ in the means by which service determination will be decided. Most states utilize a managed care approach, with services provided by commercial insurers.

Managed care organizations utilize a variety of approaches aimed at controlling expenses. These include low reimbursements and prior authorization requirements. Low reimbursement and the bureaucracy imposed by prior authorization requirements discourage practitioners from providing behavioral health services to Medicaid beneficiaries. These conditions lead to a dearth of available clinicians, too often relegating some with the greatest need for mental health and substance-use disorder services to lengthy wait periods, or simply to suboptimal care or no care at all. In addition, Medicaid often pays on a fee-for-service basis that minimally compensates medical providers for direct care and excludes compensation for the community-based approaches necessary to support recovery for those with SMI.

To better serve Americans with SMI and severe substance-use disorders, new approaches are needed to increase access to these necessary services and to ensure the best possibility for successful community living.

New models and ideas: Integrated care for serious mental illness

For several decades there has been growing recognition that mental health care, substance abuse treatment, and physical health care have been siloed, with the result being that individuals with co-occurring disorders struggle to obtain necessary care. Further, co-occurring conditions are the rule and not the exception. Physical illnesses and polysubstance misuse are common in those with mental disorders. Outcomes for this population have often been poor. For example, individuals with schizophrenia die, on average, 14.5 years earlier than the general population.[6] This loss of life expectancy is directly related to inability to access essential health care services, including psychiatric, substance abuse, and medical services.

In the USA, the response has been to move toward the establishment of systems of integrated care, termed "certified community behavioral health clinics" (CCBHCs). This model is an outgrowth of the successful federally qualified health center (FQHC) model that provides integrated medical care as well as mental health and substance-use disorder services to patients with mild to moderate behavioral health disorders. The success of the FQHC model depends on its prospective payment system, which ensures that the facility is reimbursed for all of the services provided at cost. Those services include case management, preventive services, health education, and, when needed, transportation. The mental health system in the USA, conversely, has relied on community mental health centers (CMHCs) to provide mental health services to the population with severe mental illness, and it has been poorly reimbursed using Medicaid fee-for-service billing and ancillary support from mental health block grants. The result has been a system of care that is unable to provide the necessary services to Americans with illnesses that impact their ability to carry out routine daily functions. The restrictions on CMHCs include not only low payments, but also prohibitions on case management services, no transportation services, very limited laboratory services needed to monitor responses to and adverse effects of prescribed medications, and limited substance-use disorder services. This system of care that includes basic services for those with uncomplicated behavioral health conditions in FQHCs and the dearth of necessary services for those with severe mental and substance-use disorders in CMHCs have contributed to the large numbers of Americans who experience homelessness and, increasingly, unsheltered homelessness, as well as to disproportionate numbers in jails and prisons with serious mental and substance-use disorders.

CCBHCs were established in the 2014 Protecting Access to Medicare Act. This legislation set the parameters of care for adults with SMI and children with SED. In addition to the integration of mental health, substance-use, and physical health services in one system, CCBHCs are mandated to provide other services as well (Box 25.1).

The requirement for targeted case management as well as community outreach in the form of Assertive Community Treatment (ACT) and Assisted Outpatient Treatment (AOT) will help to address the needs of those who may be too impaired

Box 25.1 Required services in certified community behavioral health clinics

Crisis services: mobile as well as brick-and-mortar facilities

Screening, assessment, diagnosis, and risk assessment

Treatment planning

Outpatient mental health and substance use services

Targeted case management

Outpatient primary care screening and monitoring

Community-based mental health care for veterans

Peer, family support, counselor services

Psychiatric rehabilitation services (including Assertive Community Treatment [ACT] and Assisted Outpatient Treatment [AOT])

by their mental illness to be able to manage their care and to get to brick-and-mortar structures for services. The requirement for 24/7 crisis intervention services will decrease emergency department overcrowding and the countertherapeutic practice of holding severely mentally ill people in these facilities with no treatment while waiting for a hospital bed to become free somewhere. CCBHCs will also offer veterans a community-based alternative to the Veterans Administration Health Centers for those who want that choice for their ongoing behavioral health needs.

The CCBHC program was first initiated by legislative mandate to the Centers for Medicare and Medicaid Services (CMS) to establish these programs in 10 states. The Substance Abuse and Mental Health Services Administration (SAMHSA) initiated a supplemental program that provided funding for specific entities in communities able to put CCBHC services in place. These programs were evaluated by the federal government and found to be successful in terms of improving health care for those with SMI.[7] Early outcomes from CCBHCs showed improvements in mental health functioning, reductions in substance use, reductions in emergency department visits and psychiatric hospitalizations, reductions in homelessness, reductions in criminal justice involvement, and an overall improvement in quality of life.[8] In 2022, the passage of the Safer Communities Act established the CCBHC program nationally with a plan for 10 states yearly to be awarded funding to establish these programs, creating a national system of integrated care for those with the most severe behavioral health conditions.

Innovative models

Substance-use disorders: The hub-and-spoke model

The hub-and-spoke model of care originated in Vermont in response to rising rates of opioid-use disorder (OUD), overdose, and overdose death. It has been adopted and expanded to include partner services in many iterations nationwide at this point. The hub-and-spoke model consists of regional "hubs" that provide intake services for those in need of medication treatment for OUD. The hubs induct and stabilize individuals with the most appropriate, US Food and Drug Administration (FDA)-approved medication for OUD and provide ancillary services during stabilization. The hubs then refer their clients to community providers, who will continue medication for OUD (MOUD), with these providers being known as "spokes." Clients who experience exacerbation of their OUD and relapse behavior can be referred to the hub for further stabilization if needed. Community providers not only continue MOUD, but also provide primary care and in some cases mental health care for those with co-occurring conditions.

The hub-and-spoke model is one that has been adopted in a number of states over the past 10 years. It is particularly appealing to community providers who do not specialize in the treatment of substance-use disorders and, without the backup provided by the hubs, would not be willing to provide MOUD and other medical/psychiatric/substance-use disorder services. This collaborative care model has been utilized to reach some marginalized and underserved populations effectively. For example, this approach has been successfully used to address the needs of incarcerated individuals returning to communities, pregnant women with OUD, individuals referred from syringe-exchange programs, and those who have sought assistance from crisis intervention services.

Hub-and-spoke programs have focused on OUD but could also expand services to include other common substance-use disorders for which FDA-approved medications are available. This would include alcohol- and tobacco-use disorders. Given the high rates of polysubstance abuse, it would make sense to screen for and provide treatment to individuals with polysubstance-use problems. Further, hub-and-spoke programs could partner with local CCBHCs to provide these services in a collaborative care setting that has relationships with local providers who serve not only as spokes but could also be sources of referral for a person with OUD to a hub/CCBHC.

These models, developed and implemented independently, provide a foundation for the integrated health care services necessary to provide seamless services to the most severely mentally ill and those experiencing the most severe substance-use disorders. In serving the most ill, we provide improvements in community living for all.

Service enhancements to improve behavioral health

Full implementation of a continuum of services that will meet the mental health needs of the most seriously ill should include additional components that can be funded through mental health or substance abuse prevention and treatment block grants as well as discretionary funding from Health and Human Services agencies and state funding to provide additional enhancements.

Many experiencing homelessness have untreated mental and/or substance-use disorders. Federal agency cooperation is an important part of the solution. For example, pairing mental health and substance-use services paid for by Medicaid and supplemented with block grant and discretionary funding from SAMHSA in partnership with housing resources provided through the Department of Housing and Urban Development (HUD) programs would be a way of providing wraparound services for high-need and high-risk individuals.

Another area of service enhancement that is important to those with the most severe mental and substance-use disorders is to address the behavioral health needs of those who are incarcerated. The unfortunate reality in the USA is that up to 20% of jail inmates and 15% of those in state prison are estimated to have SMIs.[9] Because jails and prisons do not receive Medicaid funding for health services provided to inmates, an important aim should be to provide funding for mental health services to this population. This is possible with mental health block grant dollars to states that can address the mental health needs of the incarcerated using community-based providers. This approach helps to ensure that those with SMIs leaving jails and prisons are able to seamlessly transition into community mental health services, facilitating the best outcomes for this high-risk group.

Americans with significant mental health and substance-use treatment needs who live in rural areas often struggle to get to facilities that can provide necessary care. An approach that has been successfully implemented in some areas is that of sending mobile units into rural areas to provide substance-use disorder treatment.[10] This model can also be used to provide mental health care as well. Payment for services, again, can be a function of partnerships at the federal level that extend into state systems. For example, the Department of Agriculture has programs that can fund the purchase of equipment such as vans specially outfitted for treatment services for mental and substance-use disorders. Funding for the service provision in these vehicles can be through Medicare/Medicaid, SAMHSA block grant funding, or discretionary funds to meet these special needs. Treatment providers will increasingly need to go directly into communities to ensure that those with the most serious behavioral health conditions receive essential care.

Recovery from SMI and severe substance-use disorders requires a holistic approach. Medical, psychiatric, and psychological care are components of several necessary services for those with the most severe illnesses. The ability for people to have access to community-based resources where they can spend social time with others, work on skills for employment, or return to work or school as well as obtain health support is an important part of recovery. The clubhouse model provides a setting of mutual support and activities, with the goal of maintaining healthy and productive community living for those with SMI.[11] Insurers generally do not pay for such services, but in 2019 SAMHSA made funding available for these types of programs as partners in the CCBHC discretionary grant program. Permanent partnerships between integrated health care programs such as CCBHCs and clubhouse community resources provide an ongoing source of funding for these community programs and build the needed social support system to better support the ongoing mental health of those living with SMI.

Having a continuous source of essential hospital beds for those with SMI and severe substance-use disorders is also a vital part of the safety net for this population. The lack of strong data showing the benefit of acute psychiatric hospitalization has led to the continued downward pressure on hospital lengths of stay, even for those with grave disability who have shown refractoriness to currently available treatment approaches, such that the average length of stay is now approximately 7 days.[12] The Institution of Mental Disease (IMD) exclusion, which prohibits payments by Medicaid to hospitals that have more than 16 beds for psychiatric patients, has contributed to a lack of acute care beds for psychiatric treatment, as well as to the closure of hundreds of thousands of state hospital beds. This reality contributes greatly to homelessness and ongoing severe impairment from mental disorders in people who might have been able to enter recovery if the appropriate level of care and time for intensive, monitored treatment were available to them. Lifting the IMD exclusion is an important step in building the necessary safety net for those with very debilitating behavioral health conditions. The Congressional Budget Office says that lifting the IMD exclusion would cost USD 38.4 billion over 2024–2033.[13] This is far less than the cost of mistreating the seriously mentally ill through homelessness, incarceration, and emergency department boarding, which is what happens now, at a cost of over USD 22 billion yearly. Ending the IMD exclusion is an important part of the safety net for those with the most serious behavioral health conditions and will increase public safety and quality of life within communities.

Addressing potential barriers to progress

The ability to provide behavioral health services to the American people depends on a skilled workforce that can meet their mental health and substance-use treatment needs. There are major shortages in numbers and types of behavioral health providers, and this need is greatest in mental health professional shortage areas (HPSAs). More than one-third of Americans (122 million people) live in these shortage areas, which are rural and remote areas of the country. Lack of providers and geographic challenges, in addition to the scope of practice limitations and reimbursement issues, translate into nearly half of the 59 million Americans with mental health conditions not receiving treatment.

One way to address this problem would be to prioritize the training of behavioral health providers in order to grow the workforce. Currently, the Health Resources and Services Administration (HRSA) estimates a behavioral health workforce shortage that exceeds 800,000, with over 100,000 of that shortage being in adult and child psychiatrists.[14] Loan repayment programs for service in HPSAs are currently available through the National Health Services Corps that is administered by HRSA. However, the HPSAs cover large areas and do not distinguish between rural and more remote areas. As a result, some rural towns and cities will get available practitioners while more remote areas do not attract these clinicians. States can assist in this by offering additional incentives for loan repayment to attract behavioral health providers to those areas of their jurisdictions where they know need to be greatest. Health care companies can offer incentives to attract clinicians in high-need specialties to join their workforces. The state and federal governments can increase interest in behavioral health careers through grants or loan repayment plans that incentivize the choice of a career in behavioral health. Such programs can be innovative and can target any number of specific needs of a population. Understanding on the part of leaders with the ability to legislate conditions and funding of the critical lack of workforce that can provide necessary clinical care to Americans with serious mental health and substance-use conditions is imperative. This is an area that will need to be a focus for stakeholders who serve this population of Americans and their families with great need.

Conclusion

Addressing the needs of those with SMI and severe substance-use disorders requires a multifaceted approach that encompasses psychiatric, medical, and substance-use disorder treatment as well as community supports that provide holistic care for some of our most disabled and vulnerable people. There are already in place models of care that can better coordinate and integrate services to ensure that this population gets the necessary care and community resources. Further, there are federal and state funding mechanisms that already exist to serve people with these conditions. The challenge will be to innovate in how we utilize these funds to assist some of our most severely ill in successful community living.

References

1. National Survey on Drug Use and Health 2019. Rockville, MD: Substance Abuse and Mental Health Services Administration, 2020.

2. National Survey on Drug Use and Health 2022. Rockville, MD: Substance Abuse and Mental Health Services Administration, 2023.

3. Soni A. Healthcare expenditures for treatment of mental disorders: Estimates for adults ages 18 and older, U.S. civilian population, 2019. https://meps.ahrq.gov/data_files/publications/st539/stat539.pdf. Accessed December 15, 2024.

4. Medicaid.gov. Behavioral Health Services. www.medicaid.gov/medicaid/benefits/behavioral-health-services/index.html. Accessed December 15, 2024.

5. KFF. Federal Medical Assistance Percentage (FMAP) for Medicaid and Multiplier. www.kff.org/medicaid/state-indicator/federal-matching-rate-and-multiplier. Accessed December 15, 2024.

6. Galletly CA. Premature death in schizophrenia: Bridging the gap. *Lancet* 2017;4(4):263–265.

7. Substance Abuse and Mental Health Services Administration (SAMHSA). Certified Community Behavioral Health Clinics demonstration program, Report to Congress, 2017. www.samhsa.gov/sites/default/files/ccbh_clinicdemonstrationprogram_081018.pdf. Accessed October 16, 2025.

8. Substance Abuse and Mental Health Services Administration (SAMHSA). Report to Congress on the Certified Community Behavioral Health Clinic expansion (CCBHC-E) grant program, 2020.

9. Treatment Advocacy Center. Treatment Advocacy Center homepage. https://tac.org. Accessed December 15, 2024.

10. Crumpler R. NC turns to mobile clinics to expand substance use treatment. www.northcarolinahealthnews.org/2025/09/16/nc-turns-to-mobile-clinics-expand-opioid-addiction-treatment/. Accessed October 16, 2025.

11. Fountain House. What is a clubhouse? www.fountainhouse.org/about/clubhouse-model. Accessed December 17, 2024.

12. American Psychiatric Association. The psychiatric bed crisis in the U.S., understanding the problem and moving toward solutions. May 2022. www.psychiatry.org/getmedia/81f685f1-036e-4311-8dfc-e13ac425380f/APA-Psychiatric-Bed-Crisis-Report-Full.pdf. Accessed December 17, 2024.

13. Congressional Budget Office. Budgetary effects of policies to modify or eliminate Medicaid's institutions for mental diseases exclusion. April 2023. www.cbo.gov/system/files/2023-04/58962-Medicaid-IMD-Exclusion.pdf. Accessed October 16, 2025.

14. HRSA. State of the Behavioral Health Workforce, 2024. https://bhw.hrsa.gov/sites/default/files/bureau-health-workforce/state-of-the-behavioral-health-workforce-report-2024.pdf. Accessed February 9, 2025.

A Unified Understanding of the Human Mind – A Neuroethical Perspective

Tracing the Evolution in Western Thought and the Integration with Neuroscience, Psychology, Psychiatry, and Relational Dimensions

Alberto Carrara

Introduction

The concept of the mind has been a central focus of intellectual inquiry in the Western world, with its evolution marked by a rich tapestry of philosophical, psychological, and scientific developments. From ancient Greece to the present day, the understanding of the mind has undergone significant transformations, reflecting shifts in philosophical paradigms, scientific advancements, and societal perspectives.

This article explores the historical trajectory of the concept of human mind in the Western context, leading to a contemporary synthesis that integrates neuroscientific data, psychological and psychiatric orientations, and the relational dimension. This emerging framework on the reality of the human mind represents a valuable tool to validate a specific psychiatric treatment or a concrete psychological assessment.

The human mind in history

Ancient Greece

In ancient Greece, the exploration of the mind (ψυχή) marked a foundational chapter in Western philosophical thought. Early thinkers like Thales, Anaximenes, and Heraclitus sought to unravel the mysteries of human consciousness, offering diverse theories that spanned the spectrum from materialistic to metaphysical–spiritual explanations. Thales, for instance, speculated about water as the fundamental substance underlying all existence, including mental phenomena. Anaximenes, in turn, proposed air as the essential element shaping the mind.

However, the seminal contributions of these early philosophers paved the way for a more intricate understanding of the mind through the works of Plato. The body–mind problem is one of the most fundamental philosophical questions, which concerns the nature and relationship of the human mind and body. Plato's dialogue *Alcibiades I* (On human's nature) explores this problem through the conversation between Socrates and the young and ambitious Alcibiades, who wants to become a great leader of Athens. Socrates challenges Alcibiades to examine himself and his own nature before he can rule others or engage in politics. He argues that self-knowledge is the most important and divine kind of knowledge, and that it requires looking at the soul, which is the true self of a person.[a] The dialog presents three possible solutions to the body–mind problem, which can be called the dualistic, the monistic, and the unidual solutions. The dualistic solution is based on the idea that the mind and the body are two distinct and separate entities (or substances or *res*, in Latin), and that the mind is superior to the body in every way. The mind is immortal, divine, rational, and beautiful, while the body is mortal, material, irrational, and ugly. The mind is the source of virtue and wisdom, while the body is the source of vice and ignorance. The mind is the true self, it is the human being, while the body is a mere instrument or prison for the mind.[b] The dualistic solution implies that the mind should detach itself from the body as much as possible and seek to contemplate the eternal and intelligible forms, which are the objects of true knowledge. The monistic

---

[a] Plato. Alcibiades I, 130 C: ο άνθρωπος δεν είναι τίποτε άλλο παρά η ψυχή του, id est: human being is nothing but his soul (mind).

[b] Plato. Alcibiades I, 129 A.

solution is based on the idea that the mind is not real, but it is just an epiphenomenon of the material constitution of the body. This type of monistic interpretation is called materialistic monism, and it is very present in nowadays society. Finally, the unidual solution of the mind–body problem is based on the idea that the mind and the body are not separate, but rather aspects of the same entity, which is the human being. The mind and the body are both natural and necessary parts of the human nature, and they both contribute to the human excellence and happiness. The mind is not superior to the body, but rather depends on the body for its proper functioning and development.

Plato's philosophical legacy is notably encapsulated in his theory of the tripartite soul, expounded in works such as *Phaedrus* and *The Republic*. Departing from the monistic inclinations of his predecessors, Plato introduced a dualistic perspective that delineated the mind into three distinct components: the rational, the spirited, and the appetitive. Plato's tripartite soul concept was a metaphorical construct designed to illuminate the complex dynamics of human psychology. The rational component, located in the head, represented the intellect and reason, governing logical thought processes. The spirited aspect, residing in the chest, embodied the emotional and courageous dimensions of the psyche, steering the individual toward honor and virtue. Lastly, the appetitive element, situated in the abdomen, symbolized primal desires and appetites, encompassing basic needs and passions.

Plato's dualistic framework, while rooted in abstract metaphors, laid the groundwork for later philosophical discussions on the mind–body relationship. The tripartite soul not only influenced subsequent Hellenistic and Roman philosophies but also resonated across centuries, leaving an enduring impact on Western thought. This dualistic perspective, emphasizing the interplay of reason, emotion, and desire, set the stage for future inquiries into the nature of the mind, ultimately contributing to the rich tapestry of ideas that shaped the evolution of Western philosophical and psychological thought.

Cartesian dualism

René Descartes, in the 17th century, furthered the dualistic tradition by asserting a strict separation between mind and body. Cartesian dualism posited that the mind (*res cogitans*) and the body (*res extensa*) were distinct entities, with the mind serving as the seat of consciousness and reason. This separation influenced Western thought for centuries. In the 17th century, René Descartes made a profound impact on the understanding of the mind through his formulation of Cartesian dualism, a philosophical stance that fortified and extended the dualistic tradition in Western thought. Descartes, often regarded as the father of modern philosophy, departed from the prevailing ideas of his time by asserting a rigorous and unequivocal separation between the mind and the body. Descartes' dualistic framework is encapsulated in his famous assertion, *Cogito, ergo sum* (I think, therefore I am). According to Cartesian dualism, the mind, referred to as *res cogitans* or the thinking substance, and the body, termed *res extensa* or the extended substance, were fundamentally distinct entities. The mind, in this paradigm, was conceptualized as the seat of consciousness, self-awareness, and reason, while the body was considered a mechanical, extended entity governed by physical laws. Descartes' emphasis on the separation of mind and body was motivated by a desire to establish a foundation for certain knowledge. By isolating the mind as a thinking substance, he sought to ground human certainty in the realm of reason, thereby initiating a methodical and systematic approach to understanding reality. This conceptual division also allowed Descartes to reconcile the incorporeal nature of the mind with the materialistic aspects of the body, providing a framework that aligned with the scientific inquiries of his era. The influence of Cartesian dualism extended far beyond Descartes' immediate intellectual milieu, permeating Western thought for centuries. This dualistic perspective profoundly impacted the fields of philosophy, science, and psychology, setting the stage for ongoing debates regarding the mind–body relationship. While Descartes' approach brought clarity to philosophical discourse, it also fostered a dichotomous view that hindered a more holistic understanding of human nature. Critics of Cartesian dualism argue that such a strict separation oversimplifies the complexities of the mind–body interaction, neglecting the intricate interconnections between mental and physical phenomena. Nevertheless, Descartes' legacy remains palpable in the enduring dichotomy between mind and body that continues to shape contemporary philosophical and scientific discussions. The Cartesian dualistic tradition, with its enduring impact, serves as a critical juncture in the historical trajectory of Western conceptions of the mind.

Empiricism and associationism

The empiricist tradition, championed by philosophers like John Locke and David Hume, shifted the focus from innate ideas to the mind's dependence on sensory experience. The associationist perspective, as articulated by thinkers like David Hartley and James Mill, emphasized the role of associations in mental processes, laying the groundwork for a more empirical understanding of the mind. The empiricist tradition, a pivotal chapter in the history of Western thought on the mind, emerged as a reaction against the rationalist doctrines that posited innate ideas and a priori knowledge. Spearheaded by luminaries such as John Locke and David Hume, empiricism redirected attention toward the notion that the mind is a tabula rasa, a blank slate shaped by sensory experiences and external stimuli. John Locke, often regarded as the founder of empiricism, contended that the mind at birth is void of any innate ideas and that all knowledge is derived from sensory impressions. In his *Essay Concerning Human Understanding*, Locke proposed that the mind is like an empty vessel that gradually accumulates knowledge through sensory experiences, thereby emphasizing the importance of observation, perception, and reflection in the formation of ideas. For Locke, the human person is the reasoning and self-conscious entity which is independent of the body.[1,c]

David Hume, a prominent figure in the Scottish Enlightenment, took Locke's empiricism to new heights by challenging the concept of causation and questioning the nature of reality itself. In his *A Treatise of Human Nature*, Hume delved into the idea that all knowledge is based on impressions and ideas, rejecting the existence of causally connected entities. Hume's radical empiricism undermined traditional notions of causation and fueled skepticism, reshaping the landscape of epistemology and the philosophy of mind. The associationist perspective, intricately linked with empiricism, found expression through the works of thinkers like David Hartley and James Mill. David Hartley, in his *Observations on Man, His Frame, His Duty, and His Expectations*, proposed a psychological theory based on the principle of associationism. Hartley argued that mental phenomena, including thoughts and emotions, result from the association of sensory experiences, forming complex chains of ideas. James Mill, a utilitarian philosopher and father of John Stuart Mill, further developed the associationist framework by positing that mental processes are composed of elementary ideas linked through associative principles. Mill's contributions laid the groundwork for a more systematic and empirical understanding of the mind, wherein complex mental phenomena could be dissected into simpler components governed by principles of association. The empiricist and associationist tradition, championed by Locke, Hume, Hartley, and Mill, shifted the intellectual landscape away from innate ideas toward an empirical investigation of the mind's reliance on sensory experiences and the associative processes governing mental life. This paradigmatic shift not only influenced the trajectory of philosophy but also paved the way for the empirical methods embraced by modern psychology, marking a significant transition in the evolution of Western thought on the nature of the mind.

Structuralism and functionalism

In the late 19th century, psychology emerged as a distinct scientific discipline. Structuralists like Wilhelm Wundt sought to analyze the mind's structure through introspection, while functionalists like William James focused on understanding the mind's adaptive functions. This period marked the beginnings of a more systematic and empirical approach to the study of the mind. The late 19th century witnessed the birth of psychology as a distinct scientific discipline, marking a departure from philosophical speculation to a more systematic and empirical inquiry into the intricacies of

---

[c] "This being premised, to find wherein personal identity consists, we must consider what PERSON stands for; which, I think, is a thinking intelligent being, that has reason and reflection, and can consider itself as itself, the same thinking thing, in different times and places; which it does only by that consciousness which is inseparable from thinking, and, as it seems to me, essential to it: it being impossible for anyone to perceive without PERCEIVING that he does perceive. When we see, hear, smell, taste, feel, meditate, or will anything, we know that we do so. Thus, it is always as to our present sensations and perceptions: and by this everyone is to himself that which he calls SELF:—it not being considered, in this case, whether the same self be continued in the same or divers substances. For, since consciousness always accompanies thinking, and it is that which makes everyone to be what he calls self, and thereby distinguishes himself from all other thinking things, in this alone consists personal identity, i.e. the sameness of a rational being: and as far as this consciousness can be extended backwards to any past action or thought, so far reaches the identity of that person; it is the same self now it was then; and it is by the same self with this present one that now reflects on it, that that action was done."

the mind. This transformative period gave rise to two influential schools of thought: structuralism, led by Wilhelm Wundt, and functionalism, championed by William James. Wilhelm Wundt, often regarded as the father of experimental psychology, founded the first psychological laboratory in 1879 at the University of Leipzig. Wundt's structuralist approach aimed to unravel the complexities of the mind by employing a method known as introspection. Subjects were instructed to reflect on and report their own thoughts, feelings, and sensations in response to controlled stimuli. Through these introspective analyses, Wundt sought to identify the fundamental elements, or structures, of consciousness. His emphasis on rigorous observation and experimental procedures laid the foundation for psychology as a scientific discipline. In contrast to Wundt's structuralism, William James, a pioneering American psychologist, spearheaded the functionalist movement. James shifted the focus from the mere analysis of the mind's structure to understanding the adaptive functions of mental processes. His seminal work, *The Principles of Psychology*, explored how the mind functions to help individuals adapt to their environment. James was particularly interested in the evolutionary advantages conferred by various mental phenomena, emphasizing the practical utility of consciousness and behavior. Functionalism broadened the scope of psychological inquiry, incorporating the study of emotions, habits, and practical problem-solving into the discipline. The structuralist and functionalist perspectives, though distinct, shared a commitment to empirical investigation and the scientific study of the mind. Structuralism sought to identify the elemental building blocks of consciousness, paving the way for systematic analysis. Meanwhile, functionalism focused on the adaptive roles of mental processes, aligning psychology with evolutionary principles and emphasizing the pragmatic significance of cognitive functions. This period marked a pivotal shift in the history of psychology, transitioning from speculative and introspective approaches to a more rigorous, empirical, and experimental discipline. The legacy of structuralism and functionalism endured, influencing subsequent psychological schools and shaping the development of methodologies that remain integral to contemporary psychological research. The dialectical interplay between these two schools laid the groundwork for the multifaceted and interdisciplinary nature of modern psychology, reflecting the evolving quest to comprehend the intricate workings of the human mind.

Expressive individualism

According to O. Carter Snead, a legal scholar and bioethicist, Expressive Individualism is an anthropology where the individual self is the fundamental unit of human reality. This self is not defined by its attachments or network of relations, but rather by its capacity to choose a future pathway that is revealed by the investigation of its own inner depths of sentiment. Key aspects of expressive individualism according to Snead include: (i) The self is not defined by objects of choice – whether property, a particular vocation, or even the creation of a family. (ii) The self is associated fundamentally with its will and not its body. (iii) Flourishing is achieved by turning inward to interrogate the self's own deepest sentiments to discern the wholly unique and original truths about its purpose and destiny. (iv) The truth about the self is not determined externally, and sometimes must be pursued counterculturally, over and above the mores of one's community. (v) The self is bound only to those commitments freely assumed. Does this contemporary vision reflect the full lived reality of human embodiment, with all that it entails?

Contemporary integration: Nowadays' concept of the human mind

The advent of advanced neuroimaging techniques, such as functional magnetic resonance imaging (fMRI) and electroencephalography (EEG), has allowed researchers to explore the neural correlates of mental processes. Neuroscientific data provide valuable insights into the biological underpinnings of cognition, emotion, and behavior.

Contemporary psychology and psychiatry have evolved from a neurocentric view of the human mind – born in ancient time with Alcmaeon of Croton and Hippocrates' *De morbo sacro* – to incorporate a holistic understanding. Psychodynamic, cognitive behavioral, and humanistic approaches offer diverse perspectives on mental health, considering both conscious and unconscious processes. The Diagnostic and Statistical Manual of Mental Disorders (DSM) reflects the ongoing effort to classify and understand psychiatric conditions.

According to psychiatrist and philosopher Thomas Fuchs, for example, there is a concrete and scientific-based alternative perspective to the prevailing naturalist view (or *neurocentric* view) that mental illnesses can be solely attributed to brain dysfunctions. Fuchs argues that mental illness cannot be reduced to mere brain dysfunction. His systemic and ecological account is based on three realities: (1) contextual understanding, *id est*, mental illness is inseparable from both the living organism and the patient's life world or social environment. It cannot be isolated solely within the brain; (2) circular causality, *id est*, Fuchs proposes a shift from unilinear causation to circular causality. Mental disorders result from disruptions in both vertical circular causality (interplay between lower-level processes and higher faculties of the organism) and horizontal circular causality (social relationships and responsiveness to others); and finally, (3) brain mediation, *id est*, while brain processes play a role. Mental illnesses cannot be exclusively located within the brain. Reduction of mental illnesses to brain diseases is fundamentally challenging. Nowadays neuroscientific account teaches us the interconnectedness of mental illness with the whole person, their context, and circular causal processes beyond the brain. This perspective invites us to consider a more holistic understanding of mental health and a better 360-degree therapeutic interventions.[2] The brain is interpreted as a subsystem of the person-system as a mediating organ:

> Cognitive neuroscience has been driven by the idea that by reductionist analysis of mechanisms within a solitary brain one can best understand how the human mind is constituted and what its nature is. The brain thus came to appear as the creator of the mind and the experienced world. In contrast, the paper argues for an ecological view of mind and brain as both being embedded in the relation of the living organism and its environment. This approach is crucially dependent on a developmental perspective: the brain is conceived as a plastic system of open loops that are formed in the process of life and closed to full functional cycles in every interaction with the environment. Each time a new disposition of coherent neural activity is formed through repeated experience, structures of the mind are imprinted onto the brain. The brain becomes a mediating organ or a window to the mind, for it is structured by the mind itself.[3]

Acknowledging the relational dimension involves recognizing the impact of social, cultural, and interpersonal factors on mental wellbeing. From family systems theory to attachment theory, contemporary approaches highlight the importance of relationships in shaping psychological development and mental health.

Daniel J. Siegel, a prominent psychiatrist, clinical professor, and author, is known for his pioneering work in the field of interpersonal neurobiology. His holistic approach to understanding the human mind transcends traditional disciplinary boundaries, integrating neuroscience, psychology, and the social sciences. Siegel's vision of the human mind is encapsulated in his concept of the mind itself, a term he uses to represent the embodied and relational nature of mental processes. Siegel emphasizes the idea of the mind as an emergent and embodied process that arises from the intricate interplay of the brain, the body, and the external environment. Siegel's work is deeply rooted in the interdisciplinary field of interpersonal neurobiology.[4] This approach integrates findings from neuroscience, psychology, and other disciplines to offer a comprehensive understanding of the mind. Siegel posits that the mind is not confined to the brain alone but is distributed throughout the body and is shaped by social interactions. Siegel emphasizes the embodied nature of the mind, acknowledging the interconnectedness of the brain and the body. He underscores the importance of integration, both within the brain itself (integration of different neural circuits) and between the individual and their social environment. Integration, according to Siegel, leads to a flexible and adaptive mind. The term *mindsight* refers to the capacity to perceive and understand one's internal mental processes. It involves the ability to observe one's thoughts and feelings without being overwhelmed by them. Mindsight, as conceptualized by Siegel, is crucial for mental well-being, fostering emotional regulation, empathy, and enhanced interpersonal relationships. Siegel often refers to the *triangle of wellbeing*, which highlights the interconnectedness of the mind, the brain, and relationships. This model underscores the idea that the mind is shaped by both internal and external factors, including biological processes, mental activities, and social interactions. Siegel embraces the concept of neuroplasticity, the brain's ability to reorganize and adapt in response to experience. This idea reinforces the notion that the mind is not fixed but can be shaped and transformed through intentional mental practices, relationships, and experiences.[5]

This vision of the human mind is a holistic and integrative perspective that emphasizes the embodied, relational, and dynamic nature of mental processes. By weaving together insights from various disciplines, it provides a framework for understanding how the mind emerges from the intricate dance between the brain, the body, and the social world. This contemporary account of the body–mind problem sees the human person as a unity, neither a sole brain, nor a disembodied mind, but a third "thing":

> ... [A human being] is said to be from soul and body as a third thing constituted from two things neither of which he is, for a [human] is not soul nor is he body.[6]

This medieval understanding indicates that one body plus one soul/mind equals a third, original material: the human being, which has a dual nature (not dualistic!). It is surprising that a contemporary holistic and integrative account of the human person sounds in the line of Thomas Aquinas' consideration that it is not the body (or the brain) that "contains" the mind, but the mind the body.[7]

According to the well-known Italian philosopher of science Evandro Agazzi, the human mind is a complex subsystem of the whole person-system characterized – according to psychiatrist Daniel J. Siegel, Thomas Fuchs, and Georg Northoff – as an emergent, self-organizing, embodied, and relational (embeddedness) process that regulates the flow of energy and information of the organism. This definition suggests that the mind is not confined to or localized in the brain or even the physical body but is a systemic process that emerges from both the body and our relationships with others and the environment (epigenetic causality). It also implies that the mind is capable of self-organization and plays a crucial role in regulating how energy and information flow within us and between us and our environment. This perspective allows for a more comprehensive understanding of the mind, encompassing not just our thoughts, emotions, and memories but also our connections with others and the world around us.[8]

So, what does it really mean to be *human*, to be a human *person*? In contemporary neuroethical account – neuroethics is a systematic and informed reflection dealing with neuroscience and interpretations of the same neural sciences – the human person is not considered as a "separate and distinct from the manner in which he is or is not embedded in a web of social relations," neither he/she is not identified with and defines by the exercise of their will – their capacity for choosing in accordance with their wants and desires"; the human person is not identical to the psychological conception of personhood that "decisively privileges cognition as the indispensable criterion for membership in this category of beings. In this way, it appears to be dualistic, distinguishing the mind from the body." The mind and will alone do not define the whole of the human person, and the body is not merely "a contingent instrument for pursuing the projects that emerge from cognition and choice."[9]

Public bioethics' debates prevails a kind of individualism that is classified as *expressivism*, which elevates autonomy and liberty above the fundamental human good, *id est*, human life. As expressed by many philosophers, neuroscientists, physicians, and others, "human beings experience themselves and one another as living bodies, not disembodied wills"[10]:

> the anthropology of the atomized, unencumbered, inward-directed self of expressive individualism falls short because it cannot render intelligible either the core human realities of embodiment or recognize the unchosen debts that accrue to all human beings throughout their life spans[11] [...]. Like Milton's Satan and fallen angels, the expressive individual self "know[s] no time when [it was] not as now; Know none before [it], self-begot, self-rais'd/By [its] own quickening power." A purely inward-looking and individualistic anthropology can give no intelligible or justified account of uncompensated, unconditional, and often self-sacrificial care of others. There is no warrant to give more than one could ever hope to receive. There is no imperative to give to those from whom nothing will ever be repaid in return.[12]

Benefits for psychiatric treatment and psychological assessments

This holistic, integrative, and ecological vision of the human mind helps therapeutic approaches that combine physical and mental elements, such as exercise, yoga, meditation, biofeedback, and hypnosis. These solutions are based on the idea that the mind and the body are not separate, but rather interconnected and interdependent, and that they influence each other in various ways. These solutions aim to enhance the well-being and health of both the mind and the body by addressing the psychological, emotional, social, and biological factors that affect them; also, they offer a holistic and integrative way of treating and preventing mental disorders, such as depression, anxiety, stress, and addiction. These disorders are often associated with physical symptoms, such as pain, fatigue, insomnia, and inflammation, as well as cognitive and emotional impairments, such as memory loss, low self-esteem, and negative mood. This type of dual approach to the mind–body relation can help to alleviate these symptoms, by improving the physiological and psychological functioning of the mind and the body, and it can help to promote positive mental health, by enhancing the resilience, happiness, and quality of life of individuals. The mind–body solutions can foster a sense of self-awareness, self-regulation, and self-care, by teaching individuals how to cope with stress, manage their emotions, and cultivate positive habits and attitudes. This mind–body solution can also foster a sense of connection, belonging, and meaning, by facilitating social support, interpersonal relationships, and spiritual growth.[13]

This approach is supported by scientific evidence, which shows that they can have beneficial effects on the brain, the nervous system, the immune system, and the endocrine system. These effects can modulate the neurochemical and hormonal balance, the inflammatory and oxidative stress response, and the gene expression, which are involved in the development and maintenance of mental disorders. This mind–body solution can also influence the neural pathways, the brain regions, and the brain networks, which are involved in the regulation of cognition, emotion, and behavior, and it is not meant to replace the conventional treatments for mental disorders, such as medication and psychotherapy but rather to complement and enhance them. This mind–body solution can also offer a personalized and flexible way of addressing the specific needs and preferences of each individual, by taking into account their physical and mental condition, their personality and lifestyle, and their cultural and environmental context, and it can also empower individuals to take an active role in their own recovery and well-being, by providing them with skills and tools that they can use in their daily life.[d]

Thomas Fuchs offers a systemic and ecological account as an opposing view to the naturalist idea that mental illnesses can be reduced to dysfunctions of the brain. He regards mental illness as inseparable from the living organism and the patient's life world or social environment. He introduces the notion of circular causality to replace the notion of monolinear causation in order to grasp mental disorders in their context. Fuchs identifies two types of disruptions that characterize mental illnesses: (i) vertical circular causality: this refers to the interplay between lower-level processes and higher faculties of the organism. This primarily affects a mentally ill person's relation to themselves, which continually codetermines the course of the illness; (ii) horizontal circular causality: this refers to social relationships and the ability to respond adequately to the demands and expectations of others. Disruptions here lead to negative feedback loops in sociofunctional cycles that influence the course of the illness from the very beginning. Both kinds of circular causal processes are tied to mediation by the brain but cannot exclusively be located within it. Therefore, Fuchs argues that reducing mental illnesses to diseases of the brain is in principle not possible.[14] In his article *The Brain – A Mediating Organ*, Fuchs challenges the reductionist view of cognitive neuroscience that sees the brain as the creator of the mind and the experienced world and proposes an ecological view of the mind and brain, arguing that both are embedded in the relationship between the living organism and its environment. This perspective is dependent on a developmental view: the brain is seen as a plastic system of open loops formed in the process of life and closed to full functional cycles in every interaction with the environment. Each time a new disposition of coherent neural activity is formed through repeated experience, structures of the mind are imprinted onto the brain. Thus, the brain becomes a mediating organ or a window to the mind, as it is structured by the mind itself. Fuchs presents the brain not as the seat of the mind, but as an organ that mediates our conscious experience, structured by the mind through our interactions with the world.[15]

This integrated, holistic, and ecological solution is not only important for individuals but also for society, as they can contribute to the prevention and reduction of the burden and cost of mental disorders, which affect millions of people worldwide, and it can also foster a culture of health and wellness, by raising awareness and education about the importance and benefits of the mind–body connection, and by encouraging people to adopt healthy and positive behaviors and practices. Finally, it can also foster a culture of compassion and empathy, by promoting a holistic and humanistic view of mental health, and by reducing the stigma and discrimination that often surround mental disorders.

---

[d] See the vast bibliography of neuroscientist, psychiatrist and philosopher Georg Northoff, Canada Research Chair in Mind, Brain Imaging and Neuroethics.

Conclusion

The history of the concept of mind in the Western context has seen a dynamic interplay of philosophical, scientific, and psychological ideas. The integration of neuroscientific data, psychological and psychiatric orientations, and the relational dimension offers a comprehensive framework for understanding the human mind. By embracing a multidimensional perspective, this synthesis allows for a more nuanced and holistic-ecological approach to mental health, bridging the gap between the subjective and objective aspects of the human experience. As our understanding continues to evolve, this integrated concept of the human mind holds promise for advancing both theoretical knowledge and practical applications in the fields of psychology, psychiatry, and neuroscience.

In conclusion, the unidual body–mind solution sketched in this article is important in the context of mental health because it offers a comprehensive and integrative way of enhancing the wellbeing and health of both the mind and the body by addressing the multiple and complex factors that affect them. This contemporary, anticartesian and antineurosolipsism solution – that sees the human mind both embodied and embedded, is supported by scientific evidence, and it can complement and enhance the conventional treatments for mental disorders, and it can also benefit individuals and society, by promoting positive mental health, and by fostering a culture of health, wellness, compassion, and empathy.

References

1. Locke J. *An Essay Concerning the Human Understanding.* 1690;XVII:11.

2. Fuchs T. Are mental illnesses diseases of the brain? In Choudhury S, Slaby J, eds., *Critical Neuroscience: A Handbook of the Social and Cultural Contexts of Neuroscience.* West Sussex: Wiley Blackwell; 2012:331–344.

3. Fuchs T. The brain – a mediating organ. *J Conscious Stud.* 2011;**18**(7–8):196.

4. Siegel DJ. *The Developing Mind: Toward a Neurobiology of Interpersonal Experience.* New York: Guilford Press; 1999.

5. Siegel DJ. *Mindsight: The New Science of Personal Transformation.* New York: Bantam; 2010.

6. Aquinas T. *On Being and Essence.* Trans. Ralph McInerny. Selected Writings. London: Penguin; 1998:36.

7. Kenny A. *Aquinas on Mind.* New York: Routledge; 1994.

8. Agazzi E. *Dimostrare l'esistenza dell'uomo.* Milan: Mimesis; 2023.

9. Snead OC. *What It Means to Be Human. The Case for the Body in Public Bioethics.* Cambridge, MA: Harvard University Press; 2020:69–70.

10. Snead OC. *What It Means to Be Human. The Case for the Body in Public Bioethics.* Cambridge, MA: Harvard University Press; 2020:88.

11. Snead OC. *What It Means to Be Human. The Case for the Body in Public Bioethics.* Cambridge, MAQ: Harvard University Press; 2020:88.

12. Snead OC. *What It Means to Be Human. The Case for the Body in Public Bioethics.* Cambridge, MA: Harvard University Press; 2020:90.

13. Glannon W. *Brain, Body, and Mind: Neuroethics with a Human Face.* Oxford: Oxford University Press; 2011.

14. Fuchs T. Are mental illnesses diseases of the brain? In Choudhury S, Slaby J, eds., *Critical Neuroscience: A Handbook of the Social and Cultural Contexts of Neuroscience.* West Sussex: Wiley Blackwell; 2012:331–344.

15. Fuchs T. The brain—a mediating organ. *J Conscious Stud.* 2011;**18**(7–8): 196–221.

27 A Neuroethical Approach to Human Life, Identity, and Liberty of Patients with Schizophrenia

Alberto Carrara

Introduction

Consciousness and free will are fundamental aspects that define the human experience, serving as crucial pillars that distinguish us in the natural world. Consciousness, more than just awareness, involves a complex interplay of sensory perceptions, thoughts, and emotions that allow individuals to interpret and interact with their environment in uniquely human ways. It is the lens through which we perceive the world and our place within it, facilitating nuanced understandings and deep introspections. This self-awareness is essential not only for survival but also for the pursuit of knowledge, the development of personal identity, and the cultivation of relationships. It enables us to reflect on past actions, conceive future possibilities, and engage in the moral and ethical considerations that underpin society.

Free will, on the other hand, plays a pivotal role in actualizing the potentialities presented by consciousness. It affords individuals the autonomy to make choices that reflect their desires, beliefs, and values. The exercise of free will is critical in shaping one's destiny and is intimately linked to concepts of responsibility and accountability. In a world where actions have consequences, the ability to choose freely is what empowers people to steer their lives and influence the communities around them. Together, consciousness and free will form the bedrock of human dignity and liberty, underscoring the responsibility we have toward ourselves and others in crafting a meaningful existence. Thus, in contemporary discourse, these elements are not just philosophical abstractions but practical necessities that inform legal, social, and ethical frameworks designed to uphold human rights and foster societal progress.

Neurological diseases and mental illnesses can profoundly impact consciousness, altering the very fabric of how individuals perceive, interact with, and understand their environment. Disorders such as Alzheimer's disease, schizophrenia, and severe depression can disrupt cognitive functions and emotional stability, leading to changes in awareness and a diminished capacity to respond to external stimuli. As these conditions alter the clarity and continuity of conscious thought, they inherently affect an individual's ability to make informed and intentional choices. The erosion of consciousness can thus lead to a corresponding reduction in free will, as the afflicted may no longer be able to engage with the world in a way that reflects their true intentions and desires.

This interplay between compromised consciousness and diminished free will raises significant ethical and practical challenges. It questions the extent to which individuals with severe mental impairments are responsible for their actions. In legal contexts, this can affect judgments regarding culpability and consent, necessitating a nuanced approach that considers the impact of such illnesses on free will. Similarly, in healthcare, understanding the influence of these conditions on autonomy is crucial for ethical decision-making, particularly regarding treatment and care. Ultimately, acknowledging how neurological diseases and mental illnesses can affect consciousness and free will is essential for fostering compassionate and just societies that recognize the vulnerabilities of their members and strive to support them appropriately.

This exploration of consciousness and free will builds upon and revises previous scholarly proposals by the author in 2018, 2021, and 2023, which articulated a model of human conscious stratification (The author of this contribution published in Italian and English).[1,2,3] The current discussion enriches these earlier frameworks by introducing a parallel stratification of human freedom, thereby creating a more holistic view of the human experience. This dual stratification approach offers a nuanced perspective that recognizes the layered complexities of both consciousness and free will. It posits that just as consciousness can be viewed as operating at multiple levels – from basic sensory awareness to higher-order reflective thinking – so too can free will be understood as varying in its expression depending on cognitive capabilities, external constraints, and internal psychological states.

This refined model underscores the dynamic interplay between an individual's level of conscious awareness and the degree of freedom they possess in making decisions. By mapping these dimensions together, the author provides a more comprehensive framework that accounts for the variations in human autonomy and cognitive experience seen across different mental states and in the presence of neurological disorders or mental illnesses. This approach not only advances theoretical understandings in psychology and neuroscience but also has practical implications for fields such as ethics, law, and healthcare. It prompts a reconsideration of how society measures responsibility and autonomy, particularly for those whose capacity for free will is compromised, advocating for policies and practices that are more attuned to the real conditions of human freedom and consciousness.

The author's perspective is rooted in neuroethics, a field that deals with the systematic and informed reflection on the human condition through the lens of neuroscientific evidence and its interpretations (The term "neuro-ethics" dates back to 1973, although its characterization and diffusion has been taking shape and consistency since 2002).[4,5] This approach emphasizes the ethical, legal, and social implications arising from advancements in neuroscience. By incorporating neuroscientific findings into discussions of consciousness and free will, the author seeks to bridge the gap between empirical data and the philosophical inquiries surrounding human agency and mental integrity. This integration is crucial, as it helps inform debates about the extent to which neurological and psychological conditions can influence personal autonomy and moral responsibility.

Neuroethics, therefore, serves as a pivotal framework for the author's analysis, providing the tools needed to critically examine how changes in brain function can impact conscious experience and the exercise of free will. By focusing on this intersection, the author proposes a model that is not only scientifically informed but also deeply attuned to the ethical dimensions of human freedom. Such a perspective is essential for developing sensitive and effective policies that accommodate the complexities of human behavior as revealed through neuroscience. This approach ensures that ethical considerations are not overlooked in the rush to apply new scientific knowledge, thereby safeguarding human dignity and promoting a more nuanced understanding of freedom and consciousness in the face of neurological and mental health challenges.

Multidimensional bottom-up stratification of human consciousness

In discussing consciousness, it is important to recognize that it is a polysemic term, encompassing a broad spectrum of meanings and implications. In the context of the current discourse, the term "consciousness" is explored from the very inception of human life, beginning with our constitution as biological entities. This perspective traces the arc from conception, where consciousness is considered in its nascent biological form, through the intricate process of cellular interactions that progressively build our biological body. This biological viewpoint frames consciousness not merely as a psychological or philosophical phenomenon, but as an emergent property that begins in the very early stages of life, evolving as cells multiply and differentiate, laying the groundwork for later cognitive and perceptual abilities.

This biological foundation of consciousness underlines the interconnectedness of life and consciousness, suggesting that our cognitive experiences and capacities for free will are deeply rooted in our biological origins. By tracing consciousness back to these fundamental biological processes, the discussion expands to consider how our initial cellular development might influence or correlate with later stages of cognitive consciousness and the unfolding of free will. This approach not only highlights the complexity of consciousness as a concept but also emphasizes the continuity from biological entity to sentient being, offering a comprehensive understanding that spans from the microscopic cellular interactions to the macroscopic level of human behavior and cognition.

In the organic structuring of the human body, a complex interplay of DNA activation and epigenetic factors guides the development and functioning of our biological systems. Central to this developmental journey is the emergence of interoception, which can be considered one of the earliest forms of consciousness. Interoception refers to the perception of internal bodily states rather than external events. It encompasses the body's ability to sense fundamental homeostatic needs such as hunger and thirst, which are critical for survival. This level of consciousness provides continuous feedback about our internal physiological condition, allowing us to maintain balance within our biological systems.

Interoceptive awareness represents a fundamental dimension of consciousness, establishing a kind of continuous contact with our bodily interiority. This intimate connection with the inner workings of our body not only signals our physiological needs but also potentially influences our emotional experiences and decision-making processes, integrating the biological and psychological facets of human life. Understanding interoception as a primary level of consciousness challenges and expands traditional notions of consciousness, which often focus predominantly on higher cognitive functions and external sensory inputs. Thus, interoception underscores a profound aspect of what it means to be human, reflecting a deep, intrinsic link between our biological states and our experiences of self-awareness and agency.

The second level of conscious experience, exteroception, is critical in the development of human sensory awareness. Exteroception refers to the perception of external stimuli through our sense organs, which involves a complex articulation between these organs and their neurological underpinnings. This level of consciousness is essential for interpreting the environment around us, as it encompasses the integration of sensory data – from sight, sound, touch, taste, and smell – into a coherent perceptual experience. This sensory input is processed by various neural pathways, allowing for the detailed recognition and reaction to external events, which is vital for interaction with the world.

The maturation of human sense experience through exteroception is not merely about the passive reception of stimuli but also involves active processes that enhance our understanding and interaction with our surroundings. For instance, the development of depth perception in vision, the differentiation of tones in hearing, or the complexity of taste and smell discrimination, all depend on the sophisticated integration of sensory information by the brain. These capabilities are foundational not only for basic survival but also for higher-level cognitive functions such as learning, memory, and complex decision-making. Thus, exteroception plays a fundamental role in shaping our engagement with the world, enabling us to navigate, manipulate, and ultimately transform our environment in ways that reflect our needs, desires, and knowledge.

The third dimension of consciousness, often encapsulated by the millennia-old concept of "common sense," or perception integration, is crucial in forming our own internal representation of the world. This level involves the synthesis of diverse sensory inputs into a unified and coherent whole, allowing individuals to integrate and interpret the multitude of stimuli they encounter. Common sense in this context goes beyond mere sensory perception; it involves the cognitive processes of organizing, prioritizing, and making sense of different sensory data to form a comprehensive picture of reality.

This internal representation is not simply a passive aggregation of data but an active construction that enables humans to navigate their environment more effectively. It allows for the identification of objects and situations, understanding their significance, and anticipating potential outcomes. For example, the ability to recognize a face, understand the mood conveyed by a tone of voice, or anticipate the trajectory of a moving object all depend on this complex integration. This capacity forms the basis of practical intelligence and situational awareness, underpinning not only daily survival but also sophisticated human interactions and behaviors. Through this integrated perception, individuals can apply learned knowledge and abstract reasoning to new situations, a testament to the dynamic and adaptable nature of human cognition.

Gerald Edelman, a Nobel Prize-winning neuroscientist, significantly contributed to our understanding of consciousness by delineating what he termed "primary consciousness." This level of consciousness, according to Edelman, encompasses both exteroception and perception integration, which together allow for the creation of an internal representation or "scene" of reality. Primary consciousness is described as the ability to generate a mental map of external events, providing a perceptual framework on which reasoning and subsequent actions can be based. This model underscores the brain's remarkable ability to form a coherent, momentary present from diverse sensory inputs, enabling an organism to navigate and respond to its environment effectively.

This foundational form of consciousness is crucial as it represents the preliminary stage necessary for more complex forms of conscious awareness, such as self-reflection, planning, and deliberate choice. By generating an internal scene, primary consciousness allows for immediate, yet simple, awareness of the world without the depth of past memories or future projections involved in higher consciousness. It is a real-time representation that enables adaptive behaviors essential for survival. Thus, exteroception – the sensing of external stimuli – and perception – the integration and interpretation of those stimuli – serve as the pillars of primary consciousness. These processes equip the brain to function not merely as a passive recipient of information but as an active participant in its perception, providing the groundwork upon which all higher cognitive functions are built.

The fourth dimension of consciousness, awareness, extends beyond the primary consciousness of perceiving and integrating sensory information. Awareness refers to a higher level of conscious experience that involves not only recognizing one's environment but also having self-awareness and the ability to reflect upon one's own thoughts and feelings. This form of consciousness is often the focus of neurological studies, particularly in clinical settings where altered states of consciousness, such as minimal conscious states (MCS) and vegetative states (VS), are examined.

In MCS, individuals exhibit a partial preservation of conscious awareness. They can demonstrate some behaviors that indicate a limited awareness of self or environment but do so inconsistently. For example, a person in an MCS might be able to follow an object with their eyes or respond to simple commands intermittently, suggesting some level of awareness, yet lacking the full, consistent engagement seen in fully conscious individuals.

Conversely, in a vegetative state, patients show no signs of conscious awareness despite appearing awake; they might open their eyes or exhibit reflexive responses, but they do not exhibit purposeful behavior or awareness of their surroundings. These states are particularly challenging to study and treat because the presence or absence of awareness can profoundly impact medical, ethical, and legal decisions concerning care and treatment.

The exploration of awareness, especially in these altered states, highlights the complex interplay between various brain functions and regions. Understanding awareness involves deciphering the neurological substrates that enable conscious reflection, emotional processing, and self-recognition. It also encompasses studying how these processes are disrupted, providing insight into the resilience and fragility of the human mind. Awareness is not just a passive occurrence but an active, dynamic process that integrates multiple cognitive and affective components, making it a critical area of study in both neuroscience and clinical practice.

The fifth dimension of consciousness, proprioception, refers to the body's ability to sense its own position, movement, and overall physical orientation without relying on external cues. This internal sense is sometimes described as the "sense of self" in the physical world, providing the necessary feedback for coordinating movements and maintaining balance and posture. Proprioception is a critical component of consciousness because it integrates sensory information from muscles, tendons, and joints with central nervous system inputs to create a continuous internal map of the body's position in space.

This proprioceptive awareness is fundamental to all physical activities, from basic actions like walking and standing to complex maneuvers in sports and other skilled behaviors. It allows individuals to perform movements smoothly and efficiently without the need to consciously think about each muscle and limb position. For example, proprioception enables a person to touch their nose with their eyes closed or adjust their gait to uneven surfaces without visually monitoring their feet.

In clinical contexts, the study of proprioception becomes particularly important when dealing with conditions that affect motor control and bodily awareness, such as stroke, Parkinson's disease, or injuries that involve nerve damage. Loss of proprioceptive ability can severely impact a person's quality of life, leading to challenges in performing everyday tasks and increasing the risk of falls and injuries.

Overall, proprioception is a vital aspect of consciousness that works largely unnoticed but is essential for interacting effectively with the physical environment. It exemplifies how our bodies and minds are intricately linked, contributing to our sense of self and enabling our interaction with the world around us.

In this bottom-up stratification of conscious manifestations, which maps closely to the increasing complexity of human bodily and particularly neuronal structures, a pinnacle is reached when all elements are organically well-integrated, culminating in the highest level of conscious experience: self-awareness, often referred to as phenomenal consciousness. Phenomenal consciousness represents the sophisticated ability to not only perceive and react to the environment but also to have a subjective and introspective experience of those perceptions and reactions – what is often termed the "qualia" of consciousness.

Phenomenal consciousness enables individuals to experience the world not just through sensory input and cognitive reactions but through deeply personal and unique perspectives. This form of consciousness is where sensations are not merely noted, but felt; where thoughts are not only considered but understood as part of the self's narrative. This level involves an awareness of one's existence and identity that transcends simple sensory awareness or the processing of external and internal stimuli – it includes an awareness of one's own mind and its workings.

The development of phenomenal consciousness is a testament to the intricate and highly organized structure of the human brain, particularly its neuronal architecture, which allows for such complex integrations and manifestations of consciousness. This level of consciousness is what enables humans to reflect on their past, plan for their future, and engage in abstract thinking. It represents a significant evolutionary advantage, allowing for levels of creativity, problem-solving, and social interaction that are uniquely human. Thus, in the hierarchy of consciousness as understood in a neuroscientific context, self-awareness or phenomenal consciousness stands as the most intricate and richly human of all conscious states, encapsulating the full depth and breadth of what it means to be "conscious."

Indeed, in this multidimensional stratification of consciousness, we can see how it constitutes a privileged place of unity within the human person, profoundly shaping personal identity. Each layer of consciousness, from the most basic perceptions of proprioception and interoception to the sophisticated realms of exteroception and phenomenal consciousness, contributes to a cohesive sense of self. This integration of various conscious experiences provides a continuous internal narrative that is central to personal identity.

Consciousness is not merely a passive recipient of sensations or a simple processor of inputs; it is an active, dynamic force that assembles our thoughts, feelings, perceptions, and memories into a coherent self-image. Through this unification, individuals are able to perceive themselves as distinct entities with unique histories, desires, and future aspirations. The various dimensions of consciousness interlock to create a continuous experience of being, anchoring an individual's identity over time despite changes in environment or physical state.

This conceptualization of consciousness highlights its role in not just surviving but thriving through the maintenance of a stable yet adaptable identity. It allows individuals to navigate complex social landscapes, reflect on their place in the world, and make meaningful choices that reflect their values and beliefs. In essence, the layered complexity of consciousness is what enables the rich tapestry of human experience, grounding each person's identity in a continuously evolving but fundamentally integrated perception of self.

Multidimensional bottom-up stratification of human freedom

The profound connection between consciousness, agency, and free will is elegantly captured in the words of Rita Levi-Montalcini, who highlighted how consciousness serves as a bridge linking our sense of self with our experiences.[6] This connection is crucial as it empowers us to comprehend our existence as thinking entities, thus grounding us in responsibility for our actions. Consciousness does not merely enable awareness but facilitates a deeper understanding of the implications of our actions, reflecting the core human capacity for choice and moral responsibility.

This synthesis underscores the integral role that consciousness plays in the exercise of free will. By allowing us to evaluate and choose among different options, consciousness imbues our actions with intentionality and purpose. It is this ability to deliberate and make informed choices that form the basis of personal responsibility. As such, consciousness is not just a passive state but an active process that engages with the events of the world and our possible actions within it. Through this dynamic interplay, individuals are not only aware of their actions but also possess the capacity to shape their consequences, a testament to the profound ethical dimension of human consciousness as articulated by Levi-Montalcini. This makes consciousness a foundational element in the development of personal identity and moral agency, illustrating its central role in our lives as both a cognitive and ethical force.

First and foremost, choice (in latin, *electio*) is an act of the will, or human appetitive (tendential) power, realized through a movement toward what is perceived as good, namely a chosen good. The notion of "chosen" presupposes a comparative judgment between alternatives, a preference that precedes and indeed becomes an integral part of the choice itself. This choice is predicated on what might be termed "advice," that is, a judgment (or a series of reasoning) aimed at determining a course of action. This advice reflects self-consciousness.

From a neuroscientific perspective, it is clear that a "chain" of reasoning underlies any considered decision. Furthermore, these judgments are grounded in their physical capacity to manifest and process, specifically through integration in neuronal structures, particularly in cortical networks.

Similarly, as we have discussed with consciousness, there emerges a gradual bottom-up development for free will manifested in choice. This can be seen as parallel and reflective of consciousness. Just as consciousness is built from the ground up – starting with basic sensory levels like interoception and exteroception, through to perception integration (common sense), awareness, and proprioception, culminating in the highest level of integrative judgment, which is self-aware and self-conscious – so too is the development of free will and its associated responsibility. This multidimensional stratification mirrors the stratification of consciousness and highlights the role of many unconscious processes in influencing our choices.

In this framework, each level of conscious experience has a corresponding dimension of freedom, illustrating a complex interplay between our internal states and our capacity for choice. Interoception, which is the awareness of internal bodily states, corresponds to what can be termed "intero-freedom." This is the freedom to respond to internal cues such as hunger and pain, guiding decisions that meet basic bodily needs.

Similarly, exteroception – the sensory perception of the external world – corresponds to "extero-freedom," which involves the freedom to interact with and respond to external stimuli. This type of freedom enables us to navigate and adapt to our environment effectively.

At the level of integrated perception, or what is commonly known as common sense, there arises "integrative freedom." This represents the ability to synthesize information from various sources, making informed decisions that reflect a holistic understanding of our circumstances.

The level of awareness, which includes a conscious recognition of one's environment and self, correlates with "aware freedom." This freedom is characterized by the capacity to reflect on one's situation and choices, providing a deeper layer of decision-making that considers personal values and ethical implications.

Proprioception, the sense of the relative position of one's own parts of the body and strength of effort being employed in movement, leads to "propriofreedom." This is the freedom to control one's movements and physical actions with precision, vital for skilled and deliberate activities.

Finally, self-awareness or phenomenal consciousness, where one is fully aware of oneself as a distinct entity with complex thoughts and emotions, corresponds to "self-freedom." This ultimate form of freedom manifests in the capacity for human phenomenal free action through choices that are deeply reflective, fully considered, and aligned with one's self-identity and aspirations. This layered approach to consciousness and freedom encapsulates the breadth of human autonomy, reflecting how our internal experiences shape our external choices and actions.

Life, identity, and liberty of patients with schizophrenia

In exploring the complexities of how different conditions affect the relationship between choice and action, it is insightful to consider specific neurological disorders. For instance, patients with apraxia or those suffering from anarchic hand syndrome illustrate distinct disruptions in the pathway from choice to action. Apraxic patients retain their freedom of choice – the apex of the multidimensional pyramid of consciousness and free will. However, due to their pathological condition, they struggle to translate these choices into coordinated actions. In contrast, patients with anarchic hand syndrome can make choices but find their actions do not align with these choices due to involuntary movements of the hand that act independently of their intentions.

Similarly, the condition of schizophrenia profoundly impacts the freedom of choice. Unlike the disorders affecting motor control and action execution mentioned earlier, schizophrenia can interfere with the very capacity to make coherent choices. This disruption occurs due to a variety of symptoms such as delusions, hallucinations, and disorganized thinking, which can cloud judgment and complicate the decision-making process. Patients may find themselves unable to sift through distorted perceptions and thoughts to reach a clear decision, thus affecting their free will at a fundamental level of choice rather than at the level of action execution.

These examples highlight that while the capacity to choose freely and execute those choices can be seen as separate components, they are deeply interconnected. Understanding these nuances is crucial in appreciating the full spectrum of how neurological conditions can influence different aspects of free will, from the formation of intent (choice) to the execution of that intent (action). This knowledge underscores the need for a compassionate and nuanced approach to supporting individuals with such conditions, recognizing the particular ways in which their autonomy and freedom are affected.

In conclusion, the neuroethical stratification proposed in this discussion offers a powerful framework for understanding the conditions of psychiatric patients more profoundly. By examining the different levels at which consciousness and free will can be affected – ranging from basic sensory integration to complex decision-making processes – this model helps to pinpoint where interventions might be most needed. It allows healthcare providers to tailor treatments that address specific impairments in the spectrum of cognitive functions, thereby enhancing the effectiveness of therapeutic approaches.

Moreover, this stratification underscores the essential humanity and inherent dignity of every individual, regardless of neurological or psychiatric conditions. By improving our understanding of how various disorders affect a person's freedom and decision-making capacity, we can better support their recovery and reintegration into society. This approach not only aims to restore functionality but also to reaffirm the intrinsic value of each patient, recognizing their right to autonomy and a fuller expression of their personal freedom. Such an enlightened perspective is crucial in advancing both the science and the ethics of mental health care, ensuring

that patients regain the level of freedom they deserve as beings of infinite dignity.

The principles laid out in this paper offer valuable insights into the complex relationship between consciousness, free will, and schizophrenia. Schizophrenia, characterized by impaired decision-making and distorted perceptions, poses a significant threat to an individual's sense of autonomy and self-ownership. By understanding the multifaceted nature of free will in schizophrenia, we acknowledge the profound impact this disorder has on patients' lives and the urgency of addressing their needs through comprehensive and tailored interventions.

The concept of free will is not only a philosophical abstraction but also a fundamental aspect of human dignity, as established by the UNESCO Declaration of Human Rights and Bioethics in 2005 (www.unesco.org/en/ethics-science-technology/bioethics-and-human-rights). This paper's stratification of consciousness and freedom aligns with the declaration's emphasis on preserving human dignity and autonomy (Art. 3 and Art. 5):

Article 3. Human dignity and human rights
1. Human dignity, human rights, and fundamental freedoms are to be fully respected.
2. The interests and welfare of the individual should have priority over the sole interest of science or society.

Article 5. Autonomy and individual responsibility
The autonomy of persons to make decisions, while taking responsibility for those decisions and respecting the autonomy of others, is to be respected. For persons who are not capable of exercising autonomy, special measures are to be taken to protect their rights and interests (www.unesco.org/en/legal-affairs/universal-declaration-bioethics-and-human-rights?hub=66535).

It becomes a moral duty to help patients with schizophrenia regain authentic ownership of themselves, allowing them to lead a freer and more fulfilling life. This duty extends from pharmacological interventions to encompass psychological and humanistic approaches, fostering an environment that supports the holistic well-being of these individuals.

From a neuroethical standpoint, the pursuit of restoring autonomy to patients with schizophrenia is essential for respecting their inherent dignity (*dignitas infinita*) and promoting their freedom. Is it better to help schizophrenic individuals regain their freedom, or to let them live without autonomy and dignity, languishing in the streets?

The framework outlined in this paper highlights the need for interventions that address the specific impairments affecting free will in psychiatric conditions. By providing compassionate and targeted care, we not only enhance patients' quality of life but also uphold the core principles of human rights and neuroethics, reaffirming the value of every individual and their right to a meaningful existence.

References

1. Carrara A. Breve approccio neurobioetico all'identità umana e alla responsabilità personale: un modello bio(neuro)-psico-sociale dell'integrazione antropologica che parte dalle esperienze coscienti e di volontà libera. In: Di Mieri F, Agostino D, eds. *Identità, Libertà e Responsabilità*. Series La Tavola di Vico (Vico'Tablet). Rome: Edizioni Ripostes; 2018:195–212.

2. Carrara A. The neuro-psycho-social model of anthropological integration of conscious and free will experiences: a short neurobioethical approach to human identity and personal responsibility. In: García Gómez A, Brugnoli MP, Carrara A, eds. *Bioethics & Consciousness*. Newcastle: Cambridge Scholars Publishing; 2021:23–40.

3. Carrara A. Neurobioethics of consciousness: a multidimensional stratification of human conscious experience. In: García Gómez A, Carrara A, eds. *Bioethics and Modified States of Consciousness (Second Part)*. Newcastle: Cambridge Scholars Publishing; 2023;15–24.

4. Pontius AA. Neuro-ethics of "walking" in the newborn. *Percept Mot Skills*. 1973;37(1):235–245.

5. Marcus SJ. *Neuroethics: Mapping the Field. Conference Proceedings, May 13–14, 2002*. San Francisco, CA: The Dana Foundation; 2002.

6. Levi-Montalcini R. *Have the Courage to Know*. Milan: Bur Rizzoli; 2004:25.

Neuroethics and Treatment Without Consent

Harry G. Kennedy and Mary Davoren

Introduction

Treatment without consent has always been an ethical challenge in medicine. In psychiatry and neuroethics, the problem is more complicated, because the person who must make choices and decisions about treatment – the patient, often must do so while impaired in their ability to understand and reason about the decision in hand. We are taking as our starting point, Carrara's aphorism elsewhere in this volume:

Together, consciousness and free will form the bedrock of human dignity and liberty, underscoring the responsibility we have towards ourselves and others in crafting a meaningful existence.

Carrara may be writing from the perspective of ethics grounded in philosophy of mind.[1,2] We are writing from a medical and common law perspective. In common law, the legal concept of mind has reached a consensus according to which "mind" is defined in law, not as consciousness but more simply as a collection of capacities: to know, including to perceive, to retain and recall, to reason and to make decisions, and then to form intentions and to act, including to communicate the decisions.[3–7] Current clinical ethics and legal precedents in common law jurisdictions presume free will unless there is evidence to the contrary. We propose that the ability to exercise free will and to accept responsibility for one's acts, omissions, and decisions is a definition of mental health. In order to rebut the presumption of responsibility in criminal law, some impairment of the capacity to form specific intentions must be shown; to rebut the presumption of competence to make decisions about one's person and treatment, welfare, and financial affairs in civil law, including mental health law, some impairment of mental capacities to make and communicate decisions must be shown. In Roman law, the emphasis is on consciousness, self-awareness, and personality. This is a more holistic approach, but also more

hermeneutic, subjective, and unconstrained by readily discernible signs or even symptoms. This contrasts with Wittgenstein's aphorism "an inner state is in need of an outer sign."[8]

We also assume that neuroethics is a part of bioethics. The "mind" considered here is embodied and inseparable from anatomical and physiological life and effects in the real world. In this article we will set out (i) goals as derived from legal and human rights principles. We then consider (ii) decision-making processes. This is followed by examples of practical applications to (iii) treatment decisions. We conclude with a discussion of how to apply (iv) clinical scientific evaluations to consider whether the goals are being achieved by these processes and the duty to achieve excellence through research-driven continuous improvement of health gains for patients.

Goals

Rather than discuss principles based on human rights, constitutional and legal rights, for this article on neuroethics, we commence by deriving concrete goals (specific, measurable, timed) from such principles. Our objectives are to consider the neuroethics of treatment without consent from a broader perspective and wider context than the routinely accepted starting point of functional mental capacities. Notably, in common law jurisdictions, consciousness is seldom admitted in criminal law as a topic for expert evidence of mentalistic defenses or impairments in civil proceedings. Criminal defenses specifically referring to consciousness, such as automatism and its fashionable variants somnambulism and sexsomnia, the "absence of mind," are notoriously unreliable.[9–12] Nor is dignity often considered at present except in human rights conventions and case law derived from the United Nations Convention on the Rights of Persons with Disabilities[13] or ECtHR case law concerning torture when it is often considered alongside personhood.[14]

Methods

The framework we have adopted is to consider the principles of the European Convention on Human Rights (ECHR) in relation to treatment for mental disorders, including treatment without consent, as a means of deriving goals. The ECHR and the judges of the European Court of Human Rights (ECtHR, "The Strasbourg Court") are drawn from both common law and Roman law jurisdictions, so that their interpretations and precedents may be informative concerning alternatives to strict application of capacity tests.

The European Convention on Human Rights

There are many international conventions on human rights, social, cultural, and economic rights, and related matters. The ECHR is taken here as a useful guide to the relationship between neuroethics and treatment without consent as manifested in the laws of many modern states. The ECHR has been accepted by the members of the Council of Europe (CoE, 46 member states, 675 million population), who undertake to be bound by the rulings of the European Court of Human Rights (ECtHR), often referred to as the Strasbourg Court. Central to the ECHR is a system for the rule of law. The ECtHR is widely respected as an authoritative source for interpretive case law and precedent, binding on the member states of the CoE and showing consistency, coherence, and respect for legal process and rules of evidence that is lacking in the interpretative processes of other international conventions and international bodies. The ECHR has also been incorporated into the law of the European Union (EU, 27 member states, 449.2m population) and is now being interpreted alongside the United Nations Convention on the Rights of Persons with Disabilities.[13]

Two substantive obligations arise from ECHR Article 2 (Box 28.1): a positive obligation to protect the right to life by law, which in practice requires a regulatory framework, and a negative right, the prohibition of the intentional deprivation of life, with some exceptions, and a positive obligation to prevent suicide, particularly for persons in detention. Those who are vulnerable due to mental disabilities, and those who are detained by law in hospital, require a stricter standard of protection.

ECHR Article 3, the prohibition of torture (Box 28.2), is an unqualified right. Case law of the ECtHR is enlightening: "A measure which is a therapeutic necessity from the point of view of established principles of medicine cannot, in principle, be regarded as inhuman and degrading. The Court must, nevertheless, satisfy itself that a medical necessity has been convincingly shown to exist and that procedural guarantees for the decision exist and are complied with (*Jalloh* v. *Germany* [GC], 2006, § 69)".[14] The concept of "therapeutic necessity" or "medical necessity" is a widely recognized and essential component of legal and ethical reasoning and decision-making in relation to treatment and consent generally.

In accordance with ECHR Article 5, the right to liberty (Box 28.3), there are three minimum conditions for lawful detention on the basis of unsoundness of mind: (1) the person concerned must reliably be shown to be of unsound mind, that is, a true mental disorder must be established before a competent authority on the basis of objective medical evidence; (2) the mental disorder must be of a kind or degree that warrants compulsory confinement; and (3) the validity of continued confinement must depend upon the persistence of such a disorder.

The Strasbourg Court has held that no deprivation of liberty of a person considered to be of "unsound mind" is permitted if it has been ordered without seeking the opinion of a medical expert, giving evidence that is reliable. Any other approach falls short of the required protection against arbitrariness.

> **Box 28.2 ECHR Article 3**
>
> *No one shall be subjected to torture or to inhuman or degrading treatment or punishment.*

> **Box 28.3 ECHR Article 5 § 1 (e) of the Convention provides**
>
> *Everyone has the right to liberty and security of person. No one shall be deprived of his liberty save in the following cases and in accordance with a procedure prescribed by law: [. . .] (e) the lawful detention [. . .] of persons of unsound mind*

> **Box 28.1 ECHR Article 2**
>
> *Everyone's right to life shall be protected by law. No one shall be deprived of his life intentionally.. . ..*

> **Box 28.4** ECHR Article 8
>
> *the right to respect for private and family life, home and correspondence . . . . there shall be no interference by a public authority with the exercise of this right except such as is in accordance with the law and is necessary in a democratic society in the interests of national security, public safety or the economic wellbeing of the country, for the prevention of disorder or crime, for the protection of health or morals, or for the protection of the rights and freedoms of others*

In *Winterwerp* v. *The Netherlands* (1979 6301/ 73 ECHR 4, paragraph 37),[15] the Strasbourg Court held that "the convention does not state what is to be understood by the words 'person of unsound mind'. This term is not one that can be given a definite interpretation . . . . . . it is a term whose meaning is continually evolving as research in psychiatry progresses, and increasing flexibility and treatment is developing and society's attitude to mental illness changes, in particular so that a greater understanding of the problems of mental patients is becoming more widespread." This definition may be compared with the definition in the United Nations principles for the protection of persons with mental illness,[16] principle 4 "determination of mental illness" which emphasizes the importance of international classification systems and definitions such as those of the World Health Organization International Classification of Mental and Behavioural Disorders.[17]

Notably, there is no requirement that detention on the grounds of unsound mind is exclusively for treatment. Protection of life, bodily integrity, and dignity may also be engaged. However, it is also the case that detention without treatment, for example, delaying treatment after detention pending a second hearing to determine incapacity, is harmful[18,19] and therefore unethical. Detention without treatment is merely imprisonment (Box 28.4).

ECHR Article 8 sets out the right to private life. The concept of private life covers the physical and moral integrity of the person (*X and Y* v. *The Netherlands*, 1985, § 22.)[20] Emergency medical interventions on life-saving grounds performed in the absence of the patients' consent are not incompatible with the Convention. An individual's involvement in the choice of medical care options available and consent to such treatment falls within the scope of Article 8. There is a general requirement on States to provide a legal framework of guidelines and procedures setting out the elements of informed consent and to ensure high professional standards in this area.

The ECtHR has held that mental health must be regarded as a crucial part of private life associated with the aspect of moral integrity. The preservation of mental stability is in that context an indispensable precondition to effective enjoyment of the right to respect for private life (*Bensaid* v. *United Kingdom*, 2001, § 47).[21] Compulsory medication of a mentally ill patient may be justified in some circumstances, in order to protect the patient and/or others. However, such decisions must be made against the background of clear legal guidelines and with the possibility of judicial review.

Although the right to health is not among the rights guaranteed under the ECHR or its Protocols, Contracting States are under a positive obligation to take appropriate measures to protect the life and health of those within their jurisdiction and there is also an obligation "to place the best interests of the child, and also those of children as a group, at the centre of all decisions affecting their health and development."

It can reasonably be taken that the "best interests" of persons of unsound mind, and especially those who are vulnerable due to mental disabilities and those who are detained by law in hospitals, should also be at the center of decisions affecting their health, to protect the patient and/or others.

Principled and process approaches to ethical reasoning about treatment

Legal decision-makers should not impose legal values and priorities (as distinct from lawful processes) imported from the criminal justice system into medical ethics and professional decision-making. For example, Rawls prioritizes liberty above all other values.[22] Whether Rawls's primacy of liberty is a principle or merely a conjecture is open to challenge.[23,24] In the ECHR and other similar systems of human rights, liberty is a qualified right. Medical ethics must be subject to the principles of natural justice, with respect for rights and compliance with the law. But it should not be acceptable to denigrate as "paternalism" the medical obligation to act with compassion in the best

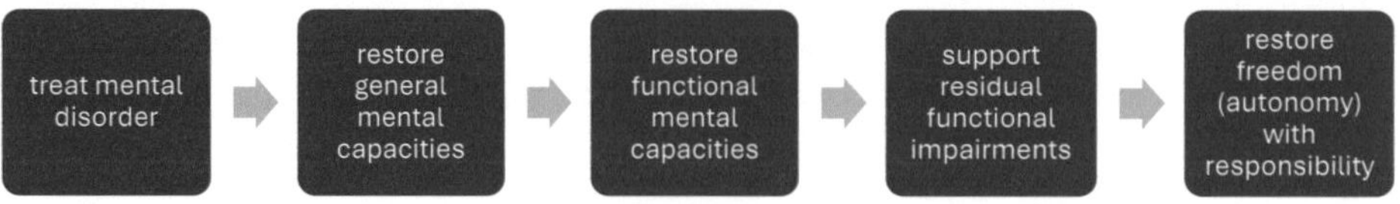

Figure 28.1 Ethics as process

interests of a vulnerable and impaired person, either professionally or as a state.

Medical, psychiatric values and priorities in decision-making can be identified with scientific values. Bronowski[25] pointed out that successful factual scientific discoveries require a commitment to values such as truth, good explanations, and openness to new ideas and change, further entailing tolerance, integrity, and openness to debate. Deutsch[26] developed a theory of moral reasoning from his scientific emphasis on the importance of "good explanations" in successful science. Good explanations are hard to vary because they are about reality and close to truth (verifiable observations in the real world, consistent with other known scientific explanations and explanatory systems, cannot simply be bent to suit some bias or vested interest), simple or elegant (make no assumptions beyond necessity), are falsifiable (constrained by existing knowledge including other good explanations), and a good explanation reaches out to explain other problems beyond the problems it was created to solve. Further, Deutsch goes on to assert that the same scientific characteristics of good explanations can be used to find solutions to moral problems.[26] Since the process of solving moral problems is ethics, this is a scientific form of ethics and is likely to be more successful in the real world than the conjectural, literary-critical, or normative approaches.

A compatibilist "process" approach may reconcile many of these apparent clashes between legal and medical decision-making. Figure 1 offers an alternative to Rawls' hierarchical principles of justice, which insist on freedom before other values and elevates this value to a principle by an act of reification. Rawls' second principle, that inequality is only to be allowed if the worse off will be better off than they might otherwise be, seems in keeping with the system proposed in Figure 28.1. In this ethical system, there can be no freedom without responsibility and no responsibility without intact functional mental capacities. Therefore, the first step and first priority is to treat mental disorders with a view to restoring capacity, thereby restoring responsibility, to whatever extent is possible. The

alleviation of suffering and restoration of dignity in the best interests of the person concerned are inseparable benefits and measurable health gains from this process.

Goals derived from principles

We propose that goals can be derived from these principles, and we propose also that goals can be ordered according to a rational process. This contrasts with principles, which are universally agreed but extremely difficult to resolve into an ordered hierarchy for decision-making. We propose that the overarching goal of treatment in neuropsychiatry is to achieve health gains for patients. This process starts with the obligation to ensure that all rights are vindicated and legal processes are complied with. Next is the duty of care to ensure a safe, violence-free therapeutic environment for patients and clinicians. This enables the next stage in a process of goal-directed activity to prioritize effective treatments over other activities. The fourth stage in the process is the evaluation of health gains achieved and the duty to continuously improve health gains through research, development, and evaluation of treatment at the individual and organizational level for specific cohorts and general populations.

Processes

Clinical decisions of great consequence are made regarding patients with severe mental illnesses. Such decisions should be made in accordance with an ethical process to ensure fairness, the right to be heard, consistency, proportionality, respect for rights, and compliance with law. The obligation to make such decisions ethically is all the greater where the patient is vulnerable and may lack the ability to make competent decisions for themselves. Among the most consequential and complex decisions are those regarding deprivation of liberty and triage to levels of care, including levels of therapeutic security,[27–29] the management of waiting lists,[30] decisions about length of stay,[31,32] and restoration of competency, conditional discharge,[33] and community treatment orders,[34] or the use of restrictive practices such as seclusion or restraint.[35] There is increasing evidence that such decisions are more reliable when a structured professional judgment instrument is used to guide the clinical assessment and decision-maker,[36–39] and when such structured professional judgments are considered within a decision-making judgment support framework such as an admissions panel, court process, or review board.[40]

Diagnosis as an ethical process in psychiatry

Establishing a diagnosis is often the first step in a process leading to treatment. The correct process of establishing a diagnosis has consequences for the evaluation of prognosis. This in turn has a large influence on decisions about the benefits and risks of treatment. The operational diagnostic criteria of the American Psychiatric Association's Diagnostic and Statistical Manual (APA DSM)[41] and the World Health Organization's International Classification of Diseases for Mental and Behavioural Disorders (WHO ICD[17]) favor a syndromal approach with operationalized criteria that works well with palliative and ameliorative treatments. The eventual emergence of disease-modifying treatments for causes will fracture these diagnostic categories. This is not to be taken as indicating the end of diagnosis.[42] Diagnosis will remain essential for assessment of prognosis and selection of treatment.[43,44]

Recent progress in the assessment and diagnosis of neurodegenerative disease with perceptual and processing disturbances (NDPPD) has focused on staging these "process" illnesses, first characterized as dementia praecox because the onset is often with decline in functional ability in late adolescence before the emergence of delusions and hallucinations sufficient to meet diagnostic criteria for schizophrenia.[45] Stage "zero" or at-risk mental state has a predictive power for the emergence of any of the NDPPD mental illnesses.[46,47] This is often bound up with substance misuse, particularly cannabis.[48,49]

A "chicken and egg" conundrum of causation arises from the circular relationship between vulnerability to substance misuse due to NDPPD (for example, schizophrenia), while early onset and severity of substance misuse also leads to the emergence of NDPPD with delusions, hallucinations, and cognitive decline, with a consensus in favor of cannabis as a causal agent.[48–52]

Hodgins[53–55] described young people with early onset of conduct disorder and substance misuse who have single or brief episodes of psychosis resembling schizophrenia with full remission of symptoms and full functional recovery after a single episode or between episodes. These are probably best described as psychoactive substance-induced psychoses because they are distinct from Kraepelin's dementia praecox and "process" schizophrenia. These are notable because they have good outcomes.[43] Other patients develop the Kraepelinian core syndrome: they typically have had no prior conduct disorder or substance misuse and develop schizophrenia with a relapsing and remitting course, progressing from stage zero (at-risk mental states) to stage 1 (a single episode with full recovery) through stage 2 (relapsing and remitting with full recovery between episodes), stage 3 (relapsing and remitting with some residual symptoms and functional impairment between episodes, gradually deteriorating over time), and stage 4 (treatment-resistant symptoms and severe functional impairment).[56,57] In this context, the benefits of preventing relapses[18,19,58] become essential for making informed decisions about treatment, particularly the use of long-acting injections and long-term treatment to prevent relapses and progression.

A critique of capacity-based tests

It is sometimes suggested that the requirement for a medically diagnosed mental disorder could be dispensed with so that legal processes could rely solely on functional mental capacity.[59,60] Assessing mental capacities to reach an opinion about a functional mental capacity is inherently a circular, self-referential process. The capacities to understand, or to reason, or to appreciate and to communicate are evident only at the level of consciousness (a high order of emergent complexity); therefore, the assessed functional mental capacity (which is at the same level of emergent complexity) is circularly related to the end assessment. Insisting on a "functional" test does not solve this circularity. Requiring an antecedent test of impairment or dysfunction at more objective "microscopic" levels of emergence – neurophysiological, neuropathological, and neuropsychological – is necessary, if only as a protection against malingering, and is also necessary as a protection against many forms of bias and error due to mind–body dualism – the impossibility of distinguishing between "will not" and "cannot." A higher-level emergent phenomenon such as consciousness is never more than the sum of the interactions and organization of lower-level entities such as normal and abnormal anatomy and physiology and the intermediate level of neuropsychology or psychopathology. Whether all properties of an emergent system can at present be explained in terms of an underlying constituent part or not, all of the known pathological processes affecting consciousness (anesthetics, intoxicants, injuries, epileptic phenomena, cerebrovascular phenomena, metabolic phenomena, neurodegenerative diseases, developmental disorders, mental diseases, and impairments of mental capacities) have been pathologies of constituent, underlying, "smaller scale" parts and systems (genetic defects, biochemical process dysfunctions, anatomical lesions, growths, and injuries). And all effective treatments (antibiotics, neuroreceptor agonists or antagonists, immunomodulators, and immunosuppressants) have been active at the level of lower-level constituent parts. By contrast, mind–body dualist approaches and "strong emergent" theories of mental disorders and incapacities depend on circular reasoning and on the reification of notions (mistaking the name of an idea for a real thing, for example, ego, id, and super-ego) that cannot be demonstrated or falsified.[61] Treatments based only on mind–body dualism cannot show any measurable benefit beyond the placebo effect.[62–64]

There are other approaches to the ethical priorities that should be considered and weighed in relation to competence to make decisions of greater consequence. The loss of human dignity and the suffering from tormenting symptoms can be effectively treated and should not be left untreated by a caring society or a conscientious, compassionate clinician. The willingness to intervene and use restrictive means to achieve health gains – alleviating suffering due to symptoms, restoring dignity through enhanced functional ability, restoring civil autonomy and responsibility, fostering recovery, and hope are necessary professional and ethical values for doctors, nurses, and other health professionals. Acting in the best interests of vulnerable persons of unsound mind is a primary ethical obligation for doctors, nurses, and allied health professionals. Avoiding the medical necessity to intervene out of scruples for legal values and priorities (as distinct from lawful processes) falls short of medical professional ethics.

The legal exclusion of family members from the processes of making decisions for incapacitated adults is one of the least democratic, least supported pieces of legal innovation of recent decades. There is little democratic support for this and much unhappiness among families and carers.

Legal processes

Precedent setting judgments have interpreted legal provisions for detention and treatment under mental health law as "purposive" and "designed for the protection of the citizen and for the promotion of the common good."[65] Any resiling from this position would be regressive. The goal of any detention due to medical necessity must be to deliver effective medical care and treatment. Detention without treatment is merely imprisonment. For example, legal structures that allow detention under mental health legislation while delaying treatment until a court hearing at some later date to determine incapacity and permit treatment without consent should be regarded as self-defeating and causing unnecessary delays to essential treatment. Delayed treatment and deliberately prolonged duration of untreated psychosis are now known to be seriously harmful.[18,19] Such unmedical and harmful delays are therefore unethical processes. This unethical delay is a good example of prioritizing liberty as a principle while failing to recognize the process and goal-directed necessity of treating to restore mental health and capacity in order to enjoy the restoration of free will, responsibility, and liberty.

Council of Europe recommendation number REC (2004) 10 is derived from the case law of the ECtHR.[66] It is often regarded as a "model mental health act," and its language has found its way into many of the mental health acts of European states.[13] It defined "treatment" as an intervention (physical or psychological) on a person with a mental disorder that, "taking into account the person's social dimension, has a therapeutic purpose in relation to that mental disorder." Treatment may include measures to improve the social dimension of a person's life, and "therapeutic purposes" includes prevention, diagnosis, control, or cure of the disorder, and rehabilitation.

Medical necessity

The following is an ordinal scale (Box 28.5) intended to allow decision-makers to weigh up "medical necessity" as a justification for intrusive or restrictive

Box 28.5 Medical neccessity as an ordinal scale

10 =necessary to save life (urgency is essential here—the doctor must act at once or as soon as possible, e.g., refusal of all fluids).

09 = necessary to preserve life (here the intervention is necessary because otherwise deterioration to a life-threatening state will be certain, and within days. This can apply also to some maintenance treatments).

08 = necessary to prevent irreversible and serious physical injury to the patient ("serious" here would mean a disability that would alter the person or personality of the patient leading to a permanent physical or mental disability. This echoes a definition of degrading treatment that might alter the character of a person).

07 = necessary to alleviate suffering that is serious and degrading for the person concerned.

06 = necessary to bring to an end the use of other compulsory restrictive practices that might otherwise continue indefinitely where such practices are themselves a cause of suffering or are degrading (e.g., long-term isolation, long-term restraint).

05 = necessary to prevent injury to others and therefore to facilitate resocialization and integration into social contact with others (interesting questions arise here concerning the rights of nursing and care staff. Some patients may injure others because they prefer to be isolated and do not experience this as suffering or degradation and so fall outside the definitions in 06 and 07).

04 = necessary to restore functional mental capacity.

03 = necessary to achieve the least restrictive legal and social situation – either to be discharged from detention or to move to a minimally restrictive regime.

02 = necessary to restore or preserve dignity. For example, a patient with behavior that makes socialization difficult might benefit from treatment to enable resocialization and integration with others. (Some patients repeatedly scream, strip, rush about, intrude on others. . .).

01 = necessary to achieve and enjoy full potential in life. For example, a person may on achieving remission gain a much better quality of life in ways beyond the preservation of life or alleviation of suffering. Self-actualization through creativity, self-transcendence through meaningful socialization, regaining hope – these are all potential benefits of clozapine (and some other) treatments.

practices or compulsion – including compulsory detention. These "weights" should be considered in the balance against the parallel scale assigning weights to the possible adverse consequences (Box 28.6). Examples might include nasogastric feeding in life-threatening anorexia nervosa and other forms of compulsory medication, including by intramuscular injection or in rare cases, by nasogastric tube. The scale ranges from the immediate need to preserve life (arguably a right under international covenants on human rights) through to the necessity of treatment in order to restore dignity and mental capacity (according to the principle of reciprocity – no deprivation of liberty without providing treatment necessary to restore autonomy or dignity) to necessity because without treatment the right to enjoy the full potential of life may be lost.

It must be emphasized that any form of intrusive, restrictive, or compulsory intervention without consent can be justified only where the person concerned lacks the functional mental capacity to give or withhold consent. Therefore, any such intervention without consent must end when capacity is restored. In practice, however, such intrusive and restrictive interventions should always be ended earlier than the restoration of capacity on recovery and safety grounds. The prevention of imminent and serious violence to others, preserving the therapeutic milieu for all patients, and exercising the duty to keep vulnerable patients safe may also be invoked as a medical necessity.[67]

Interesting questions arise concerning the balancing of the rights of staff not to be assaulted while caring for violent patients and the necessity of preserving therapeutic relationships.[68] Medical necessity may in some circumstances be taken as a reason to intervene and treat without consent, whether there is capacity or not. In such cases, a hierarchy of necessities and a hierarchy of consequential risks are to be weighed in the balance.

Box 28.6 Adverse consequences as an ordinal scale

10 = restraint and procedures (e.g., passing of a nasogastric tube) may be fatal due to restraint asphyxia or cardiac events during a struggle.

09 = misadventure may occur (e.g., aspiration pneumonia may occur due to an incorrectly placed NG tube).

08 = known side effects of the intervention (e.g., ECT, clozapine, or other medication) may be serious though rare, and in most cases treatable (anesthetic adverse events, agranulocytosis, pulmonary embolism, megacolon. . .).

07 = the procedure may itself cause pain and gagging.

06 = the procedure may itself cause suffering due to humiliation and shame.

05 = others may be injured in the course of the procedure itself. This may include exposure of clinicians to biohazards.

04 = eventual engagement in a process of informed consent and therapeutic engagement may be made more difficult due to the alienating effect of the intervention.

03 = other processes of therapeutic engagement and negotiation may be prevented or inhibited while the process is ongoing and subsequently.

02 = the procedure may be inherently undignified while it is happening.

01 = the procedure may be experienced as traumatic, and this may shape long-term cognitive sets and perceptual biases concerning mental health treatments in a way that is against the person's best interests.

Box 28.7 Criteria for assessing functional mental capacity to give consent to treatment

Understanding
Reasoning – comparative and consequential
Appreciation
Communicating a decision

Consent to treatment

Functional mental capacity is not the only way to assess competence, nor is it the sole consideration even in jurisdictions that prioritize it.[69] Psychiatrists are accustomed to assessing the functional mental capacity to give consent to treatment. We are accustomed also to the need to ensure that consent is obtained free of duress and on the basis of having fully informed the patient of the benefits and risks of the available treatment choices. Box 28.7 sets out the most widely accepted criteria for assessing functional mental capacity to give consent to treatment.

The problem with legal reasoning about functional mental capacity is the legal belief that different functional mental capacities are independent of each other. A person who lacks the functional mental capacity to give consent to treatment for a psychosis may nonetheless be held to have the functional mental capacity to make a will or to marry. While it is reasonable to accept this when the decisions concerned are different in complexity, legal reasoning often appears to be based on mind–body dualism and a naïve acceptance of expressed will and preference, though only where this accords with the legal decision-maker's own beliefs.

Variable thresholds for capacity and competence: complexity and information overload

The difficulty arises that to give more than basic amounts of information is often enough to render the severely mentally ill patient unable to make a choice or communicate a decision.[70–72] Complex decisions are often beyond the functional mental capacities of the severely mentally ill, while relatively simple decisions are within mental capacities to understand, reason, appreciate, and communicate a decision. Lawyers attempt to gloss over this difficulty by saying that even a fleeting period of apparent capacity may allow a competent decision to be made, even if later the person makes a different choice or repeatedly changes their decision. This appears to the psychiatrist to be legal casuistry when all such fleeting decisions should be regarded as the products of an unstable and unreliable mental state. ECHR Article 8 has been interpreted to mean that the preservation of mental stability is an indispensable precondition to effective enjoyment of the right to respect for private life (*Bensaid* v. *United Kingdom*, 2001, § 47).[21] Indeed, there is a trend among legal decision-makers to accept this and instead accept "will and preference," whether capacitous or not, if it is reasonably stable, consistent with personality and preferences when well, and of no serious or life-changing consequence.

Variable thresholds for capacity and competence: seriousness of consequences

The more serious the consequences of the decision, the higher the level of functional mental capacity that should be required. For this reason, Appelbaum and his group were careful to avoid stating any threshold or cutoff score above or below which a patient did or did not have functional mental capacity. Our group offered sensitivity and specificity threshold scores for a "standardised" test (three choices, one of which is "do nothing; two pieces of information for and two against each option"), but in practice this cannot easily be extrapolated to other more complex real-life decisions about mental health.[73]

The Common Law approach privileges a particular set of common law precedents regarding functional mental capacity. The use of Appelbaum's formulation of functional mental capacity in terms of understanding, reasoning, and appreciation[74] and the related development and validation of the Mac-CAT on this basis,[75,76] are correctly regarded as the gold standard in the research literature. This is derived from the Common Law concept of "mind" as a collection of capacities.[8] This is reductive in order to eliminate the phenomenologically mysterious and subjective aspects of consciousness. These functional capacities are available for clinical examination and judicial consideration.

The Common Law approach to functional mental capacities has limitations. The Mac-CAT family of structured professional judgment instruments for assessing capacity to consent to treatment or to consent to research is demanding. A large proportion of mentally ill persons in hospitals is unable to complete the assessment and is excluded from research samples.[70,72]

This problem is compounded by the relative simplicity of the test task – having to retain two items of information about the advantages of a proposed treatment and two items of information about the disadvantages or side effects, repeated for three options. When extra information is given, an even larger proportion of mentally ill persons are unable to complete the task.[72] So for "real world" complex choices and decisions faced by clinicians and their severely mentally ill patients, the Mac-CAT instruments are limited in the extent to which their research validation can be generalized.

A method combining interviews where possible and observation in all cases based on Appelbaum's formulation (understanding, reasoning, appreciating, and communicating a choice) has the advantage of greater inclusivity because observational rating scales can be completed on all patients no matter how disturbed.[36] This is both ethically more inclusive and scientifically more valid because it does not exclude a large proportion of patients who are too ill (too functionally impaired) to complete the interview assessment.[36]

The basic concept of functional mental capacity is not the only approach to protecting the rights of the mentally ill or cognitively impaired person. The Roman Law concept of "imputability" is derived from a less reductive concept of mind. This recognizes that a mental illness resulting in delusions, hallucinations, thought disorder, and other changes in neuropsychological function,[77–80] metacognition,[81] and moral reasoning[82,83] may all impact and impair competence to make decisions about one's person and health, welfare and dignity, estate and finances, and capacity to form specific intentions.

Elsewhere, Carrara has argued[1,2] that any impairment of consciousness is an impairment of mental capacity to make responsible decisions that is generalizable and not function-specific. This is in keeping with modern neurophysiology and neuropsychology and contrary to the implicit mind–body dualism of legal concepts of functional mental capacity.

A layered concept of consciousness, from the neurophysiological to the neuropsychological and from the neuropsychological to personality or symptoms of dysfunction such as delusions, may allow a more correct assessment of capacity to make competent decisions, in the same way that "imputability" allows a different approach to criminal responsibility.

The difficulty is then to set the threshold for legal incompetence or diminished responsibility. For example, it is unlikely that personality could amount to an impairment of consciousness that mitigated or reduced either the capacity to make decisions or the responsibility for criminal acts. Kenny's critique of circular reasoning and nominalism (reification) as false justification for such opinions regarding personality and responsibility is helpful here.[4, 6] Kenny illustrates his view with an account of a case law precedent in which a defendant was convicted of causing death by witchcraft.[7]

Treatment

The overarching goal of treatment is to achieve health gains for patients. Saving life and prolonging life while enhancing quality of life are implicit within this. Health gains can be measured under four broad categories of "recovery": symptomatic recovery and the duty to prevent suffering; functional recovery and the obligation to restore or enable as much self-determination, independence, and choice as possible within the person's abilities; civil recovery of the ability to exercise legal autonomy and responsibility; and personal recovery, the ability to produce or co-produce one's own care and treatment plan, to have one's voice heard, and to have hope.[34]

The goal of achieving health gains may have been achieved at one time through conservative measures, waiting and supporting; in long-term care for untreatable or progressively degenerative diseases, through ensuring quality of life, dignity and providing the "scaffolding" of supportive care for basic biological functions and activities of daily living to ensure dignity, sensitivity to preferences in the absence of capacity, and freedom from symptomatic suffering. At its highest level, this structured care and treatment can facilitate higher functions such as self-actualization (the expression of the self as a person) and self-transcendence (the experience of being an active part of one's family and community).

In modern times, treatment in oncology, cardiology, and respiratory medicine has led to ever-improving 5-year survivals and lengthening life expectancy. During the same period, standardized mortality ratios have progressively worsened for NDPPDs such as schizophrenia and bipolar affective disorder,[84] with a measured 16-years loss of life expectancy in NDPPD.[85–87] Health gains such as life expectancy and the four recoveries, symptomatic, functional, civil, and personal recovery are as important in psychiatry as they are in any other area of medicine.

Variable thresholds and the effectiveness of treatments: palliative, ameliorative, and disease-modifying treatments

All treatment decisions involve weighing the consequences of untreated disease, the benefits of treatment, and the possible side effects of treatment, then making a decision in the balance. It is the responsibility of the patient to make the decision, but there is a strong professional responsibility on the doctor to give the advice needed for an informed decision.

Some treatments are more effective than others. In psychiatry and medicine generally, treatments can be divided into palliative, ameliorative, and disease-modifying. Palliative treatments do no more than alleviate troublesome symptoms and suffering. Ameliorative treatments may interrupt or delay a disease process for example, excising a tumor to relieve obstruction or using a diuretic to relieve congestive cardiac failure. Disease-modifying treatments act on the causative pathological process. For example, treatments in oncology can be divided into palliative treatments, for example, pain relief; ameliorative treatments, such as surgery to prevent bowel obstruction; and disease-modifying treatments, for example, surgical excision, radiotherapy, and chemotherapy combined with monoclonal antibodies to target cancerous cells. In rheumatology, there has been a dramatic change from palliative and ameliorative drugs – non-steroidal anti-inflammatory and immunosuppressive drugs to disease-modifying drugs[88] particularly biological agents.[89] Loss of hand function due to rheumatoid arthritis is now seldom seen in developed countries. Similar progress with disease-modifying treatment has occurred in Crohn's disease, ulcerative colitis, Sjogren's syndrome, and other inflammatory diseases. In congestive cardiac failure, diuretics, vasodilators, and surgery will have ameliorative effects on the secondary pathophysiology of a failing heart, but only treatments that address causes will have disease-modifying effects, for example, cardiac valve replacement when the cause is stenosis or regurgitation.

At present, almost all treatments available for NDPPD are palliative or ameliorative, alleviating the secondary effects of disease processes (symptoms, suffering) and possibly ameliorating patterns of relapse, but with no unequivocal disease-modifying effects on the earliest and most disabling stages of neurocognitive impairment and later cognitive decline.[90] However, there is emerging evidence that longer duration of untreated first-episode psychosis predicts poor long-term outcomes with worse symptoms, impaired global function, and neurocognitive abilities.[18,19] It follows that earlier intervention and the use of relapse-preventing medicines, such as long-acting injections of receptor-blocking medication are disease-modifying. The long-term prospective studies concerning the duration of untreated relapses (second and subsequent episodes) are not available,[18,19] but a relevant finding is that the benefit of treatment to prevent relapses (long-acting injections of receptor-blocking medication) is sustained over very long periods, with relapses occurring after discontinuation as much as 8 years later.[58]

The balancing of risks and benefits will be very different for a disease that is inconvenient or uncomfortable when compared to a disease that causes suffering, is life-shortening, or disabling. We must now recognize that NDDPDs such as schizophrenia and bipolar disorder are life-shortening diseases[87] as well as disabling and causes of suffering. The additional consideration arises that the threshold for intervening without consent will vary according to the risks and effectiveness of the treatment, even when this treatment is long-term use of long-acting injections of antipsychotic medication.[58,87,91,92]

Disease-modifying treatment and variable thresholds for early intervention when treating without consent

Whether or not early intervention with the treatments currently available can prevent progression of NDPPDs such as schizophrenia, it is foreseeable that disease-modifying treatments will soon be available. Such treatments are emerging for Alzheimer's disease and some genetically determined neurological disorders. Similar treatments may emerge for the early stages of neurocognitive decline in adolescents with early-stage schizophrenia. This will present a different set of ethical considerations when deciding when to offer voluntary treatment and what the information and advice should be that constitutes informed consent.

The ethical justification for treatment without consent where the treatment is disease-modifying may be more in favor of early intervention the stronger the evidence is for disease modification.

This raises the question of "medical necessity," a necessary condition for many forms of treatment or therapeutic interventions without consent in those who lack functional mental capacity or general mental capacity due to severe mental illnesses or other forms of mental disorder[14] (Box 28.5). Whether a disease-modifying treatment that addresses loss of life expectancy, prevents impairment of, or restores functional mental capacities can be interpreted as a medical necessity or a lesser justification for treatment without consent will probably require legal adjudication and precedent.

One candidate for disease-modifying treatment in NDPPD may be the permanent editing of genes (CRISPR). Since illnesses such as schizophrenia appear to be polygenic in predisposition, this may not be a way forward, though a greater concentration on the genes responsible for early neurocognitive decline may lead to interventions in the earliest stages of disease. Any permanent change in a gene that is vital to some aspect of neurocognitive function may be seen as a permanent change to the personality, temperament, or disposition. This will raise ethical problems since treatments that cause permanent changes to personality may be interpreted as inhuman, degrading, or even dehumanizing, although there is a complex counterbalance concerning medical necessity.[14] Epigenetic editing by switching genes on and off reversibly is more likely to be an ethically acceptable disease-modifying treatment.

Evaluation

There is an ethical duty to evaluate the outcomes of treatments and the delivery of treatments in models of care more generally.[93] This is essential since otherwise goals that were set in order to ensure that ethical principles are observed may be taken for granted. The aphorism "if you can't count it, you can't see it, and if you can't count it, it may not be real" applies here. There is an additional obligation in medical values to ensure that outcomes and health gains for patients are continuously improved through the virtuous circle of excellence: research, development, teaching, and training.[94]

Principled ethical barriers to research progress in psychiatry

In research on interventions that have low or negligible levels of medical necessity as described in Box 28.5, there are inevitably no adverse consequences as described in Box 28.6 and it is sufficient to rely on "will and preference" as a standard for competence to consent, whether a functional mental capacity test can be completed or not. But these "low necessity" interventions are generally either placebos or at best palliative, seldom ameliorative, and never disease-modifying.

Psychiatry has much to learn from oncology. The success of oncology arises from the systematic organization of international multicenter randomized controlled trials in which "treatment as usual" is compared to "treatment as usual plus." The result has been steady, incremental improvement in outcomes year by year. This has not yet happened in psychiatry.[94–97]

Due to ethical reliance on tests of functional mental capacity, research on treatment usually excludes all those who lack functional mental capacity to consent and all those who are detained under mental health legislation due to the obvious implied duress inherent in such a situation. Research on treatment is therefore biased by excluding the most severely ill. Excluding the most severely mentally ill is an ethical error, unfairly depriving them of the benefits of the best research. The result is not just lack of progress but worsening standardized mortality ratios and worsening 5-year survivals.[11] We do not know of any published attempt to examine and weigh the arguments for and against these conflicting ethical considerations.

In the absence of any prospect of randomized controlled trial research leading to incremental improvement, we are obliged to rely on prospective observational cohort studies, which should be inclusive and naturalistic. These can be powerful and informative. We are also obliged to wait for stepwise "break through" scientific progress. For example, if new biological treatments prove to be effective in Alzheimer's disease or multiple sclerosis, then NDPPD, such as schizophrenia, may be considered as possible additional beneficiaries if enough is known about the underlying pathophysiology to infer similarity. Inflammatory bowel diseases now benefit from the biological disease-modifying treatments for rheumatoid arthritis.[98] This approach is, however, inherently slower and less productive.

An unfortunate consequence of the right to privacy has been the burdens imposed on access to population data for medical research. The Scandinavian countries have shown the enormous advantages for progress in diagnosis and treatment from ensuring that the right to data privacy is qualified and limited for the purposes of medical research.[99–101]

Conclusions: Beyond paternalism and best interests

Characterizing as "paternalism" the compassionate duty to intervene actively in the best interests of a mentally disordered person is a pejorative rhetorical device. There is a duty to intervene with effective treatments that restore functional mental capacities, restore clear consciousness, awareness, and reality testing, restoring free will, responsibility, and autonomy. To refrain from intervening because of Rawls's theory-based prioritizing of liberty over all other principles or processes would be contrary to scientific realism, medical values, and medical ethics.

There is a difference between violence (coercion) and force, according to Hannah Arendt. Violence is destructive, even when it is state-authorized; force can be constructive, transforming routine and repetitive labor into creative and lasting work. Arendt held that it should be possible to use the power of the state as a form of force creatively and not as a vehicle of violence, which can only be destructive.[102–104] For example, it is methodologically possible to show that restrictive interventions are used proportionately and in accordance with law in a psychiatric intensive care setting to prevent imminent violence.[35]

An analogy can be drawn from Schrodinger's account of the distinguishing features of the living cell, from chaos to order, from order to disorder and decline into entropy and death.[105] In psychopathology and phenomenology, mental illness is destructive by its pathological nature. Judgment is impaired so that bad decisions are made, with outcomes that are against the best interests of the person concerned. But at a remove, what is happening is that the accumulated information and wisdom of the developed adult, the ability to adapt to the physical and social environment, is dissipated in entropy. Organization and systems that make the conscious personality, the integration of appetites and impulses with the deliberative restraint of long-term goals, are coarsened and degraded in fear and anger, shame and disgust,[106] entropy and chaos.

In the psychiatric treatment of delirium, psychosis, mania, or severe depression, treatments are effective if they restore the pre-existing organized and developed personality and consciousness – this is more than the simple restoration of some level of functional capacity, though it may require as a first step the restoration of general mental capacity, or at least the partial restoration, or the halting of further mental disintegration. Re-conceptualizing all of this as a process of opposing entropy with organization, confusion with perception, metacognitive errors with reason, and disinformation with information offers a conceptual structure with which to reason ethically about the use of legal compulsion (Arendt's "force") to prevent violence and reverse destruction.

Future directions

At the beginning of this essay, the capacity-based approach to legal concepts of mind in common law jurisprudence and forensic psychiatry was noted as distinct from Carrara's approach based on layered consciousness, described elsewhere in this collection. The connection between consciousness, agency, and free will as described in that system corresponds more closely with the Roman law concept of imputability. The system of layered consciousness described by Carrara is firmly embodied in neuroscience, anatomy, neurophysiology, and epigenetics. Carrara's system allows an approach to higher functions, including personality and identity. The two systems are therefore completely compatible at the level of embodiment and amenable to scientific modeling and hypothesis testing in the clinic as well as the laboratory, at least at the embodied levels.

Scientific theories cannot be proven or disproven in the courts, although courts can ignore science if they wish. Courts may accept non-scientific expert evidence because of the current or local social perception of cultural and artistic merit. Courts may accept expert evidence based on mind–body dualism and the related beliefs of postmodernism, critical theory, and denial of concepts of truth and fact in social discourse or even in science. Such non-scientific approaches will not sustain the dignity and respect due to the law, and such non-scientific approaches generally fall short of sustaining the dignity of the severely mentally ill person.

A system of laws concerning mental health, autonomy, and the law should be subject to critical review concerning its values, the elevation of values to principles, and subsequent prioritizing of principles. We prefer the scientific values of Bronowski[25] and Deutsch[26] and the ethical process described in Figure 28.1. There can be no individual liberties without personal mental health. There can be no practice

of medicine without the ethical principle of best interests. Dignity should be given prime position among the rights and values. Respect for human dignity demands compassionate social responsibility for our neighbors and fellow citizens.

Carrara's emphasis on the importance of consciousness as evidence of competence or impairment appears more robust than a narrow approach to functional mental capacity. Capacity, whether general or functional, remains amenable to rules of evidence and legal judgment at the expense of increasingly excessive simplification and circularity. Carrara's emphasis on the inherent dignity of the person as a neuroethical guide to the use of treatment without consent appears most in keeping with modern human rights principles.

References

1. Carrara A. A unified understanding of the human mind—a neuroethical perspective: tracing the evolution in western thought and the integration with neuroscience, psychology, psychiatry, and relational dimensions. *CNS Spectr.* 2024;**30**(1):e5.

2. Carrara A. A neuroethical approach to human life, identity, and liberty of schizophrenic patients. *CNS Spectr.* 2024;**30**(1):e4.

3. Kenny A. *The Metaphysics of Mind.* Oxford University Press; 1992.

4. Kenny A. The psychiatric expert in court. *Psychol Med.* 1984;**14**(2): 291–302.

5. Kennedy H. Limits of psychiatric evidence in civil courts and tribunals: science and sensibility. *Med-L J Ireland.* 2004;10.

6. Kenny A. *Freewill and Responsibility (Routledge Revivals).* Taylor & Francis; 2011.

7. Kenny A. *The Ivory Tower: Essays in Philosophy and Public Policy / Anthony Kenny.* Oxford; New York: B. Blackwell; 1985.

8. Grounds A. On describing mental states. *Br J Med Psychol.* 1987;**60**(4): 305–311.

9. Fenwick P. Automatism, medicine and the law. *Psychol Med Monogr Suppl.* 1990;**17**:1–27.

10. Fenwick PB. Brain, mind, insanity, and the law. *BMJ.* 1991;**302**(6783): 979–980.

11. Broughton R, Billings R, Cartwright R, et al. Homicidal somnambulism: a case report. *Sleep.* 1994;**17**(3):253–264.

12. Holoyda BJ, Sorrentino RM, Mohebbi A, et al. Forensic evaluation of sexsomnia. *J Am Acad Psychiatry Law.* 2021;**49**(2):202–210.

13. European Union Agency for Fundamental Rights (FRA). *Involuntary Placement and Involuntary Treatment of Persons with Mental Health Problems*. FRA European Union Agency for Fundamental Rights, Vienna, Austria 7 June 2012. https://fra.europa.eu/sites/default/fi les/involuntary-placement-and-involuntary-treatment-of-persons-with-mental-health-problems _en.pdf.

14. Council of Europe. *Guide on Article 3 of the European Convention on Human Rights: Prohibition of Torture*. Strasbourg: Council of Europe; 2024.

15. *Winterwerp* v. *The Netherlands*. BAILLI: ECHR; 1979.

16. United Nations General Assembly. Principles for the Protection of Persons with Mental Illness and the Improvement of Mental Health Care. In: (1991–1992) UGAts, editor. 2002.

17. World Health Organization. *International Classification of Diseases Eleventh Revision (ICD-11)*. ICD-11. 11th Revision ed. Geneva: World Health Organization; 2022:388–594.

18. O'Keeffe D, Kinsella A, Waddington JL, Clarke M. 20-year prospective, sequential follow-up study of heterogeneity in associations of duration of untreated psychosis with symptoms, functioning, and quality of life following first-episode psychosis. *Am J Psychiatry*. 2022;**179**(4):288–297.

19. Nkire N, Kingston T, Kinsella A, Russell V, Waddington JL. Mixed-effects models reveal prediction of long-term outcome by duration of untreated psychosis (DUP) and illness (DUI) varies with quantile gradation but is invariant with time across 7 years in the Cavan-Monaghan First Episode Psychosis Study (CAMFEPS). *Schizophr Res*. 2022;**248**:124–130.

20. *X and Y* v. *The Netherlands*, (Application no. 8978/80, ECtHR 26 March 1985) HUDOC. https://hudoc.echr .coe.int/fre?i=001-57603

21. *Bensaid* v. *United Kingdom*, (Application no. 44599/98, ECtHR 6 February 2001, final 06/05/2001) HUDOC. https://hudoc.echr.coe.int/

22. Rawls J. *A Theory of Justice*. Harvard University Press; 2009.

23. Sen A. *Inequality Reexamined*. Oxford University Press; 1995.

24. Nickel JW. Rethinking Rawls's theory of liberty and rights. *Chi-Kent L Rev*. 1993;**69**:763.

25. Bronowski J. *Science and Human Values*. London: Faber and Faber Ltd; 2008: 94.

26. Deutsch D. *The Beginning of Infinity: Explanations that Transform the World*. Penguin UK; 2011.

27. Freestone M, Bull D, Brown R, et al. Triage, decision-making and follow-up of patients referred to a UK forensic service: validation of the DUNDRUM toolkit. *BMC Psychiatry*. 2015;**15**:239.

28. Williams HK, Senanayke M, Ross CC, Bates R, Davoren M. Security needs among patients referred for high secure care in Broadmoor Hospital England. *BJPsych Open*. 2020;**6**(4):e55.

29. Davoren M, Byrne O, O'Connell P, et al. Factors affecting length of stay in forensic hospital setting: need for therapeutic security and course of admission. *BMC Psychiatry*. 2015;**15**:301.

30. Daniels N, Sabin JE. *Setting Limits Fairly: Learning to Share Resources for Health*. Oxford University Press; 2008.

31. Davoren M, O'Dwyer S, Abidin Z, et al. Prospective in-patient cohort study of moves between levels of therapeutic security: the DUNDRUM-1 triage security, DUNDRUM-3 programme completion and DUNDRUM-4 recovery scales and the HCR-20. *BMC Psychiatry*. 2012;**12**:80.

32. Davoren M, Hennessy S, Conway C, et al. Recovery and concordance in a secure forensic psychiatry hospital—the self rated DUNDRUM-3 programme completion and DUNDRUM-4 recovery scales. *BMC Psychiatry*. 2015;**15**:61.

33. McCullough S, Stanley C, Smith H, et al. Outcome measures of risk and recovery in Broadmoor High Secure Forensic Hospital: stratification of care pathways and moves to medium secure hospitals. *BJPsych Open*. 2020;**6**(4):e74.

34. Kennedy HG. Models of care in forensic psychiatry. *BJPsych Adv*. 2022;**28** (1):46–59

35. Kennedy HG, Mullaney R, McKenna P, et al. A tool to evaluate proportionality and necessity in the use of restrictive practices in forensic mental health settings: the DRILL tool (Dundrum restriction, intrusion and liberty ladders). *BMC Psychiatry*. 2020;**20**(1):515.

36. Moynihan G, O'Reilly K, O'Connor J, Kennedy HG. An evaluation of functional mental capacity in forensic mental health practice: the Dundrum capacity ladders validation study. *BMC Psychiatry*. 2018;**18**(1):78.

37. Jeandarme I, Habets P, Kennedy H. Structured versus unstructured judgment: DUNDRUM-1 compared to court decisions. *Int J Law Psychiatry*. 2019;**64**:205–210.

38. Habets P, Jeandarme I, Kennedy HG. Applicability of the DUNDRUM-1 in a forensic Belgium setting. *J Forensic Psychol*. 2019;**21**(1):85–94.

39. Lawrence D, Davies T-L, Bagshaw R, et al. External validity and anchoring heuristics: application of DUNDRUM-1 to secure service gatekeeping in South Wales. *BJPsych Bulletin*. 2018;**42**(1): 10–18.

40. Kennedy H. Models of care in forensic psychiatry. In: Davoren M, Kennedy HG, eds. *Seminars in Forensic*

Psychiatry. College Seminars Series. 2nd ed. Cambridge: Cambridge University Press; 2024:176–207.

41. American Psychiatric Association. *Diagnostc and Statistical Manual of Mental Disorders: DSM-5-TR*: American Psychiatric Association Publishing; 2022.

42. Chen ZS, Kulkarni P, Galatzer-Levy IR, et al. Modern views of machine learning for precision psychiatry. *Patterns.* 2022;**3**(11):100602.

43. Stürner L, Ross T, Traub HJ. Elusive cases in forensic psychiatry? Exploring subgroups of schizophrenia spectrum disorder patients in Germany. *Int J Law Psychiatry.* 2024;**93**:101971.

44. Silva RF, Plis SM. How to integrate data from multiple biological layers in mental health? In: Passos IC, Mwangi B, Kapczinski F, eds. *Personalized Psychiatry: Big Data Analytics in Mental Health.* Cham: Springer International Publishing; 2019: 135–59.

45. Keshavan MS, Anderson S, Pettergrew JW. Is schizophrenia due to excessive synaptic pruning in the prefrontal cortex? The Feinberg hypothesis revisited. *J Psychiatr Res.* 1994;**28**(3):239–265.

46. Yung AR, Phillips LJ, Yuen HP, et al. Psychosis prediction: 12-month follow up of a high-risk ("prodromal") group. *Schizophr Res.* 2003;**60**(1):21–32.

47. McGorry PD, Yung AR, Phillips LJ. The "close-in" or ultra high-risk model: a safe and effective strategy for research and clinical intervention in prepsychotic mental disorder. *Schizophr Bull.* 2003;**29**(4): 771–790.

48. D'Souza DC, DiForti M, Ganesh S, et al. Consensus paper of the WFSBP task force on cannabis, cannabinoids and psychosis. *World J Biol Psychiatry.* 2022;**23**(10):719–742.

49. Di Forti M, Quattrone D, Freeman TP, et al. The contribution of cannabis use to variation in the incidence of psychotic disorder across Europe (EU-GEI): a multicentre case-control study. *Lancet Psychiatry.* 2019;**6**(5): 427–436.

50. Schoeler T, Theobald D, Pingault JB, et al. Continuity of cannabis use and violent offending over the life course. *Psychol Med.* 2016;**46**(8):1663–1677.

51. Schoeler T, Theobald D, Pingault JB, et al. Developmental sensitivity to cannabis use patterns and risk for major depressive disorder in mid-life: findings from 40 years of follow-up. *Psychol Med.* 2018;**48** (13):2169–2176.

52. Wainberg M, Jacobs GR, di Forti M, Tripathy SJ. Cannabis, schizophrenia genetic risk, and psychotic experiences: a cross-sectional study of 109,308 participants from the UK Biobank. *Transl Psychiatry.* 2021;**11**(1):211.

53. Brennan PA, Mednick SA, Hodgins S. Major mental disorders and criminal violence in a Danish birth cohort. *Arch Gen Psychiatry.* 2000;**57**(5): 494–500.

54. Hodgins S. Violent behaviour among people with schizophrenia: a framework for investigations of causes, and effective treatment, and prevention. *Philos Trans R Soc Lond B Biol Sci.* 2008;**363**(1503):2505–2518.

55. Hodgins S, Piatosa MJ, Schiffer B. Violence among people with schizophrenia: phenotypes and neurobiology. *Curr Top Behav Neurosci.* 2014; **17**:329–368.

56. McGorry PD, Hartmann JA, Spooner R, Nelson B. Beyond the "at risk mental state" concept: transitioning to transdiagnostic psychiatry. *World Psychiatry.* 2018;**17**(2):133–142.

57. Lavoie S, Polari AR, Goldstone S, Nelson B, McGorry PD. Staging model in psychiatry: review of the evolution of electroencephalography abnormalities in major psychiatric disorders. *Early Interv Psychiatry.* 2019; **13**(6):1319–1328.

58. Tiihonen J, Tanskanen A, Taipale H. 20-year nationwide follow-up study on discontinuation of antipsychotic treatment in first-episode schizophrenia. *Am J Psychiatry.* 2018;**175**(8):765–773.

59. Law Commission. Mental incapacity, Item 9 of the forth programme of law reform: mentally incapacitated adults. *Law Com No 231.* 1995.

60. Law Reform Commission. *Vulnerable Adults and the Law.* Law Reform Commission; 2006.

61. Shepherd M. *Sherlock Holmes and the Case of Dr Freud.* Tavistock Publications; 1985.

62. Wampold BE. The good, the bad, and the ugly: a 50-year perspective on the outcome problem. *Psychotherapy.* 2013;**50**(1):16–24.

63. Wampold BE, Imel ZE, Minami T. The placebo effect: "relatively large" and "robust" enough to survive another assault. *J Clin Psychol.* 2007;**63**(4): 401–403.

64. Wampold BE. How important are the common factors in psychotherapy? An update. *World Psychiatry.* 2015;**14**(3):270–277.

65. *T. O'D.* v. *Clinical Director of the Central Mental Hospital, the Health Service Executive, the Mental Health Commission.* [2007] IEHC 129, [2007] 3 IR 698, 25 April 2007. URL: https://www.bailii.org/ie/cases/IEHC/2007/H129.html

66. Council of Europe. Recommendation Rec(2004)10 of the Committee of Ministers to Member States concerning the protection of human rights and dignity of persons with mental disorder and its Explanatory Memorandom. *Council of Europe. Committee of Ministers.* 2004;**22**(09):67.

67. *MR* v. *Byrne and Others* [2007] 3 IR 211, [2007] IEHC 73, (03 March 2007). https://www.bailii.org/ie/cases/IEHC/2007/H73.html

68. Kirchebner J, Lau S, Kling S, Sonnweber M, Günther MP. Individuals with schizophrenia who act violently towards others profit unequally from inpatient treatment-Identifying subgroups by latent class analysis. *Int J Methods Psychiatr Res.* 2021;30(2): e1856.

69. Ganzini L, Volicer L, Nelson WA, Fox E, Derse AR. Ten myths about decision-making capacity. *J Am Med Dir Assoc.* 2004;5(4):263–267.

70. Rutledge E, Kennedy M, O'Neill H, Kennedy HG. Functional mental capacity is not independent of the severity of psychosis. *Int J Law Psychiatry.* 2008;31 (1):9–18.

71. Dornan J, Kennedy M, Garland J, Rutledge E, Kennedy HG. Functional mental capacity, treatment as usual and time: magnitude of change in secure hospital patients with major mental illness. *BMC Res Notes.* 2015;8:566.

72. Kennedy M, Dornan J, Rutledge E, O'Neill H, Kennedy HG. Extra information about treatment is too much for the patient with psychosis. *Int J Law Psychiatry.* 2009;32(6):369–376.

73. Fernandez C, Kennedy HG, Kennedy M. The recovery of factors associated with decision-making capacity in individuals with psychosis. *BJPsych Open.* 2017;3 (3):113–119.

74. Grisso T, Appelbaum PS. *Assessing Competence to Consent to Treatment: A Guide for Physicians and other Health Professionals.* Oxford University Press; 1998.

75. Grisso T, Appelbaum PS. Comparison of standards for assessing patients' capacities to make treatment decisions. *Am J Psychiatry.* 1995;152(7): 1033–1037.

76. Grisso T, Appelbaum PS, Hill-Fotouhi C. The MacCAT-T: a clinical tool to assess patients' capacities to make treatment decisions. *Psychiatr Serv.* 1997; 48 (1):1415–1419.

77. O'Reilly K, Donohoe G, Coyle C, et al. Prospective cohort study of the relationship between neuro-cognition, social cognition and violence in forensic patients with schizophrenia and schizoaffective disorder. *BMC Psychiatry.* 2015; 15:155.

78. O'Reilly K, Donohoe G, O'Sullivan D, et al. Study protocol: a randomised controlled trial of cognitive remediation for a national cohort of forensic mental health patients with schizophrenia or schizoaffective disorder. *BMC Psychiatry.* 2016;16:5.

79. Richter MS, O'Reilly K, O'Sullivan D, et al. Prospective observational cohort study of 'treatment as usual' over four years for patients with schizophrenia in a national forensic hospital. *BMC Psychiatry.* 2018; 18(1):289.

80. O'Reilly K, O'Connell P, Ryan A, et al. Deficit not bias: a quantifiable neuropsychological model of delusions. *Schizophr Res.* 2020; 222:496–498.

81. Naughton M, Nulty A, Abidin Z, et al. Effects of group metacognitive training (MCT) on mental capacity and functioning in patients with psychosis in a secure forensic psychiatric hospital: a prospective-cohort waiting list controlled study. *BMC Res Notes.* 2012;5:302.

82. O'Reilly K, O'Connell P, Corvin A, et al. Moral cognition and homicide amongst forensic patients with schizophrenia and schizoaffective disorder: a cross-sectional cohort study. *Schizophr Res.* 2018;193: 468–469.

83. O'Reilly K, O'Connell P, O'Sullivan D, et al. Moral cognition, the missing link between psychotic symptoms and acts of violence: a cross-sectional national forensic cohort study. *BMC Psychiatry.* 2019;19(1):408.

84. Lomholt LH, Andersen DV, Sejrsgaard-Jacobsen C, et al. Mortality rate trends in patients diagnosed with schizophrenia or bipolar disorder: a nationwide study with 20 years of follow-up. *Int J Bipolar Disord.* 2019; 7 (1):6.

85. Uhrskov Sørensen L, Bengtson S, Lund J, Ibsen M, Långström N. Mortality among male forensic and non-forensic psychiatric patients: matched cohort study of rates, predictors and causes-of-death. *Nord J Psychiatry.* 2020; 74(7):489–496.

86. Ojansuu I, Forsman J, Kautiainen H, et al. Association of duration of treatment on post-discharge mortality in forensic psychiatric patients in Finland. *Front Psychiatry.* 2024;15: 1372687.

87. Tiihonen J, Lönnqvist J, Wahlbeck K, et al. 11-year follow-up of mortality in patients with schizophrenia: a population-based cohort study (FIN11 study). *Lancet.* 2009;374(9690):620–627.

88. Hughes CD, Scott DL, Ibrahim F. Intensive therapy and remissions in rheumatoid arthritis: a systematic review. *BMC Musculoskelet Disord.* 2018;19(1):389.

89. Abbasi M, Mousavi MJ, Jamalzehi S, et al. Strategies toward rheumatoid arthritis therapy; the old and the new. *J Cell Physiol.* 2019;234(7): 10018–10031.

90. Allott K, Wood SJ, Yuen HP, et al. Longitudinal cognitive performance in individuals at ultrahigh risk for psychosis: a 10-year follow-up. *Schizophr Bull.* 2019;45(5):1101–1111.

91. Tiihonen J, Haukka J, Taylor M, et al. A nationwide cohort study of oral and depot antipsychotics after first hospitalization for schizophrenia. *Am J Psychiatry.* 2011;168(6):603–609.

92. Tiihonen J, Mittendorfer-Rutz E, Majak M, et al. Real-world effectiveness of antipsychotic treatments in a nationwide cohort of 29 823 patients with schizophrenia. *JAMA Psychiatry.* 2017;**74**(7):686–693.

93. Glancy G, Choptiany M, Jones R, Chatterjee S. Measurement-based care in forensic psychiatry. *Int J Law Psychiatry.* 2021;**74**:101650.

94. Kennedy HG, Simpson A, Haque Q. Perspective on excellence in forensic mental health services: what we can learn from oncology and other medical services. *Front Psychiatry.* 2019;**10**:733.

95. Kennedy HG, Mohan D, Davoren M. Forensic psychiatry and Covid-19: accelerating transformation in forensic psychiatry. *Ir J Psychol Med.* 2020: 1–26.

96. Sørensen LU, Pedersen ML, Brandt-Christensen M, Kennedy HG. *Excellence Networks in Denmark.* 2020. University Library of Southern Denmark SDU https://portal.findresearcher.sdu.dk/en/publications/excellence-networks-in-denmark

97. McLaughlin P, Brady P, Carabellese F, et al. Excellence in forensic psychiatry services: international survey of qualities and correlates. *BJPsych Open.* 2023;**9**(6):e193.

98. Benjamin O, Goyal A, Lappin S. Disease-modifying antirheumatic drugs (DMARD) [Updated 2023 Jul 3]. StatPearls [Internet]. 2023.

99. Ludvigsson JF, Håberg SE, Knudsen GP, et al. Ethical aspects of registry-based research in the Nordic countries. *Clin Epidemiol.* 2015; **7**:491–508.

100. Andreassen OA. eHealth provides a novel opportunity to exploit the advantages of the Nordic countries in psychiatric genetic research,building on the public health care system, biobanks, and registries. *Am J Med Genet B Neuropsychiatr Genet.* 2018;**177**(7):625–629.

101. Petersen C, Boyd AD. Precision medicine and the ethics of electronic health records and genomics. *Comprehensive Precision Medicine* 2024;**2**: 334–350.

102. Arendt H. *The Human Condition.* 2nd ed. Chicago: University of Chicago Press; 2018.

103. Runciman D. *Confronting Leviathan.* London: Profile Books Ltd; 2021: 288.

104. Arendt H. *On Violence.* Harvest Books; 1970: 106.

105. Schrodinger E. *Nature and the Greeks and Science and Humanism.* Cambridge: Cambridge University Press; 2014:184.

106. Rozin P, Lowery L, Imada S, Haidt J. The CAD triad hypothesis: a mapping between three moral emotions (contempt, anger, disgust) and three moral codes (community, autonomy, divinity). *J Pers Soc Psychol.* 1999;**76**(4):574.

Advance Directives in Patients with Schizophrenia

Jacob M. Appel

Introduction

The second half of the twentieth century witnessed a "seismic shift towards autonomy in medical ethics" that transformed clinical care and physician–patient relationships.[1] A widespread consensus emerged in the United States by the late 1970s that patients with decisional capacity should be meaningfully informed about their illnesses and therapeutic options and should possess the authority to manage their own treatment. These principles were notably reflected in the *Belmont Report* (1978), Beauchamp and Childress's seminal text, *Principles of Biomedical Ethics* (1979), and Dennis Novack's survey of changing physician attitudes toward divulging patients' cancer diagnoses (1979).[2] In contemporary allopathic medicine, empowering capable patients to guide their own treatment has become the nearly universally accepted standard of care. Over the past 50 years, legal mechanisms have also been established to protect the autonomy of patients who have lost decisional capacity. Most notably, advance directive (AD) statutes in all 50 states have enabled capable patients to specify their medical choices for potential times of future incapacitation.[3] The Patient Self-Determination Act of 1990 compels health care institutions to inform patients about ADs and document their preferences.[1] The decisions outlined in such documents are generally binding. Patients may specify particular choices through living wills and/or appoint agents, sometimes termed health care proxies or health care powers of attorney, to effectuate their preferences during incapacitation. One of the principal goals of such advance directives is to maximize the autonomy of patients by ensuring that, even when they are incapacitated, their care remains consistent with their underlying values and preferences.[4]

For a range of reasons – some artefactual, some logistical, some reflective of a higher concern for safeguarding the rights of individuals with mental illnesses – patients in many jurisdictions have historically not been able to guide their future psychiatric treatment in the same manner as their general medical care. Psychiatric advance directives (PADs), or "psychiatric wills," proposed in the early 1980s by Thomas Szasz and others, sought to apply the general principles of ADs to patients with psychosis.[5] Szasz, a leading and controversial critic of nonconsensual psychiatric treatment, even believed that the "use of psychiatric wills might thus put an end to the dispute about involuntary psychiatric interventions."[6] In practice, although a significant number of states now have statutes authorizing PADs, and Centers for Medicare & Medicaid Services' rules from 2006 require participating hospitals to "comply with these directive," extraordinarily broad exceptions significantly limit their applicability and utility.[7] Sociologist Jeffrey W. Swanson and colleagues have noted that current PAD statutes "give doctors wide discretion to ignore them" by allowing patients' preferences to be overridden without fear of liability in cases where their choices differ from the accepted standard of care.[8] At the same time, considerable evidence (discussed below) suggests that PADs remain a largely untapped mechanism for addressing the distinctive needs of patients with schizophrenia and other severe disorders of thought. At a minimum, their increased use may prove helpful in distinguishing patients whose psychosis clouds their judgment with regard to treatment choices from those – likely a much smaller number – who possess a sincere and authentic objection to certain forms of life-preserving care. PADs also hold out the promise of empowering individuals with schizophrenia to feel invested in their own medical treatments and to increase their sense of agency with regard to their relationships with physicians and the health care system. What follows is a discussion of the legal, evidentiary, and ethical issues that arise in the use of PADs in individuals with schizophrenia.

Legal background

The terminology on the subject of PADs is evolving and often still lacks consistency. Elizabeth Gallagher offers a useful definition of a PAD, also known as a "psychiatric advance statement" in the United Kingdom, as a document that "sets forth a person's wishes concerning psychiatric treatment in anticipation of the event that he or she may later become incompetent to make informed health care decisions."[9] One form of PAD is a Ulysses contract, described by Ryan Spellecy as a document that "enable[s] persons to commit themselves now to a particular course of treatment at a future time if they suspect they will not be willing or able to follow that course of treatment at that future time."[10] Similarly, Claire Henderson and colleagues define Ulysses contacts as forms of PADs that "request that care or treatment be given during a future period of incapacity, even over the possible later objection or resistance of the person during a crisis."[11] The concept takes its name from an episode in the Homeric epic, *The Odyssey*, in which the title character, Odysseus (Latin: Ulysses) seeks to hear the music of humanlike creatures, Sirens, whose mellifluous songs lure sailors to their deaths. To prevent such a fate, Odysseus orders his sailors to bind him to the mast of his ship, to place beeswax in their own ears, and to ignore his entreaties to release him until the ship has passed the Sirens' shores – allowing him to enjoy their melodies free from peril. The purpose of Ulysses contracts is to prevent succumbing to what the Ancient Greeks called "Akrasia" or so-called "weakness of the will," which, in the case of PADs, refers to current preferences that undermine earlier, supposedly more authentic ones.[12] The following discussion will follow the definitions used by Gallagher, Spellecy, and Henderson.

American law has historically proven highly unsympathetic to Ulysses contracts. The first known effort to authorize such an agreement in the United States appears to be New York State legislation from 1857 that allowed alcohol use disorder patients to commit themselves voluntarily for 1 year to the New York State Inebriate Asylum. When patient Walter Baker sought to depart before completing this previously approved term, and the facility objected, the New York State Supreme Court ordered him released.[2] Similarly, in *Ex Parte Lloyd*, a federal district court in Kentucky adopted a constricted view of the Narcotic Farms Act of 1929, also known as the Porter Act, which on the surface seemed to allow substance users to voluntarily enroll themselves in treatment irrevocably. Emery Lloyd, who had agreed to such terms, later asked to be discharged, and the court conceded that he had a constitutional right to be released.[3] As a general rule, courts until recently viewed Ulysses contracts through the negative lens of contracts for self-enslavement or involuntary servitude and proved unsympathetic.

After Szasz raised the possibility of a "psychiatric will" in 1982, Timothy Howell, Ron Diamond, and Dan Wilder attempted to operationalize PADs with a proposed form.[13] Starting with Minnesota in 1991 and Hawaii in 1992, states began to enact statutes that authorized PADs.[14] Yet these statutes were largely designed to allow patients to *agree to* future treatment, not to *reject* future treatment. They arose after a series of court cases from the 1960s through the 1980s that required judicial review before the administration of neuroleptics or ECT to psychiatric patients, delaying care and increasing the administrative burden upon providers, even in situations in which patients did not object to such treatments but only lacked capacity to offer consent. For instance, the "Minnesota advance psychiatric directive statute allows patients to give advance consent to intrusive mental health treatments," but if the patient refuses such interventions, "Minnesota courts... require... the usual hearings for the forced administration of intrusive mental health treatments."[15] That approach has been adopted widely by states that have formally authorized PADs, effectively limiting the scope to Ulysses contracts (i.e., documents that authorize, rather than reject, future care.) Patients can bind themselves to future treatment but cannot reject interventions consistent with the standard of care; rather, in the latter circumstances, they are subject to the underlying laws of their states. For example, New Jersey's PAD statute is binding except in cases in which honoring the directive would "violate the accepted standard of mental health care or treatment under the circumstances of the patient's mental health condition," "violate a court order or provision of statutory law," or "endanger the life or health of the patient or another person."[4] Similarly, Illinois's PAD statute, the Mental Health Treatment Preference Declaration Act of 1996, contains the caveat that a "declaration does not limit any authority... either to take a person into custody or to admit, retain, or treat a person in a health care facility."[5] These statutes, with their broad exceptions, are highly representative of state PAD laws.[16] Any role they serve in limiting unwanted care likely occurs indirectly, as judges are permitted, albeit not required, to review such documents to guide their decision-making regarding requests for care refusal.

A seminal federal court case, *Hargrave v. Vermont* (2002), called these statutory limits on PADs into question.[6] That case involved Nancy Hargrave, a woman with a diagnosis of paranoid schizophrenia, who executed a durable power of attorney for health care ("DPOA") in 1999 in which she stated that she did not wish to receive "any and all anti-psychotic, neuroleptic, psychotropic or psychoactive medications" in the future.[7] Of note, no available evidence indicated that she lacked capacity to effectuate this document, essentially a PAD, at that time. Her attorneys then sought a court order to prevent any future treatment contrary to this directive. In doing so, they argued that Vermont's existing PAD statute, Act 114, violated Title II of the Americans with Disabilities Act of 1990. Both the federal district court for Vermont and the Second Circuit Court of Appeals, whose jurisdiction covers the states of Connecticut, New York, and Vermont, agreed – in essence, enabling the enforcement of treatment-rejecting PADs within the state's boundaries.[8,9] As Paul Appelbaum explained, "*Hargrave*, then, stands for the proposition that the state, having established a statutory basis for medical advance directives, cannot exclude involuntarily committed psychiatric patients from its coverage."[17] Appelbaum warned that the ruling might "chill enthusiasm for psychiatric advance directives among many clinicians" and that *Hargrave*'s legacy may be to inhibit the use of this once-promising tool."[18] In contrast, Michael Allen of the Bazelon Center hoped *Hargrave* might prove a "fresh beginning" that would lead to increased "trust building, peer support, talk therapy, and other naturalistic supports" in the patient–psychiatrist relationship and a path for "people with psychiatric disabilities [to] achieve long-term recovery and greater satisfaction with their quality of life."[19]

In practice, *Hargrave* has not led to meaningful change. That may be, in part, as some claim, because "[a]t a practical level it is most unlikely that many patients who are involuntarily hospitalized ... have the knowledge or the resources or the motivation to execute such a will."[20] However, one must note that providers and institutions have the ability to provide this knowledge and these resources to patients; data

(discussed below) suggests that the motivation already exists but merely remains untapped. At the same time, the ruling has not led to similar cases in other American jurisdictions, nor has the legal landscape evolved significantly on the subject. More than two decades after Nancy Hargrave's lawsuit, PADs remain underutilized and subject to extensive caveats in most states, restrictions that render both their utility and their appeal to patients extremely limited. In short, the potential of PADs to improve the lives of individuals with schizophrenia remains largely untested.

Evidence base

Despite their limited implementation to date, the evidence supporting the value of PADs is increasing.[21] A systematic review and meta-analyses conducted by Emma Molyneaux and colleagues reported that PADs can reduce such involuntary commitments by 25%.[22] Similarly, another meta-analysis by de Jong et al. found "advance statements," which included PADs and crisis plans, to reduce involuntary commitments by 23% – more effective than community treatment orders.[23] The expanded use of PADs outside the United States affords a valuable source of data in this regard.[24] For instance, a multicenter French study led by Aurélie Tinland found that among patients with schizophrenia, schizoaffective disorder, and bipolar I disorder, PADs facilitated by peer workers led to "significantly fewer compulsory admission."[25] Beyond evidence for efficacy, PADs remain highly popular among stakeholders. An analysis by Scholten et al., using "comparisons between the empirical findings... using a structured expert consensus process, found that stakeholders from three European nations expressed meaningful support for the use of PADs and Ulysses contracts in particular.[26] They reported that "stake-holders did not confirm the fundamental ethical and legal concerns raised by ethicists and legal scholars" and voiced few or no worries about an increase of coercion or the invalidity of SBDs due to a lack of identity between past and present self or outdated consent."[27]

Joint crisis plans, advance directives negotiated by patients and providers that share many attributes of PADs, have shown promise in enhancing the physician–patient relationship in the United Kingdom, France, and Germany.[28-31] Benefits of PADs have also been recorded in low resource settings, such as the Indian state of Tamil Nadu.[32] Moreover, broader research on the value of enhanced autonomy for psychiatric patients in treatment outcomes is robust. As noted by Debra S. Srebnik and John Q. La Fond, "research suggests that having choice and control over important life decisions, such as the selection of treatment or housing, is critical to physical and psychological well-being."[33] In contrast, fear of coercion and pressure to relinquish autonomy have been shown to reduce engagement with care among patients with schizophrenia.[34]

The strongest data supporting PADs in the United States derives from the extensive work of Swanson at Duke University. In a large study of 147 PAD completers versus 92 non-completers, with follow-ups at 6 months, 1 year and 2 years, Swanson's team found that PADs were "significantly associated with fewer coercive crisis interventions" and cut in half the odds of coercive acts such as "transport by police for mental health evaluation, use of handcuffs during transport, involuntary commitment, use of locked seclusion, use of physical restraints in the hospital, and forced medication."[35] Michelle Easter, working with Swanson and colleagues, reported the benefits of using PADs with Assertive Community Treatment teams in the United States as well.[36] Assuming that reductions in coercive interventions are desirable – and no evidence to date suggests a concomitant increase in suicides, violence, or other negative outcomes that might have justified such interventions – this data strongly supports incorporating PADs into routine clinical practice.[37]

Patients with psychiatric illnesses across diverse populations are highly open to the prospect of effectuating PADs.[38,39] For instance, a study of five groups of stakeholders (including clinicians, administrators, patients, family members, and mental health advocates) in the state of Virginia found that more than 90% agreed with the statement that "[a]dvance directives that include mental health care will give people with serious mental health problems more control over their lives" and similar percentages believed that PADs "will lead to a better understanding by providers of what consumers want for treatment in both crisis ... and outpatient settings..., and to an improved quality of life for consumers."[40] In fact, a meta-analysis conducted by Esther Braun et al. found that while [e]mpirical evidence suggests that PAD completion rates remain very low... [u]sers of mental health services are highly interested in PADs and regard them as tools to improve their involvement in care."[41] She also reported that such consumers "generally prefer legally binding PADs that can be revoked only when users are competent to consent."[42] Similarly, Marcus Sellars has observed that while "the majority of patients support PADs and would want the opportunity to complete one" and although "family members and clinicians [are] generally... supportive of PADs," nonetheless "the majority of patients in jurisdictions with the relevant legislation do not complete one."[43] This striking disconnect between preference and practice calls not only for a systemic review of the barriers creating this divide but also innovative thinking to explore how PADs might prove most helpful to patients with severe disorders of thought such as schizophrenia.

A potential path forward

A range of explanations has been offered for the low rates at which PADs are utilized.[44] These reported barriers include, among others, fear of liability on the part of providers and lack of knowledge on the part of patients.[45,46] Yet two key related factors that likely play a significant role in the underuse of PADs are providers' fears of so-called "complete treatment refusals" and patients' lack of trust that their PADs will be honored.[47] Clinicians may worry that patients with limited insight will attempt to execute PADs that decline *all* care – although empirical evidence suggests that is not actually the case.[48] At the same time, a review by Laura Shields and colleagues of 30 studies from a range of countries found that patients are "apprehensive to tell their doctor they have a PAD" and that they suspect "even mentioning the existence of a PAD" might lead to "a negative response from the doctor or involuntary treatment during future hospitalizations."[49] The majority of patients believe their preferences will be ignored or overruled.[50] State statutes that do not permit individuals with mental illnesses to opt out of the standard of care or that constrain the legal authority of PADs are unlikely to reassure psychiatric patients in this regard. In short, patients – whether informed or unwittingly, based upon general suspicions – are accurately responding to the state of the current legal landscape.

This outcome is not inevitable. The ability to accept or reject the standard of care, or even life-preserving interventions, need not be an all-or-nothing proposition. Instead, offering individuals with psychiatric illnesses the ability to generate nuanced and even conditional PADs is worth exploration. PADs offer an untapped tool that might benefit patients with schizophrenia in meaningful ways. In the case of Nancy Hargrave, she created such a nuanced PAD, in effect binding herself to long-term hospitalization rather than psychiatric medication. Her choice, one must emphasize, might have proven inconvenient for the state and consumed resources, but it did not place her life or the lives of others in direct jeopardy. (Needless to say, funds expended upon Hargrave's long-term institutionalization are funds not spent on the care of others, but whether long-term hospitalization is actually more expensive than the revolving door of treatment-and-release that many patients with schizophrenia endure, even ignoring its existential implications, remains entirely unclear.) Within the context of the resources and options available to her, Hargrave was able to ensure a safe and reasonable outcome more consistent with her own values than the alternative proposed by the state.

Psychiatrists and patients, working together to complete such documents, should they prove binding, might actually increase mutual trust and also drive systemic change. If even a fraction of the 122,000 street homeless individuals in the United States created such a conditional PAD, and these PADs proved binding, one imagines supportive services and scatter-site housing opportunities might expand quickly.[51]

Ethical considerations

Many ethical challenges that apply to PADs, such as the phenomenon of "bargaining down" and the question of whether the individual who creates an AD is truly the same person subject to one after loss of capacity, apply to all ADs.[52] For instance, Rebecca Dresser has criticized Ulysses contracts as a form of "selfpaternalism."[53] A systemic review of 50 articles by Stephenson et al. found concern that Ulysses contracts in particular might "be intended as a tool to increase service user autonomy," but "would ultimately diminish autonomy" and reported arguments that PADs should be "void and non-enforceable" because patients "would forfeit the very liberty that underlies the validity of the document[s]."[54] Yet, as noted above, this finding is inconsistent with patients' own reported concerns.[55] These are important issues, but they have been addressed extensively elsewhere in the literature and are beyond the scope of this paper.[56] However, the issue of concerns regarding complete opt-out is unique to behavioral health and requires further consideration.

The debate surrounding PADs too often conceptualized the options as binary: either a patient will accept care or they will refuse *all* treatments. This framing ignores the prospect for considerable space between these two extremes. In fact, evidence shows that many patients view PADs as a mechanism for steering care rather than rejecting it. Although many providers express concerns that fully enforceable PADs will lead large numbers of patients with severe mental illness to forgo all psychiatric care, existing evidence does not support this apprehension.[57] A meta-analysis by Anne-Sophie Gaillard et al. found that complete care refusals are rare: for instance, across 42 studies, only 0.3% of participants "used their PAD to refuse hospital admission under any circumstance." Rather, respondents often specified particular interventions they did not want (e.g., "group-based therapy") or noted limits to when certain interventions were acceptable to them (e.g., ECT only "[w] hen I have suicidal thoughts").[58] The fear that large numbers of patients will executive blank refusals is, quite frankly, counterintuitive. Patients executing PADs must meet established decisional capacity standards to do so. These are governed by statute in the vast majority of states.[59] The number of individuals who meet such capacity standards and wish to make choices that endanger others at the expense of care is likely to be exceedingly small; in addition, since this is volitional behavior in the setting of capacity, such acts – like any other volitional, clear-minded acts of violence – should be matters for the criminal justice system, not behavioral health providers. Similarly, the number of individuals who meet capacity standards and still wish to accept significant risks to their own safety, even when offered effective care, is also likely to be minute. Such unusual cases may involve patients with extensive histories of existential suffering due to severe mental illness who, in periods of full stabilization, make an informed choice not to endure such suffering in the future.[60] Anyone who works closely with patients with schizophrenia recognizes that such cases are likely to be rare outliers; fears of such complete care refusals by capacitated patients should not stand in the way of using PADs to assist and empower the vast majority of patients with schizophrenia or other severe psychiatric conditions. Moreover, since PADs in the United States operate so that the default is full care – unless a patient has executed a PAD to opt out – the risk of widespread opt-out, especially by those most in need of treatment, is minimized even further.

Patients with schizophrenia, when they are stabilized and possess relevant decisional capacity, do not want to reject all care. Rather, what they want is *effective* care. Or care different from, but not inherently worse, than what has previously been offered to them. As important, they want this care in the context of a social safety network that ensures their other basic needs – food, shelter, emotional support – are met. PADs offer patients an opportunity to collaborate with providers to spell out conditions for care that are consistent with basic human dignity and well-being. Achieving buy-in may require that states honor PADs to the same extent that they honor other medical advance directives, through which patients with capacity are able to reject unwanted future care – even at the expense of their own safety or criminal sanction. Yet the tradeoff may actually prove to be many lives saved and even more lives improved, as the trust engendered by such collaboration toward PADs will lead increasing numbers of patients with schizophrenia to receive care that is more consistent with their own underlying values and preferences.

Conclusions

In light of the empirical evidence favoring PADs discussed above, a strong argument exists for following the lead of the Second Circuit Court of Appeals and giving binding effect to PADs – both Ulysses contracts and those that reject various forms of future care. Such legal validity would likely result in many psychiatrists discussing PADs with their patients and even facilitating their completion; beyond the specific benefits of the future guidance offered by these PADs in upholding patients' autonomy and underlying values, such discussions are likely to improve the therapeutic relationship, patient engagement with care, and overall trust between patients with schizophrenia and the mental health care system. Providers may gain a better understanding of their patients' needs and concerns, while patients themselves may feel heard and empowered.

The embrace of unrestricted PADs is bound to prove controversial. Some critics may even view such an approach as a gamble. As with any other significant reform, changes should be piloted with small populations of patients and studied carefully before being enacted on a larger scale. After all, no policy's efficacy can ever be guaranteed prior to its implementation. However, based upon extensive existing evidence, the risks from such an intervention appear to be relatively low. In contrast, with 122,000 undomiciled individuals with schizophrenia and other severe psychiatric illnesses living on American streets, the current system is clearly not serving the interests or protecting the welfare of this vulnerable population. Unrestricted PADs offer the prospect for systemic change – and such change is long overdue.

References

1. Saad TC. The history of autonomy in medicine from antiquity to principlism. *Med Health Care Philos.* 2018;**21**(1):125–137.

2. Novack DH, Plumer R, Smith RL, et al. Changes in physicians' attitudes toward telling the cancer patient. *JAMA.* 1979;**241**(9):897–900.

3. Olick RS. Defining features of advance directives in law and clinical practice. *Chest.* 2012;**141**(1):232–238.

4. Appel JM. A values-based approach to capacity assessment. *J Leg Med.* 2022;**42**(1–2):53–65.

5. Szasz T. The psychiatric will: a new mechanism for protecting persons against "psychosis" and psychiatry. *Am Psychologist.* 1982;**37**:762–770.

6. Szasz T. The psychiatric will: a new mechanism for protecting persons against "psychosis" and psychiatry. *Am Psychologist.* 1982;**37**:762–770.

7. Federal Register. 2006;**71**(236).

8. Swanson JW, McCrary SV, Swartz MS, Elbogen EB, Van Dorn RA. Superseding psychiatric advance directives: ethical and legal considerations. *J Am Acad Psychiatry Law.* 2006;**34**(3):385–394.

9. Gallagher EM. Advance directives for psychiatric care: a theoretical and practical overview for legal professionals. *Psychol Pub Policy Law,* 1998;**4**:746.

10. Spellecy R. Reviving Ulysses contracts. *Kennedy Inst Ethics J.* 2003;**13**(4):373–392.

11. Henderson C, Swanson JW, Szmukler G, et al. A typology of advance statements in mental health care. *Psychiatr Ser.* 2008;**59**(1):63–71.

12. Brenna CTA, Chen SS, Cho M, McCoy LG, Das S. Steering clear of Akrasia: an integrative review of self-binding Ulysses contracts in clinical practice. *Bioethics.* 2023;**37**(7):690–714.

13. Howell T, Diamond R, Wilder D. Is there a case for voluntary commitment? In: Beauchamp T, Walters L, eds. *Contemporary Issues in Bioethics,* 2nd ed.; 1982.

14. Miller RD. Advance directives for psychiatric treatment: a view from the trenches. *Psychol Public Policy Law.* 1998;4(3):728–745.

15. Cuca R. Ulysses in Minnesota: first steps toward a self-binding psychiatric advance directive statute. *Cornell L Rev.* 1993;73:1152.

16. National Resource Center on Psychiatric Advance Directives. Available from: https://nrc-pad.org/states/ (April 10, 2024) PAD-NRC, North Carolina.

17. Appelbaum PS. Advance directives for psychiatric treatment. *Hosp Community Psychiatr.* 1991;**42**:983–984.

18. Appelbaum PS. Advance directives for psychiatric treatment. *Hosp Community Psychiatr.* 1991;**42**:983–984.

19. Allen M, Hargrave V. Vermont and the quality of care. *Psychiatr Serv.* 2004; **55**(9):1067.

20. Chodoff P, Peele R. The psychiatric will of Dr. Szasz. *Hastings Cent Rep.* 1983;**13**(2):11–13.

21. Murray H, Wortzel HS. Psychiatric advance directives: origins, benefits, challenges, and future directions. *J Psychiatr Pract.* 2019;**25**(4):303–307.

22. Molyneaux E, Turner A, Candy B, et al. Crisis-planning interventions for people with psychotic illness or bipolar disorder: systematic review and meta-analyses. *BJPsych Open.* 2019;**5**(4):e53.

23. De Jong MH, Kamperman AM, Oorschot M, et al. Interventions to reduce compulsory psychiatric admissions: a systematic review and meta-analysis. *JAMA Psychiatr.* 2016;**73**(7):657.

24. Scholten M, Gieselmann A, Gather J, Vollmann J. Psychiatric advance directives under the convention on the rights of persons with disabilities: why advance instructions should be able to override current preferences. *Front Psychiatr.* 2019;**10**:631.

25. Tinland A, Loubière S, Mougeot F, et al. Effect of psychiatric advance directives facilitated by peer workers on compulsory admission among people with mental illness: a randomized clinical trial. *JAMA Psychiatr.* 2022;**79**(8):752–759.

26. Scholten M, Efkemann SA, Faissner M, et al. Opportunities and challenges of self-binding directives: A comparison of empirical research with stakeholders in three European countries. *Eur Psychiatr.* 2023;**66**(1):e48.

27. Scholten M, Efkemann SA, Faissner M, et al. Opportunities and challenges of self-binding directives: A comparison of empirical research with stakeholders in three European countries. *Eur Psychiatr.* 2023;**66** (1):e48.

28. Szmukler G, Dawson J. Commentary: toward resolving some dilemmas concerning psychiatric advance directives. *J Am Acad Psychiatr Law.* 2006;**34**(3):398–401.

29. Henderson C, Flood C, Leese M, et al. Effect of joint crisis plans on use of compulsory treatment in psychiatry: single blind randomised controlled trial. *BMJ.* 2004;**329**:136.

30. Lequin P, Ferrari P, Suter C, et al. The joint crisis plan: a powerful tool to promote mental health. *Front Psychiatr.* 2021;**12**:621436.

31. Rixe J, Neumann E, Möller J, et al. Joint crisis plans and crisis cards in inpatient psychiatric treatment: a multicenter randomized controlled trial. *Deutsches Ärzteblatt Int.* 2023;**120**:125–132.

32. Shields LS, Pathare S, van Zelst SD, et al. Unpacking the psychiatric advance directive in low-resource settings: an exploratory qualitative study in Tamil Nadu, India. *Int J Ment Health Syst.* 2013;**7**(1):29.

33. Srebnik DS, La Fond JQ. Advance directives for mental health treatment. *Psychiatr Serv.* 1999;**50**(7):919–925.

34. Swartz MS, Swanson JW, Hannon MJ. Does fear of coercion keep people away from mental health treatment? Evidence from a survey of persons with schizophrenia and mental health professionals. *Behav Sci Law.* 2003;**21**(4):459–72.

35. Swanson JW, Swartz MS, Elbogen EB, et al. Psychiatric advance directives and reduction of coercive crisis interventions. *J Ment Health.* 2008;**17**(3):255–267.

36. Easter MM, Swanson JW, Robertson AG, Moser LL, Swartz MS. Impact of psychiatric advance directive facilitation on mental health consumers: empowerment, treatment attitudes and the role of peer support specialists. *J Ment Health.* 2021;**30**(5):585–593.

37. Srebnik DS, Russo J. Consistency of psychiatric crisis care with advance directive instructions. *Psychiatr Serv.* 2007;**58**:1157–1163.

38. Van Dorn RA, Swanson JW, Swartz MS. Preferences for psychiatric advance directives among Latinos: views on advance care planning for mental health. *Psychiatr Serv.* 2009;**60**(10):1383–1385.

39. Hotzy F, Cattapan K, Orosz A, et al. Acceptance of psychiatric and somatic advance directives: a comparison in psychiatric patients and professionals. *Psychiatr Prax.* 2020;**47**(6):319–325.

40. Wilder CM, Swanson JW, Bonnie RJ, et al. A survey of stakeholder knowledge, experience, and opinions of advance directives for mental health in Virginia. *Adm Policy Ment Health.* 2013;**40**(3):232–239.

41. Braun E, Gaillard AS, Vollmann J, Gather J, Scholten M. Mental health service users' perspectives on psychiatric advance directives: a systematic review. *Psychiatr Serv.* 2023;**74**(4):381–392.

42. Braun E, Gaillard AS, Vollmann J, Gather J, Scholten M. Mental health service users' perspectives on psychiatric advance directives: a systematic review. *Psychiatr Serv.* 2023;74(4):381–392.

43. Sellars M, Fullam R, O'Leary C, et al. Australian psychiatrists' support for psychiatric advance directives: responses to a hypothetical vignette. *Psychiatr Psychol Law.* 2016;24(1):61–73.

44. Shields LS, Pathare S, van der Ham AJ, Bunders J. A review of barriers to using psychiatric advance directives in clinical practice. *Adm Policy Ment Health.* 2014;41(6):753–766.

45. Shields LS, Pathare S, van der Ham AJ, Bunders J. A review of barriers to using psychiatric advance directives in clinical practice. *Adm Policy Ment Health.* 2014;41(6):753–766.

46. Backlar P, McFarland BH. A survey on the use of advance directives for mental health treatment in Oregon. *Psychiatr Serv.* 1996;47:1387–1389.

47. Shields LS, Pathare S, van der Ham AJ, Bunders J. A review of barriers to using psychiatric advance directives in clinical practice. *Adm Policy Ment Health.* 2014;41(6):753–766.

48. Backlar P, McFarland BH, Swanson JW, Mahler J. Consumer, provider, and informal caregiver opinions on psychiatric advance directives. *Adm Policy Ment Health.* 2001;28(6):427–441.

49. Shields LS, Pathare S, van der Ham AJ, Bunders J. A review of barriers to using psychiatric advance directives in clinical practice. *Adm Policy Ment Health.* 2014;41(6):753–766.

50. Srebnik, DS, Russo J. Use of psychiatric advance directives during psychiatric crisis events. *Adm Policy Ment Health.* 2008;35(4):272–282.

51. Cobern J, Westman N. Number of homeless people with mental illness increased slightly in recent years, but experts say they are more visible: analysis. Available from: https://abcnews.go.com/Health/amount-homeless-people-mental-illness-increased-slightly-recent/story?id=103751677 (April 1, 2024).

52. Appel JM. Decisional capacity after dark: is autonomy delayed truly autonomy denied? *Camb Q Healthc Ethics.* 2023;33:260–266.

53. Dresser RS. Ulysses and the psychiatrists: a legal and policy analysis of the voluntary commitment contract. *Harv Civ Rights Civil Lib Law Rev.* 1982;16(3):777–854.

54. Stephenson L, Gieselmann A, Gergel T, et al. Self-binding directives in psychiatric practice: a systematic review of reasons. *Lancet Psychiatry.* 2023;10(11):887–895.

55. Scholten M, Efkemann SA, Faissner M, et al. Opportunities and challenges of self-binding directives: a comparison of empirical research with stakeholders in three European countries. *Eur Psychiatry.* 2023;66(1):e48.

56. Mitchell M. An analysis of common arguments against advance directives. *Nurs Ethics.* 2012;19(2):245–251.

57. Appelbaum PS. Advance directives for psychiatric treatment. *Hosp Community Psychiatr.* 1991;42:983–984.

58. Gaillard AS, Braun E, Vollmann J, et al. The content of psychiatric advance directives: a systematic review. *Psychiatr Serv.* 2023;74:44–55.

59. Appel JM. The statutory codification of decisional capacity standards. *J Am Acad Psychiatry Law.* 2023;51(4):506–519.

60. Appel JM. A suicide right for the mentally ill? a Swiss case opens a new debate. *Hastings Cent Rep.* 2007;37(3):21–23.

Dignity Restored
The Power of Treatment First

Jhilam Biswas

"I couldn't tell where my body ended and the world began. Voices were speaking to me from the television, telling me I was doomed."

In *The Quiet Room: A Journey Out of the Torment of Madness*, Lori Schiller, who lives with a diagnosis of Schizoaffective Disorder, vividly recounts her intense struggles with psychosis. Schiller's narrative provides profound insight into the unsettling and often terrifying world caused by this condition, characterized by feelings of isolation and being inundated with fear and distressing delusions.[1] Psychosis, far from harmless, carries a significant burden of trauma, evidenced by the tragically high suicide rates among individuals diagnosed with diseases associated with psychosis. The battle with intrusive perceptual disturbances and paranoia presents a relentless test of human endurance, and this painful state requires alleviation through many modalities and, importantly, medical treatment.

The symptom of anosognosia, or lack of insight and awareness of the disease, can make it challenging to provide care as the patient is not aware they are ill. This symptom is a common symptom of schizophrenia, and this lack of insight often results in stopping and starting medications, frequent hospitalizations, chronic illness, and increasing risk of homelessness and incarceration.[2] Without a thorough and data-driven assessment of the patient, psychiatric providers may misdiagnose anosognosia symptoms as an ambivalence to care. Some researchers think that the psychoanalytic ideas of denial and defense mechanisms, which historically have played a prominent role in psychiatric education, may make it harder for clinicians to spot anosognosia correctly[3] as it could be misconstrued as defensiveness. Beyond clinical observation, recent brain imaging studies linking cognitive awareness problems in the neurocircuitry of the brain to mental illness,[4,5] as well as blood gene expression biomarkers,[6] have also led to supporting evidence of anosognosia in schizophrenia. These studies are explained in more detail elsewhere in this book.

This chapter explores the challenges of delivering timely psychiatric treatment and its vital role in restoring health and dignity in individuals with serious mental illness. The piece examines potential pitfalls in international organizations' training materials that label certain psychiatric interventions as human rights violations. A case study from a state in the United States demonstrates how rights-based legal models in psychiatric care that adhere to similar ideas illustrated in the international training materials have increased access barriers to care and increased adverse events to both patients and health care staff.

The chapter discusses how compulsory yet necessary psychiatric interventions when used appropriately and administered respectfully for patients with severe illnesses who have been determined to lack decision-making capacity, can improve well-being, restore a patient's dignity, and reduce caregiver fatigue and demoralization.[7] Failure to provide necessary psychiatric interventions due to stigma around psychiatric treatment raises serious ethical concerns about healthcare access, equity, and delivery.[8]

The global mental health policy landscape and the stance on intensive psychiatric interventions

Global perspectives on psychiatric care and treatment vary widely as many countries continue to navigate the complex socioeconomic challenges of providing care in varying legal contexts.[9] Although standardization is difficult to achieve globally, the United Nations Convention on the Rights of Persons with Disabilities (CRPD) and the World Health Organization (WHO) initiatives have articulated policies to integrate important human rights principles into global mental health. The organizations have advocated for equal and non-discriminatory practices, rights to informed consent, the right to rehabilitation and recovery, access to justice, the right to privacy, and participation in public life.[10] More recently, organizational efforts have led to the development of training modules that are aimed at reducing human rights violations in treating individuals with mental illnesses.

In 2019, the World Health Organization (WHO) QualityRights Initiative released training materials to guide improved mental health care.[11] These training modules cover several topics, such as patient-centered recovery, supportive communication, and de-escalation techniques, to reduce abuse and neglect in mental health practices. The training modules have many positive aspects and aim to reduce a variety of abuses that have been documented to occur in low-resourced settings that are attempting to provide mental health care.[12] However, the training module content does critique acute and necessary psychiatric interventions. The modules portray psychiatric providers and psychopharmacology in a stigmatizing manner by equating medically necessary interventions – which physicians and other providers use as part of evidence-based practice to restore health and well-being – with violence and abuse.

The initiative includes five core training modules focused on human rights, mental health, and human rights, legal capacity and the right to decide, recovery, and the right to health, as well as freedom from coercion, violence, and abuse. Specifically, in the materials for "Freedom from coercion, violence, and abuse," the training explicitly states that practices such as using involuntary medications in the inpatient unit, forced admissions to psychiatric units, and forced treatments in the community constitute "examples of violence and coercion."

While these training modules incorporate crucial safeguards to improve mental healthcare, they also introduce a paradox. The challenge lies in reconciling the QualityRights Initiative's advocacy for rehabilitation and recovery with its simultaneous classification of potentially necessary interventions, like brief involuntary treatments for recovery, as violations. This dichotomy highlights the ongoing debate within mental health care about balancing protective measures for autonomy with the clinical realities faced by medical professionals and caregivers in treating serious mental illness.[13]

In an editorial in the British Journal of Psychiatry, two physicians describe the negative portrayal of psychiatry and psychopharmacology in the WHO QualityRights training module, stating:

> Psychiatrists are mentioned at least 16 times, 13 of those references are negative. Practitioners are portrayed as unsympathetic, dismissive, and heavy-handed in prescribing medication. This is stigmatizing of the profession and could create a further barrier to individuals accessing healthcare.
>
> Similarly, psychotropic medication is represented in a highly negative light. There are multiple references to the adverse effects of medication; at least 14 references to medication were identified, none of which mentioned the advantages of pharmacological interventions. Psychotropics have the potential to dramatically improve the quality of an individual's life. Although they are associated with both risks and benefits, this is true of all medications. Their depiction in the training materials does not reflect their robust evidence base.[14]

Classifying essential psychiatric interventions in acute care settings as human rights violations is highly problematic. While global instances of misuse certainly need addressing, such classifications may impact health systems making evidence-based decisions and good-faith efforts to provide treatment. Medications are an essential part of the recovery from psychosis, mania, and other debilitating symptoms of mental illness. Stigmatizing these essential treatments and how they are administered as human rights violations risks undermining their legitimacy and effectiveness at restoring a person's dignity, right to healthcare, and freedom from a distressing emotional state.

There is a significant gap in international policy-making discussions concerning biological disease processes and the management of agitated psychosis and other severe conditions when they become unpredictable, dangerous, and resistant to treatment. This is particularly notable in the context of policies that criticize the use of involuntary neuroleptic treatment, and the ethics of its use require multilayered conversations with all stakeholders.[15,16]

One example of the excessive use of adversarial legal frameworks to protect the right to refuse treatment for severe and acute mental illness in one state in the United States is called the Rogers Guardianship Hearing. This court hearing, used in Massachusetts, adheres to the substituted judgment principles. The case law that led to this procedure and its aftermath illustrate the potential stigmatization of medication and the delays to treatment that can arise from solely relying on legal mechanisms to dictate already scarce medical care.

The Massachusetts experiment: The Rogers case decision and its impact

In 1970, the Massachusetts legislature established that admission to a psychiatric hospital did not necessarily equate to incompetence around treatment. This decision set the stage for the legal and ethical stance that a formal assessment of incompetence in medical decision-making is required before treatment can be administered against a patient's will to protect the patient's right to refuse medications. Massachusetts ended up with a complex process called the Rogers Guardianship, resulting from a series of legal battles that began in 1975 and culminated in a series of district, state, and Supreme Court decisions over eight years. Starting with the case named *Rogers* v. *Okin*, the final decision and following precedent were made in 1983 in a district court in the case called *Rogers* v. *Commissioner*,[17] *Rogers* v. *Okin*,[18] *Mills* v. *Rogers*,[19] *Rogers* v. *Commission of the Department of Mental Health*.[20]

This case became an important precedent and, in forensic psychiatry literature, represented the rights-driven model in state case law for psychiatric care. Notably, the Rogers case highlighted employing the substituted judgment approach over a best-interests model for decisions on necessary treatment for individuals suffering acute mental illness. This method asks a judge, rather than a doctor, to discern whether the patient, deemed incompetent, would agree to take antipsychotic medication if they could make medical decisions for themselves. This exercise introduced a paradoxical dilemma in psychiatric contexts: if incompetence is due to a mental condition that improves with medication, making the patient competent, then theoretically, the now-competent individual would not require the medication. Taken to its logical extreme, this would suggest that involuntary treatment could never be justified, irrespective of the apparent need.[21,22]

However, case law decisions made at the time of the Rogers ruling did not all reduce physicians' expertise to clinical testimony in scenarios involving compulsory treatment. The following cases represented case law in the treatment-driven model. In the 1982 case of *Youngberg* v. *Romeo*, the U.S. Supreme Court tackled the issue of rights for individuals with intellectual and developmental disabilities under state care. The case examined the patient's right to safe confinement conditions, protection from unnecessary bodily restraint, and access to sufficient medical care and habilitation. The Court emphasized that, in deciding what qualifies as "reasonable" care, courts must rely on the expertise and professional judgment of qualified specialists. Soon after, in the same year, in *Rennie* v. *Klein*, the Federal District Court of New Jersey acknowledged that decisions by independent psychiatrists regarding forced treatment should be respected, provided they stem from appropriate professional evaluation.

Given the Rogers statute, in Massachusetts, access to antipsychotic medications over objection requires the court to commit an individual to an inpatient treatment setting, which is followed by a psychiatrist's treatment petition to the court, called a "Rogers Treatment Plan (MGL Ch. 123 §8B)." This treatment petition awaits an adversarial hearing, and the patient remains in a locked setting until the hearing date. As background, the United States is a common-law country and uses the adversarial court system, where two lawyers represent their positions for the plaintiff and respondent in front of an impartial judge and/or jury. The treatment petition undergoes the same adversarial process as other matters would in the criminal courts. It is important to note that treatment cannot be administered if the patient and their counsel contest or dispute the commitment to the hospital. The treatment petition will be put on hold until the commitment status is determined, thereby denying access to care.

Since the Rogers case decision in Massachusetts, multiple studies have illustrated the costs, adverse events, and negative impact of delaying antipsychotic treatment for those suffering from acute illness while awaiting adversarial hearings.[23,24] The process of arranging and conducting this hearing takes time, often months while healing, stabilization, and recovery for the sickest patients stall. A study by Schouten and Gutheil published in the American Journal of Psychiatry highlighted the human and economic toll of postponing necessary psychiatric treatment to protect the right to refuse medications legally. The study looked at 2,216 Rogers Guardianship petitions that the Massachusetts Department of Mental Health had submitted for patient treatment over an 18-month period. The data showed that the court eventually approved 99.1% of them. Meanwhile, a burdensome and expensive process resulted in significant delays in administering this treatment to patients.[25] A study published in 2023 on the Rogers Guardianship also showed similar results and documented adverse medical events.

Data published from a strict security forensic hospital in Massachusetts revealed, on average, that it took 61 days, and often longer, to treat patients with medication for serious mental illness due to statute and court-related delays in the Rogers Guardianship pathway for forensic patients. Such a delay in care displayed serious consequences for a patient with a severe mental illness and criminal charges. The study showed that emergency restraints, as well as adverse events, like patient-on-patient assaults, staff assaults, self-harm behaviors, and acute psychotic symptoms like paranoia, persecutory delusions, and hallucinations, decreased significantly in forensic patients once they were finally able to get consistent treatment with a psychiatric treatment provider.[2] Of the guardianship petitions reviewed in Court, 99.2% were approved, thereby rendering the legal process that caused the treatment delays more of an obstacle than protecting patient decision-making autonomy.

Also, Massachusetts does not permit mandated court-ordered treatment or assisted outpatient treatment in the community, relying instead on Rogers Guardianships. In contrast, almost all other states in the United States allow for mandated court-ordered treatment, particularly for individuals connected to the criminal justice system. However, despite such laws, there is a significant shortage of clinical facilities that provide the necessary specialized services. This shortfall makes it challenging to meet the demand for care among these underserved populations.[26]

Timely psychiatric treatment improves healthcare equity and reduces healthcare staff burnout and demoralization

The postponement of care due to the Rogers Guardianship process illustrates the high price of solely protecting the autonomy of patients refusing medications who are suffering from severe mental illness.[27] This cost of delay in treatment not only exacerbates the worsening of the illness by preventing recovery but also increases disparities in healthcare access and increases the cycle of homelessness and incarceration among those who are most vulnerable and least able to bear such burdens. Studies show that mentally ill individuals are much more likely to interact with law enforcement.[28,29] Multiple factors contribute to the involvement of individuals with mental illness in the criminal justice system.[30] However, a significant factor is that their active illness is often undertreated or not treated at all, effectively criminalizing mental illness.[31–33]

Equitable care means being fair, inclusive, and timely around access while providing necessary care to patients. While it has been established that timely treatment brings important lifesaving benefits to the individual patient and allows them to live more independently in the community rather than in locked settings, it also promotes equity in under-resourced communities where larger populations of racial diversity stand to gain the most.[34–36] Certainly, arrest and incarceration should not be the entry point to long-term psychiatric care. Yet, if barriers to accessing care persist, the ongoing trend of doubly stigmatizing the mentally ill through criminal involvement will continue.[37] Criminalizing mental illness represents a subtle but serious human rights violation in the care of the mentally ill, especially when intensive psychiatric interventions, which the WHO QualityRights initiative currently labels as abuse, are too challenging to implement effectively and in a standard and well-resourced manner.

Timely psychiatric treatment for SMI in the community and shorter bursts in psychiatric units reduce the cycle of homelessness, crime, and incarceration, as well as the negative impacts of long-term institutionalization among those with chronically undertreated psychosis. Treatment in a monitored setting is also important, as these medications require psychiatric expertise to administer, and there should be options to titrate up, taper down, and change medications as the person improves or develops side effects. Proper and adequate treatment can only happen when patients are supported with wraparound services and healthcare staff are supported with resources and feel safe physically, mentally, and legally providing care.

The United States Surgeon General has identified healthcare provider burnout to be on the brink in the 21st century, and in May 2022, he declared the healthcare worker burnout crisis a national priority and called the nation's stakeholders to action. He cited workplace violence as one major factor contributing to the problem.[38] In 2019, the WHO defined burnout as an "occupational phenomenon" in the International Classification of Disease (ICD-11)[39] and noted that up to 38% of healthcare workers have experienced workplace violence and experienced burnout due to these experiences.[40] A New England Journal of Medicine review article reported that workplace violence against healthcare workers leads to missed workdays, general dissatisfaction, reduced productivity, and burnout. The review identified psychiatric inpatient settings as having the highest risk of workplace violence. It also found that the most common perpetrators of workplace violence are individuals with altered mental status or decompensated mental illness.[41]

Inpatient units, where much of the involuntary treatments take place, often involve a concentration of untreated patients, which may create a hazardous working condition for staff.[41,42] A clinician's ability to provide compassionate care is closely tied to feeling safe at their job. When staff feel unsafe, the quality of care they can provide can deteriorate. Additionally, healthcare equity becomes compromised, particularly in areas with more scarce healthcare resources, as healthcare workers are even more susceptible to burnout. Research indicates that burnout in clinical providers can reduce the improvements seen in patients. Timely treatment and reduced barriers to care to accelerate recovery for patients with acute mental illness not only grant them access to equitable and higher-quality care but also enhance working conditions and mitigate burnout among healthcare staff.[43]

Conclusion

There needs to be a balanced approach to the consideration of administering psychiatric interventions involuntarily to deliver life-saving and dignity-restoring care to patients with SMI who need it. While there are many mental healthcare inequities and abuses that do occur globally and should be addressed with sound policies, labeling intensive psychiatric interventions as abusive and violent is problematic. As illustrated by the Rogers Guardianship case example, when psychiatric treatment is postponed or withheld to provide for prolonged legal maneuvering, we risk overlooking the core objectives of mental healthcare. While every effort should be made within a short period of time to determine the capacity for medical decision-making in an individual, this pursuit should not irreversibly deteriorate the patient's condition in the process of waiting.

Prompt treatment not only helps to restore a patient's decision-making capacity and their ability to live in less restrictive settings, but it also allows them to live with their dignity intact.[7] Additionally, timely treatment enhances the common goal for healthcare equity and boosts healthcare staff morale, well-being, and a professional clinician's capacity to deliver compassionate and safe care.

In conclusion, it is paramount that national and global policy acknowledge the need for essential psychiatric care in serious mental illness and actively destigmatize its utilization. Without medication, certain mental illnesses have little chance of recovery. Psychiatric physicians and other mental health professionals find no joy in using involuntary methods in care, yet they ethically weigh this decision against graver consequences. As discussed, these consequences include prolonged and refractory illness, confinement in locked and restrictive settings, diminished access to care for the individuals and those around them, heightened risk of homelessness and incarceration, and the demoralization of healthcare staff and caregivers. The ethical imperative is clear: destigmatizing psychiatric treatment is essential within global policy frameworks if we are to restore the dignity of those living with mental illness.

References

1. Schiller L, Bennett A. *The Quiet Room*. Grand Central Publishing; 2008.

2. Biswas J, Drogin EY, Gutheil TG. Treatment delayed is treatment denied. *J Am Acad Psychiatry Law*. 2018;**46**(4):447–453. https://doi.org/10.29158/JAAPL.003786-18

3. Amador X. Denial of anosognosia in schizophrenia. *Schizophr Res*. 2023;**252**:242–243. https://doi.org/10.1016/j.schres.2023.01.009

4. Gerretsen P, Chakravarty MM, Mamo D, et al. Frontotemporoparietal asymmetry and lack of illness awareness in schizophrenia. *Hum Brain Mapp*. 2013;**34**(5):1035–1043. https://doi.org/10.1002/hbm.21490

5. Kletenik I, Gaudet K, Prasad S, Cohen AL, Fox MD. Network localization of awareness in visual and motor anosognosia. *Ann Neurol*. 2023;**94**(3):434–441. https://doi.org/10.1002/ana.26709

6. Hill MD, Gill SS, Le-Niculescu H, et al. Precision medicine for psychotic disorders: objective assessment, risk prediction, and pharmacogenomics. *Mol Psychiatry*. 2024;**29**(5):1528–1549. https://doi.org/10.1038/s41380-024-02433-8

7. Buchanan A. Respect for dignity and forensic psychiatry. *Int J Law Psychiatry*. 2015;**41**:12–17. https://doi.org/10.1016/j.ijlp.2015.03.002

8. Trestman RL. The treatment of mental illness is a human right. *J Am Acad Psychiatry Law*. 2018;**46** (1):2–4.

9. Davidson G, Brophy L, Campbell J, et al. An international comparison of legal frameworks for supported and substitute decision-making in mental health services. *Int J Law Psychiatry*. 2016;**44**:30–40. https://doi.org/10.1016/j.ijlp.2015.08.029

10. United Nations. *Convention on the Rights of Persons with Disabilities and Optional Protocol*; 2006. www.un.org/disabilities/documents/convention/convoptprot-e.pdf

11. WHO. WHO QualityRights Tool Kit. www.who.int/publications/i/item/9789241548410

12. Mahdanian AA, Laporta M, Drew Bold N, Funk M, Puras D. Human rights in mental healthcare; A review of current global situation. *Int Rev Psychiatry*. 2015;**35** (2):1–13. https://doi.org/10.1080/09540261.2022.2027348

13. Dawson J. A realistic approach to assessing mental health laws' compliance with the UNCRPD. *Int J Law Psychiatry*. 2015;**40**:70–79. https://doi.org/10.1016/j.ijlp.2015.04.003

14. Hoare F, Duffy RM. The World Health Organization's QualityRights materials for training, guidance and transformation: preventing coercion but marginalising psychiatry. *Br J Psychiatry*. 2021;**218**(5):240–242. https://doi.org/10.1192/bjp.2021.20

15. Wickremsinhe MN. Global mental health should engage with the ethics of involuntary admission. *Int J Ment Health Syst*. 2021;**15**(1):20. https://doi.org/10.1186/s13033-021-00448-0

16. Appelbaum PS. Protecting the rights of persons with disabilities: an international convention and its problems. *Psychiatr Serv*. 2016;**67**(4):366–368. https://doi.org/10.1176/appi.ps.201600050

17. *Rogers v. Okin. 478 F.2d 650* (United States Court of Appeals, First Circuit 1980). https://casetext.com/case/rogers-v-okin

18. *Rogers v. Okin. 634 F.2d 650* (United States Court of Appeals, First Circuit 1980). https://casetext.com/case/rogers-v-okin-2

19. *Mills v. Rogers, 457 U.S. 291.* (U.S. Supreme Court 1982).

20. *Rogers v. Commissioner of Department of Mental Health.* 390 Mass. 489 (Mass. 1983) 458 N.E.2d 308 (Supreme Judicial Court of Massachusetts. Suffolk 1983). https://casetext.com/case/rogers-v-commissioner-of-department-of-mental-health

21. Appelbaum PS, Gutheil TG. "Rotting with their rights on": constitutional theory and clinical reality in drug refusal by psychiatric patients. *Bull Am Acad Psychiatry Law*. 1979;7(3):306–315.

22. Gutheil TG. The right to refuse treatment: paradox, pendulum and the quality of care. *Behav Sci Law*. 1986;**4**:265–277.

23. Hoge SK, Appelbaum PS, Lawlor T, et al. A prospective, multicenter study of patients' refusal of antipsychotic medication. *Arch Gen Psychiatry*. 1990;**47**(10):949–956. https://doi.org/10.1001/archpsyc.1990.01810220065008

24. Kasper JA, Hoge SK, Feucht-Haviar T, Cortina J, Cohen B. Prospective study of patients' refusal of antipsychotic medication under a physician discretion review procedure. *Am J Psychiatry*. 1997;**154**(4):483–489. https://doi.org/10.1176/ajp.154.4.483

25. Schouten R, Gutheil TG. Aftermath of the Rogers decision: assessing the costs. *Am J Psychiatry*. 1990;**147**(10):1348–1352. https://doi.org/10.1176/ajp.147.10.1348

26. Pro G, Horton H, Tody B, et al. National and state-level trends in the availability of mental health treatment services tailored to individuals ordered to treatment by a court: United States, 2016, 2018, and 2020. *Soc Psychiatry Psychiatr Epidemiol*. 2024;**59**(10):1815–1824. https://doi.org/10.1007/s00127-023-02589-8

27. Weissman AR, Candilis PJ. Humane forensic practice serves social justice. *J Am Acad Psychiatry Law*. 2018;**46**(4):454–457. https://doi.org/10.29158/jaapl.003796-18

28. Hirschtritt MR, Binder RL. Interrupting the mental illness-incarceration-recidivism cycle. *JAMA*. 2017;**317**(7):695. https://doi.org/10.1001/jama.2016.20992

29. Fazel S, Baillargeon J. The health of prisoners. *Lancet*. 2011;**377**(9769):956–965. https://doi.org/10.1016/s0140-6736(10)61053-7

30. Green TM. Police as frontline mental health workers. The decision to arrest or refer to mental health agencies. *Int J Law Psychiatry*. 1997;**20**(4):469–486. https://doi.org/10.1016/s0160-2527(97)00011-3

31. Magee LA, Fortenberry JD, Rosenman M, et al. Two-year prevalence rates of mental health and substance use disorder diagnoses among repeat arrestees. *Health Justice*. 2021;**9**(1):2. https://doi.org/10.1186/s40352-020-00126-2

32. Robst JM, Constantine R, Petrila J. Association of involuntary psychiatric examination with probability of arrest of people with serious mental illness. *Psychiatr Serv*. 2011;**62**(9):1060–1065. https://doi.org/10.1176/ps.62.9.pss6209_1060

33. Constantine R, Andel R, Petrila J, et al. Characteristics and experiences of adults with a serious mental illness who were involved in the criminal justice system. *Psychiatr Serv.* 2010;61(5):451–457. https://doi.org/10.1176/ps.2010.61.5.451

34. Allison S, Bastiampillai T, Fuller DA. Mass incarceration and severe mental illness in the USA. *Lancet.* 2017;390(10089):25. https://doi.org/10.1016/s0140-6736(17)31479-4

35. Wildeman C, Wang EA. Mass incarceration, public health, and widening inequality in the USA. *Lancet.* 2017;389(10077):1464–1474. https://doi.org/10.1016/s0140-6736(17)30259-3

36. Forrester A, Hopkin G. Mental health in the criminal justice system: a pathways approach to service and research design. *Crim Behav Ment Health.* 2019;29(4):207–217. https://doi.org/10.1002/cbm.2128

37. Roskes E. Arrest: the "Front Door" to long-term care? *Psychiatr Serv.* 2011;62(11):1394–1394. https://doi.org/10.1176/ps.62.11.pss6211_1394

38. Murthy VH. Confronting health worker burnout and well-being. *N Engl J Med.* 2022;387(7):577–579. https://doi.org/10.1056/nejmp2207252

39. World Health Organization. Burn-out an "occupational phenomenon": International classification of diseases. World Health Organization. Published May 28, 2019. www.who.int/news/item/28-05-2019-burn-out-an-occupational-phenomenon-international-classification-of-diseases

40. World Health Organization. Preventing violence against health workers. Published 2022. www.who.int/activities/preventing-violence-against-health-workers

41. Phillips JP. Workplace violence against health care workers in the United States. *N Engl J Med.* 2016;374(17):1661–1669. https://doi.org/10.1056/nejmra1501998

42. Lehmann LS, McCormick RA, Kizer KW. A survey of assaultive behavior in veterans health administration facilities. *Psychiatr Serv.* 1999;50(3):384–389. https://doi.org/10.1176/ps.50.3.384

43. Caruso R, Roffanin T, Folesani F, et al. Violence against physicians in the workplace: trends, causes, consequences, and strategies for intervention. *Curr Psychiatry Rep.* 2022;24(12):911–924. https://doi.org/10.1007/s11920-022-01398-1

The Four Principles of Bioethics in Cases of Anosognosia

Rennie Burke and Katherine Warburton

Introduction

When a person rejects treatment for a condition that may literally be killing them due to reasons that are bizarre, irrational, or even delusional, how should we proceed? Psychosis presents a unique bioethical challenge. Anosognosia – the term for a person having impaired insight into the fact that they are ill – frequently afflicts those who suffer from psychotic illness. This lack of insight makes treatment much more ethically complicated. The central issue is the extent to which the doctor weighs the patient's *autonomy* against their own sense of *paternalism*. Simply put: How do doctors balance the patient's treatment goals against the doctor's when there is disagreement? Psychiatrists have embraced both approaches throughout the course of the field's history, and, as we will see, the current absolutist trend toward autonomy may ultimately be causing more harm than good. Before exploring this question in depth, however, some context is necessary. Why is autonomy important to medical ethics, and where did the idea come from?

While there are multiple approaches to bioethics, the one that has achieved primacy in American medical school education – and which therefore permeates the thinking of many health care professionals – is principlism.[1] Principlism, as the name suggests, is the application of a set of principles to help solve moral problems. While these principles vary, the most popular formulation was developed by the bioethicists Tom Beauchamp and James Childress. This model proposes four core principles for medical ethics: autonomy, beneficence, nonmaleficence, and justice. Though there are other models that include principles such as utility, truthfulness, fidelity, and confidentiality, it is Beauchamp and Childress's formulation that reigns supreme. The challenge of principlism is not so much what principles one chooses as ethical pillars but in applying those principles. Inevitably, principles come into conflict. For the purposes of this chapter,

the most widely embraced bioethical principles of autonomy, beneficence, nonmaleficence, and justice will be examined through several cases to explore the treatment of patients with anosognosia.

Case 1: Nonmaleficence

A 43-year-old man arrives at the emergency room by ambulance looking disheveled and emaciated. He was found lying behind a convenience store dumpster rambling incoherently, wearing four sweaters despite the 102°F (38°C) weather. Routine blood-work reveals severe anemia as well as several electrolyte abnormalities related to severe dehydration. He can provide his name and knows the date and his current location, but he does not understand the situation he is in. A review of his medical records indicates that he has a diagnosis of schizophrenia and a long history of taking multiple antipsychotics, most notably the powerful antipsychotic clozapine. He refuses to drink water because it has not been "operated upon." Instead, he requests only coffee and energy drinks, which he calls "life liquids."

Nonmaleficence has a long history in medicine, stretching back to Hippocrates in ancient Greece.[2] In essence, it holds that a doctor should do no harm, which seems straightforward. Harm, or the potential for harm, is an inevitable part of all medical treatment. Every surgery, medication, or even laying on of hands may have a negative consequence for the patient, even if not intended. Nevertheless, if the balance comes out to be on the side of the patient's well-being, and an effort has been made to minimize the harms, then a physician has abided by the principle. Psychiatric treatment in this respect is no different from other fields. The side effects of antipsychotics – which can include weight gain, movement disorders, and other harms – must be accounted for and tailored to the patient's unique situation.

Complexity stems from whether doing harm requires actually *doing* something. Can doing *nothing* constitute a harm? In Case 1, one could simply treat the patient's dehydration and electrolyte abnormalities and release him back to the community. Though not *doing* anything actively harmful or cruel to the man, discharging him without treating his underlying condition might be construed as a harm. Indeed, in this scenario, the patient may simply return to the exact same circumstances that led him to the emergency room, only with more lethal results. The Hippocratic exhortation against doing harm, then, may not be as simple as it initially seems. "Not doing" may result in doing harm.

To be sure, there is a dark side to nonmaleficence. For centuries, paternalism was the order of the day in medicine. The Hippocratic justification for medicine's paternalistic practices was closely intertwined with the notion of not doing harm. Doctors routinely withheld information from patients or decided themselves what was the best course of action on the basis of potential harms. You may have entered a surgery intending to have your appendix removed, but you could wake up bereft of a gallbladder, too, if a doctor determined that the organ needed to go. If allowing a patient to make a harmful decision or even telling a patient about their condition might cause harm, then the physician could not do it. Paternalism, then, has been embedded in medicine from its very foundations, and its conflict with nonmaleficence is not new.

Many ethical principles, nonmaleficence included, are understood to operate on a sliding scale. If a patient has a cold and declines symptomatic treatment, the doctor can rest easily knowing that not treating those symptoms is unlikely to result in a seriously harmful outcome. In other scenarios, when not doing anything may be the difference between life and death, application of the principle becomes thornier. As we will see, in the practice of psychiatry, the principle of nonmaleficence frequently comes into conflict with autonomy as well as the other principles. When insight is absent, and physicians uncritically uphold a patient's right to choose harmful outcomes for themselves, nonmaleficence comes squarely into conflict with autonomy.[3]

Case 2: Beneficence

A 33-year-old man presents to the psychiatric emergency room rambling incessantly about the "Alpha and the Omega" and "Judgment Day." His religious realizations were prompted in part by the voice of God, which he states had spoken directly to him and commanded him to share a new revelation with humanity. He is difficult to interrupt and redirect, though he is able to engage to some degree on religious topics. He appears well-groomed and states he is housed, has a romantic partner, and had a job he recently quit so that he could spread his religious teachings. He states that though he felt stable on his past medications, he wanted to try living without them. After stopping his medications, he experienced his religious epiphanies. Though obviously psychotic and reluctant to take medication, he is open to trying something that will make him "think more clearly." His decision required a long conversation and a significant amount of persuasion. A chart review indicates that he has a history of schizoaffective disorder, bipolar type, and has historically done well on medications, with long periods of lucidity and employment. An antipsychotic that he has done well on in the past is prescribed, and within 2 weeks he has returned to a nondelusional baseline. He is thankful for having been treated and states that he will be more diligent about taking his medication in the future.

Beneficence – the idea that a doctor's actions should have a positive effect on the patient – may also depend on action or inaction. Beneficence can be justified on the grounds of its outcome – does the action maximize the amount of good that can be done for a person? Called *consequentialism*, the idea that an act is moral because its consequences are good has been a way of evaluating the morality of an act since the time of the ancient Greeks.[4] This is not the only way to understand beneficence, however: It can also be based on the intrinsic value of doing good regardless of the outcome. This concept of morality, which is equally ancient, is embodied in the law codes – both holy and secular – that bar murder or exhort truth-telling irrespective of the consequences. Whether by divine mandate or by Immanuel Kant's "Categorial Imperative" for rational subjects to act only according to principles they would want to be universal, *deontology* holds equal influence in the world of bioethics.[5]

Regardless of whether it is based on the outcome or the intrinsic nature of doing good, beneficence is a cornerstone principle of modern medical practice. In Case 2, a patient with a history of living independently in the community while taking psychiatric medications arrived at the hospital in a highly decompensated state after he stopped taking them. Though he is highly psychotic and seems to lack insight into the relationship between his medications and his delusional and religiously preoccupied state, he is still able to consent to taking medications that would restore him to a state of insight. The most obvious act of beneficence in this case would be to provide him with these medications.

What amount of persuasion is appropriate, and at what point should we allow him to persist in his delusional and hallucinatory state knowing that he has a track record of doing well while taking medication? Paternalism again rears its head depending on how one views the nature of the persuasion that occurred.[6] As with the case of nonmaleficence (i.e., Case 1), the principle of autonomy may clash with beneficence. The extent of the clash depends on how much one chooses to accept "no" for an answer to the question of taking medication. When exactly a doctor's efforts at persuasion become inappropriate is a complex question. Again, the appropriateness of this persuasion is on a sliding scale: The more consequential the decision, the more avid the persuasion is likely to be. Though psychotic illnesses may very well be akin to dementia in terms of its neurodegenerative effect, American culture's respect for autonomy entails treating the initial "no" to medication as the final word, no matter how psychotically motivated.[7] This standard of care, which eschews assessment of capacity for imminent danger to one's self or others, is the subject of our next discussion.

Case 3: Justice

A disheveled woman arrives at the psychiatric emergency room after climbing onto a golf course and attacking an empty golf cart. She has been seen roaming the woods behind the golf course before, at times sleeping there, and has also been observed eating out of the trash can behind the snack bar. Though the weather is quite cold, she is wearing light, thin clothing. Her thinking is highly disorganized, and she arrives by ambulance screaming and refusing to participate in any staff attempt to interact with her. In her private room at the emergency department, she is demanding to leave and return "home," but she cannot provide an address. She is adamant that there is nothing wrong with her. Her worried family arrives at the emergency department and describe increasingly bizarre behavior, which now includes wandering from the house at night and not coming home. After a workup, she is given a diagnosis of neurodegenerative disease: Alzheimer's. A social worker meets with the family

to help connect them to the multiple resources available through the Alzheimer's Association and local nonprofits. They are given a pamphlet describing dementia care practice recommendations, which outlines the comprehensive, person-centered biopsychosocial standard of care for this condition. The compassionate staff members give the family a list of locked memory care facilities and recommend placement in a locked environment if she continues to wander. They describe the typical medication algorithms that are recommended to slow the progression of her disease and to help her overcome her agitated mood. Due to her anosognosia, she will now have a family member help make the decisions about when she will go to a memory care center, perhaps locked, and will authorize doctors to start a medication to help preserve her memory.

Imagine if this patient's diagnosis was schizophrenia, a condition now also understood to be a neurodegenerative disorder. In that case, she would be allowed to leave the emergency department with no treatment or resources. Her family would be told that there is nothing that the hospital staff can do to help her because she doesn't want treatment and is not dangerous to herself or other people. They will be told that sleeping in thin clothes in the woods behind the golf course during inclement weather doesn't rise to the level of dangerousness needed for them to intervene; neither will her behavior of eating out of trash cans at the golf course. Even if these behaviors cause her to be arrested and incarcerated, the hospital staff would still not be able to intervene. Why does our society treat these two neurodegenerative disorders so differently? Is this justice?

The ethical principle of justice concerns fairness, and this is especially salient in discussions about the way we have distributed our resources to treat mental illness.[8] For our purposes, justice also includes how we allocate other, equally precious resources: our attention and compassion. A tragically common feature of life in American cities is a disheveled person with a psychotic illness talking to themselves in the street as passersby ignore them. That this person is clearly suffering makes no difference to how much care the world at large chooses to give them. This same attitude can permeate health care interactions, too. Our attention – and who we give it to – is tragically limited.

The explanation for this striking disparity may lie in a contrast with the treatment of that other large group of patients with anosognosia: those with dementia. These patients are often treated with dignity and understanding. Patients with schizophrenia, by contrast, are often denied the same dignified treatment because of perceptions about the alienness of their thinking, talking, and acting. Providers are likely not completely conscious of the inequitable distribution of their care because a psychotic patient's protests may not even register – some patients who have prominent "negative symptoms" of social withdrawal and disorganized thought can only register their discontent in the most indirect ways. Moreover, their distorted relationship with reality and the behaviors it can lead to at times provoke strong feelings of fear and even dislike from providers. Yet if we hold up justice as a value worth striving for, this inequitable distribution of care should be unacceptable.

There is also a striking disparity in the way we evaluate the ability to make decisions by patients who lack insight. Patients with dementia routinely undergo evaluations of whether or not they can make decisions about their health, and there are widely followed conventions and regulations about how to involve them in this process.[9] The traditional criteria for evaluating capacity, set forth by ethicist Paul Appelbaum, consists of the ability to understand information, to appreciate the consequences of acting or not acting, to reason about the information provided, and the ability to communicate a decision.[10] If a patient lacks one of these abilities, then they are said to lack capacity to make a specific medical decision. Capacity can wax and wane as people recover or lose their faculties, as in delirium.[11] In some instances, when there is a global decline in capacity – as with dementia – a person can be found to lack competence and have all medical decision-making taken away. In Case 3, the patient lacks capacity to make treatment decisions, if not competence entirely. Her cognition and her insight into her condition are impaired by illness, as judged by a medical professional.

With mental illness, a different standard is routinely employed: that of dangerousness. If a patient is behaving in a way that may endanger themselves or others due to their mental illness, then they may have their ability to make their own medical decisions stripped from them. In practice, this is a much higher standard. Even in instances in which their presenting condition may be driven by an underlying psychotic – and, indeed, neurodegenerative – process, they are allowed to make their own decisions so long as they are not overtly "dangerous."[12] With our patient in Case 3, eating out of the trash and living lightly clothed in cold outdoor weather were not dangerous enough to rise to the level of a legal hold. The reasoning often goes that there are people with no illness who pursue this lifestyle out of choice, so why should doctors be able to deprive patients of that life choice? In many instances, the patient will continue to deteriorate until there is a life- or limb-threatening condition, at which point they will be placed on a legal hold. In many instances, this is too little, too late. Is this allocation of our mental energies toward capacity assessments for dementia patients and dangerousness assessments for the mentally ill just? Or is there an asymmetry between these two similar groups of patients that has gone unexamined?

Whether it is financial resources, time, or our hearts, there is a clear miscarriage of justice with respect to the care of people with psychotic illness. Unlike neurodegenerative dementia disorders, whose progress can only be slowed and not reversed, patients with schizophrenia can be restored to levels of function that had previously been lost. Currently, individuals with severe psychotic illnesses might cycle through forensic hospitals, carceral settings, and the open streets when they could be – with proper treatment – living in the community and flourishing. The present situation violates the ethical principle of justice on an individual and a systemic level, but there are ways forward. Models of care developed in other countries show that people with severe psychotic illness and low insight can live in the community and lead meaningful, rich lives.

Case 4: Autonomy

A 27-year-old man arrives at a hospital in the custody of a local official, complaining that there is a gang of people controlling his thoughts and behaviors with an "air loom," a gigantic weaving device whose invisible threads have become attached to his body. The "air loom gang" did not just attack him, however: They use their contraption's gases and rays to control politicians around the world and are inspiring wars and revolutions. This conviction led him to disrupt the proceedings of the national legislature in spectacular fashion. His speech is replete with odd phrasing and neologisms, and he is tormented by his paranoia. His only seeming wish is that the operators of the air loom be tracked down and brought to justice. He declines psychiatric help and insists that the real problem is the existence and activities of the "air loom gang."

James Tilly Matthews, the subject of this case study, was first admitted to hospital on January 28, 1797. A record of his delusions and treatment comprises what may be the first case study of schizophrenia ever published, first appearing in London, England, in 1810.[13] Matthews lived much of the remainder of his life in Bethlem Royal Hospital in London. Though relatively harmless, he was perceived to be a "maniac," and he was committed over the objections of his family, who fought through the legal system to keep him free and living with them. Doctors of the time felt that treating him required involuntary commitment. Ultimately, after significant agitation by his family, he was transferred to a private asylum in 1814, and he died one year later, in 1815.[14]

Matthews's experience encapsulates the debate about how much autonomy should be accorded patients with anosognosia – a debate that continues to this day. Would Matthews meet the criteria for hospitalization now? According to a strict legal definition, he most likely would not: He was eating, clothing himself, and living independently (and thus not "gravely disabled"), though in the community he was causing disruptions to the British parliament and experiencing extreme, psychotic paranoia. Nevertheless, there is an attitude among some that patients such as Matthews can only improve if they are committed to an inpatient unit, possibly indefinitely.

To place a patient such as Matthews on an inpatient unit indefinitely would represent – then as now – a failure of care. First, it would be unjustified. Unlike Cases 1–3, Matthews was not gravely disabled, nor was he a threat to his own life or the lives of others, despite his erratic behavior. Proactive treatment in the community and connections to resources that would allow him to continue independent living would be the ideal. This was the promise of twentieth-century legislation regarding mental health, justifying in part the drive for deinstitutionalization that resulted in state hospitals being closed. Unfortunately, the promised community treatment never materialized. Patients like Matthews suffered, as did patients such as those in Cases 1–3.

As the case of Matthews shows, anosognosia has been evident in society in some recognizable form for hundreds of years, and likely much longer. It is in this context – in which patients might not be able to clearly articulate their wishes – that the appeal of paternalism is strongest. Indeed, it *has been* strong. Psychiatry, it should be acknowledged, has had an ugly history of paternalism. Asylums born of a progressive, reforming instinct rapidly became overcrowded and sites of forced procedures to "cure" mental illness. From insulin shock therapy (in which patients were put into hypoglycemic comas) to the notorious lobotomy,(which shredded the neural connections in the prefrontal cortex), these treatments were generally ineffective and often barbaric. Yet this was not the perspective of mainstream medicine: The lobotomy's inventor, Antonío Egas Moniz, won the Nobel Prize in Medicine for its discovery.[15] In one instance, a psychiatrist in New Jersey's state hospital system took the notion of psychosurgery to such an extreme that he began removing tonsils, gallbladders, appendices, teeth, and ultimately sections of the colon to cure mental illness.[16] The historical record of people who have suffered at the hands of paternalistic psychiatrists who saw themselves as benevolent is indeed long.

A number of factors transformed the paternalistic approach over the course of the twentieth century. The Nuremburg Trials of Nazi war criminals revealed the routine, barbaric violation of the autonomy of concentration camp inmates in the name of "research," though the experiments themselves were often mere pretexts for cruelty. These violations led to the promulgation of an ethical code for medical research: the Nuremburg Code, which enshrined patient autonomy as its first principle.[17] Though an extreme example, this laid bare the coercion that was inherent in many contemporary medical practices, including the much more mundane. The medical world was rocked again when Dr. Henry Beecher released a landmark paper outlining violations of patient rights in various medical experiments in the years after Nuremburg. Comfortable in their conviction that they were far removed from the Nazis in time, geography, and behavior, the medical establishment continued to routinely violate patient autonomy and indulge its worst paternalistic impulses.[18] The current standards for medical research ethics, 1964's Helsinki Declaration and 1979's Belmont Report, are routinely updated in light of changing technology – and continued violations of medical and research ethics.[19,20]

Given the horrors that were visited on many people with mental illness, the arc of development of the last 75 years has been toward restoring autonomy to psychiatric patients. While some of this was spurred on by a growing antipsychiatry movement, supporters came from across the political spectrum. This advocacy resulted in legislation such as the federal Community Mental Health Act and bills like California's Lanterman–Petris–Short Act.[21,22] Psychiatric patients who had once been institutionalized found themselves able to exercise autonomy over their lives and health. Yet, as we explored earlier, the effects of this have often been negative for patients themselves. As their neurodegenerative diseases progress untreated, their situations can become increasingly desperate, and many find themselves in significant danger that they lack the insight to recognize or abate. Has the pendulum swung too far in the direction of autonomy?

Balancing autonomy and paternalism is especially vexing in psychiatry. As in the cases described earlier, individuals with psychotic disorders do not always recognize the extent to which their symptoms impact their lives, or even whether they have a disease at all. This need not be inconsistent with autonomy; regardless of how psychotic a patient may be, they may still maintain their core perspectives on life and death and be able to articulate them fluently. Yet when it comes to whether or not they should take medication, enter the hospital, or even have the ability to make decisions about where they live, mental health professionals and patients with anosognosia may find themselves at odds.

In protecting patients from their lack of insight, we must be careful to respect their autonomy and maintain a high standard for treatment against their will. In our case series, we saw people whose insight was impaired to the point that it made it impossible for them to live successfully in the community with our present resources. But we also saw Matthews, who similarly lacked insight but had survived without issue with his family's support prior to his lengthy institutionalization in Bethlem Royal Hospital.[22] As it is with people who have insight, we must have a high standard for overriding a patient's autonomy and abandoning hope that they could live in the community. Matthews did not seem to meet this criterion, but the norms of the time mandated that someone as paranoid and psychotic as he was be institutionalized. We must be careful not to make the same mistakes.

As noted earlier, twentieth-century legal developments concerning severe psychosis have been in the direction of greater autonomy. Patients who had formerly dwelt in state hospitals were released to the community in part because this was thought to be less of a constraint on their autonomy. This could have been a positive development. Exposés about the nature of asylums are numerous, and the inhumane treatment and overcrowding necessitated reform if not revolution. But current outcomes for people living with schizophrenia suggest that there may have been an overcorrection. Patients like those described earlier are routinely in danger, or they might endanger others. Their seemingly autonomous decisions are not actually autonomous, but rather weighed down by decades of mental illness, often untreated. Respecting their desire not to drink water or to eat trash behind a golf course on the grounds of respecting their autonomy does a disservice to them and to their community. There are a range of options currently available, from intensive mandated or voluntary outpatient treatment to inpatient hospitalization of varying durations (including indefinitely), but all of these solutions have in common one thing: paternalism. The echoes from the medical past therefore remain with us. What is needed is a way forward that both respects a patient's autonomy but also gives them the best chance to utilize their autonomy in the community in all of the ways that make life meaningful. Models of community-based care from elsewhere in the world serve as examples that could one day influence how care is delivered in the USA.

Conclusion

Finding a balance between the push and pull of autonomy and paternalism for patients with anosognosia will not be easy. The answer may lie in incorporating other principles outside of Beauchamp and Childress's original four, as well as more observable changes in a patient's well-being and our own inner feelings. All of these factors could resolve some of the tensions that the existing principles have with one another in the case of psychosis with anosognosia.

We explored in this chapter how patient autonomy often runs afoul of the paternalistic impulses of doctors who want to treat a problem even if it's against a patient's wishes. In a different vein, beneficence and nonmaleficence come into conflict with justice when resources are limited and one cannot do an equal amount of good for all parties involved.

And most notably, as it is the basis of some of the cases presented earlier, beneficence and nonmaleficence conflict with autonomy when respecting the desires of a patient with anosognosia leads to conditions that may result in severe harm or even death to a patient. In all of these cases, the four chief principles of bioethics are in tension. What can we do to resolve this conundrum?

One answer may be to consider other principles in conjunction with our four discussed in this chapter. Transparency and truth-telling are two principles that could be helpful. Through a commitment to transparency, discussions around voluntary or even compelled treatment would become more collaborative, as the decision-making is laid bare to the patient and the scope of who is involved in care is dramatically expanded. The approach of "Open Dialogue" promises just this. In Open Dialogue, the approach of dialogic practice entails creating a broad, interdisciplinary, and intercommunity team that includes a patient's friends and family.[23] This group discusses a patient's situation with the patient in an effort to foster an appreciation for multiple perspectives, not just those of the clinicians. This even includes discussions of things the patient may lack insight into, such as hallucinations or delusional systems. Transparently sharing perspectives and experiences between the two parties respects the patient's autonomy regardless of their level of insight.

Beyond the realm of principles, improving quality of life in concrete ways may also inform our conceptions of beneficence, justice, autonomy, and nonmaleficence. In the USA, many thousands of people living unhoused experience mental illness. An important first step, then, could be working to provide housing for this population as a prerequisite to treatment. The stability that housing affords could immeasurably improve quality of life. So too could employment, as patients with severe mental illness report enhanced quality of life through employment.[24] Though these may also be proxies for other factors such as social connectedness, enhancing the material conditions of patients in and of itself could be a principle to strive for.

Over and above the principles we have explored, a robust sense of compassion would do well in serving the principles of justice and beneficence. As we alluded to earlier, there is a disparity in the distribution of emotional energy in the treatment of patients with psychotic patients who have anosognosia. A compassion that derives not from a condescending sense of noblesse oblige but instead relating to a patient's experiences, however different, would enhance the quality of care delivered and go a long way toward addressing the asymmetries of care in treatment. Compassion is a force amplifier that enhances the positive effects of treatment and aligns well with the principles that undergird medical treatment.

Ultimately, guaranteeing better treatment for patients with anosognosia will require a broader array of resources than we currently employ. Yet, this need not be *more* resources. The USA spends significant amounts of money incarcerating patients with anosognosia in prisons and jails, remanding them to indefinite stays in inpatient facilities and hospitals, and attempting to provision numerous services to them in nonideal settings such as the street. Yet, around the world, there are numerous people with serious mental illness and anosognosia who live successfully in the community. Models such as that followed in Italy (see Chapter 17) show that this is not simply a speculative dream, but a reality that can be emulated. It will be up to us to build a brighter future.

References

1. Beauchamp TL, Childress JF. *Principles of Biomedical Ethics*, 8th edition. Oxford University Press; 2019.

2. Hippocrates. The Internet Classics Archive | Of the Epidemics by Hippocrates. https://classics.mit.edu/Hippocrates/epidemics.1.i.html

3. Varkey B. Principles of clinical ethics and their application to practice. *Medical Principles and Practice.* 2020;30(1):17–28. https://doi.org/10.1159/000509119

4. Demosthenes. Olynthiac 1, section 11. 2025. www.perseus.tufts.edu/hopper/text?doc=Perseus%3Atext%3A1999.01.0070%3Aspeech%3D1%3Asection%3D11

5. Kant I, Ellington JW. *Grounding for the Metaphysics of Morals With, on a Supposed Right to Lie because of Philanthropic Concerns.* W. Ross Macdonald School Resource Services Library; 2017.

6. Pelto-Piri V, Engström K, Engström I. Paternalism, autonomy and reciprocity: Ethical perspectives in encounters with patients in psychiatric in-patient care. *BMC Medical Ethics.* 2013;14(1):49. https://doi.org/10.1186/1472-6939-14-49

7. Stone WS, Phillips MR, Yang LH, et al. Neurodegenerative model of schizophrenia: Growing evidence to support a revisit. *Schizophrenia Research.* 2022;243:154–162. https://doi.org/10.1016/j.schres.2022.03.004

8. Beauchamp TL, Childress JF. *Principles of Biomedical Ethics*, 8th edition. Oxford University Press; 2019:250.

9. National Institute for Health and Care Excellence (NICE). *The Health and Social Care Act 2008 (Regulated Activities) Regulations.* NICE;2018.

10. Appelbaum PS, Grisso T. Assessing patients' capacities to consent to treatment. *New England Journal of Medicine.* 1988;**319**(25):1635–1638. https://doi.org/10.1056/nejm198812223192504

11. Soriano MA, Lagman R. When the patient says no. *American Journal of Hospice and Palliative Medicine*®. 2011;**29**(5):401–404. https://doi.org/10.1177/1049909111421163

12. Disability Rights California. Understanding the Lanterman–Petris–Short (LPS) Act. Disability Rights California. January 8, 2018. www.disabilityrightsca.org/publications/understanding-the-lanterman-petris-short-lps-act

13. Haslam J. Illustrations of madness: Exhibiting a singular case of insanity and a no less remarkable difference in medical opinion . . . with a description of the tortures experienced [by the patient, James Tilly Matthews, in hallucinations]. Wellcome Collection. 2024. https://wellcomecollection.org/works/e6n82yw6/items

14. Jay M. Illustrations of Madness: James Tilly Matthews and the Air Loom. The Public Domain Review. https://publicdomainreview.org/essay/illustrations-of-madness-james-tilly-matthews-and-the-air-loom/

15. Tierney AJ. Egas Moniz and the origins of psychosurgery: A review commemorating the 50th anniversary of Moniz's Nobel Prize. *Journal of the History of the Neurosciences.* 2000;**9**(1):22–36. https://doi.org/10.1076/0964-704x(200004)9:1;1-2;ft022

16. Scull A. *Madhouse: A Tragic Tale of Megalomania and Modern Medicine.* Yale University Press; 2007.

17. The University of North Carolina at Chapel Hill. Nuremberg Code. UNC Research. 2025. https://research.unc.edu/human-research-ethics/resources/ccm3_019064/

18. Beecher HK. Ethics and clinical research. 1966. *Bulletin of the World Health Organization.* 2024;**79**(4):367.

19. World Medical Association. WMA Declaration of Helsinki – Ethical Principles for Medical Research Involving Human Participants. December 13, 2024. www.wma.net/policies-post/wma-declaration-of-helsinki/

20. Office for Human Research Protections. The Belmont Report. US Department of Health and Human Services. 1979. www.hhs.gov/ohrp/regulations-and-policy/belmont-report/read-the-belmont-report/index.html

21. United States Congress. Mental Retardation Facilities and Community Mental Health Centers Construction Act of 1963. 1963. www.congress.gov/bill/88th-congress/senate-bill/1576/text

22. Lanterman–Petris–Short Act. Codes: Code Search. leginfo.legislature.ca.gov. https://leginfo.legislature.ca.gov/faces/codes_displayexpandedbranch.xhtml?tocCode=WIC&division=5.&title=&part=1.&chapter=&article=

23. Sekikula J, Arnkil TE. *Open Dialogues and Anticipations: Respecting Otherness in the Present Moment.* National Institute for Health and Welfare; 2014.

24. Bouwman C, de Sonnevile C, Mulder, CL, Hakkaart-van Roijen L. Employment and the associated impact on quality of life in people diagnosed with schizophrenia. *Neuropsychiatric Disease and Treatment.* 2015;**11**:2125–2142. https://doi.org/10.2147/NDT.S83546

Complexities of Competency and Informed Consent as Applied to Individuals with Symptoms of Anosognosia

Nina M. Labovich

Introduction

"As if the symptoms of schizophrenia were not devastating enough in themselves, nature has added a cruel joke, a seemingly valueless yet powerful barrier between the sufferer and professionals reaching out to help. The cruel joke is called anosognosia."[1]

Imagine you are a sophomore in college. You have been diagnosed with a serious mental illness and take medication to manage your symptoms. At first, you check in with your family and keep them updated on your condition, therapy, and medications. Several successful months on medication later, however, you know that you can control your own symptoms and medication. You stop taking your medication because you are fine and you do not have a mental illness – how could your family or doctor know more than you about *your* condition? Your family visits and begs you to get back on your medication. You refuse. Your doctor finds that you have the medical capacity to refuse treatment because you can understand the risks and benefits of the treatment, even though you cannot see that you are sick. You refuse medication, and eventually, you drop out of college due to your lack of control over your symptoms. You are not violent, so the state does not impose involuntary commitment. But you eventually become homeless, disconnected from family, and have worsening symptoms due to lack of medication.

This representative story demonstrates how anosognosia may impact an individual living with mental illness. Anosognosia may render a person unable to see that they are sick, which can snowball into refusing medication, worsening symptoms, and, unfortunately, homelessness or incarceration.[2] Separate from the devastating personal implications of anosognosia, the symptom may have critical legal implications as well.

Although medication may be, arguably, the best option for a patient with schizophrenia and anosognosia, prior to administering medication, the doctor must explain the pros and cons of accepting the treatment and ask for the patient's informed consent.[3] Informed consent occurs when a patient either accepts or declines treatment, following a doctor's explanation of risks involved in the procedure.[4] For an individual to give informed consent, a doctor must first find that the person can make medical decisions.[5]

If there is a dispute concerning a person's capacity to make medical decisions, a judge may be required to make a legal competency determination, or in other words, determine whether the individual is considered competent to refuse treatment under the governing state statute. Medical capacity and legal competency findings have some overlap, as both require a careful analysis of an individual's ability to make decisions, but the focus of this article is on the legal competency analysis. Although it may seem logical that a person who cannot see his or her illness cannot give informed consent, the law is inconsistent – in some jurisdictions, denial of illness warrants incompetency, but in others, it does not.

This chapter attempts to develop (or at minimum, articulate the challenges of developing) a legal solution, via a model definition of "competent," to the question of competency for individuals living with anosognosia. As is obvious from the history of mental health treatment in the United States – ranging from overinstitutionalization to wholly ignoring people living with mental illness – no solution is perfect and the path forward is muddy; however, at a bare minimum, the law should evolve with the science.

Informed consent and theories of competency

The doctrine of informed consent is grounded in an essential premise of the U.S. legal tradition – all individuals have the right to make their own choices.[6,7] As a result, in most circumstances, a doctor cannot ignore the individual's choice, even if the doctor thinks it is unwise.[6] There are narrow exceptions to this rule, such as in an emergency or, as is most relevant here, when a judge finds a patient legally incompetent to consent to treatment.[8] This article only considers competency to refuse treatment, not, for example, competency to stand trial; there are a variety of types of competency, each requiring different elements and legal tests.

Generally, adults are considered competent to make their own treatment decisions under the law. If a patient's legal competency is questioned, a physician must assess whether the patient has the medical capabilities to make decisions, often referred to as determining a patient's capacity.[9,10] Note that the medical capacity test is different from legal competency, although in crafting definitions of competency or incompetency, theorists and legislatures will consider the elements and extent of medical capacity required to be considered competent under their law.[10] With respect to medical capacity, doctors generally base that determination on the patient's ability to do the following: understand the situation, communicate a choice to the physician, appreciate the potential outcomes, and reason or rationalize (in other words, weigh the pros and cons) generally.[11]

When patients dispute a physician's determination of medical capacity, a judge may be required to make a legal competency determination; there is, however, no general consensus among approaches to competency determinations and definitions, with statutes varying across the country, state by state.[10] In any event, upon a finding of incompetence, an individual will not be able to make treatment decisions directly, requiring a surrogate to make decisions on the patient's behalf.[12]

At a minimum, experts have identified four prominent legal theories of competency, although there are certainly others.

The patient can articulate a choice

The first theory, the mere "ability to communicate a choice," requires the least rigorous review of the patient's capabilities: when a patient can communicate a decision, the patient is deemed competent.[10] In effect, only patients in comas or vegetative states would be deemed incompetent under this theory.[10] Although this theory of competency arguably may be

the most dependable theory (because it is subject to the least amount of interpretation), it is insufficient to establish competency alone.[9,10] Rather, the ability to communicate a choice often is one component of existing theories.[10]

The patient can understand – but cannot appreciate – the information presented

A second theory – often applied in the United States – tests whether a patient can understand the information presented.[10,13] In jurisdictions that use this theory, courts require an individual to "comprehend the concepts involved," but the patient need not *fully appreciate* the situation.[10] As applied, a patient would solely need to understand what a disease or symptom is, but not appreciate that the symptom or disease is *applicable* to the patient themself.[10] For example, Idaho adopts the "understanding" theory, defining "[l]acks capacity to make informed decisions" as the "inability … to achieve a rudimentary understanding of the purpose, nature, and possible risks and benefits of a decision."[14]

The patient can understand and appreciate the information

A third, more stringent theory requires the patient to both understand the information presented and to understand that the information is applicable to the patient.[10,13] In jurisdictions using this theory, to be deemed competent the patient must understand the information and appreciate the fact that the information applies to the patient and may carry certain consequences for the patient.[10] State statutes incorporating this theory may vary; for example, in Alaska, the relevant statute explicitly requires patients to appreciate that they have an impairment to be deemed competent,[15] whereas in Tennessee, the statute merely requires that patients are "able to understand and appreciate the nature and consequences" of their treatment decisions.[16]

The patient understands, appreciates, and makes a rational decision

Finally, some theories of competency require that a patient can understand and appreciate the information provided, *and* make a rational decision concerning treatment.[10,13] This approach examines whether the patient is capable of logically deciding on treatment by considering all of the information offered and weighing the pros and cons of the proposed treatment.[10] As one example, in Alabama, individuals are considered "incapacitated person[s]" when they become impaired such that they "lack[] sufficient understanding or capacity to make or communicate responsible decisions."[17]

Applying legal theories of competency to people with anosognosia

Scholars, courts, and legal practitioners disagree about the competency of individuals with schizophrenia and symptoms of or like anosognosia. Due to the patchwork legal framework in the United States, and the reliance upon individual judges and triers of fact to apply the legal standards in a variety of circumstances, it is difficult to cleanly silo court decisions and legal theories into one category or another. The following section summarizes three approaches, over a broad time period, and is meant to be illustrative, not exhaustive.

An individual with a lack of insight is competent

In 1994, in *In re Virgil D.*, the Supreme Court of Wisconsin held that an individual with schizophrenia who was unable to recognize his illness was competent to refuse antipsychotic medication, reversing the decision of the Court of Appeals of Wisconsin that had found the patient's inability to understand his illness warranted incompetency under state law.[18] Applying the plain language of the statute, which merely required a patient to understand the effects, benefits, and risks of a particular treatment, the Supreme Court of Wisconsin concluded that it was of no moment that the patient could not understand or accept his sickness; he merely needed to understand the particulars of the *treatment*.[18]

There are notable benefits to finding an individual with anosognosia competent. For one, given the misunderstanding of individuals living with mental illnesses, patients that repeatedly deny their illness may not be suffering from anosognosia, but instead could be avoiding the stigma of being diagnosed with mental illness.[13] In addition, finding patients incompetent any time they denied a supposed illness could have severe implications. In theory, and at its most extreme extension, permitting denial of a mental illness to warrant a finding of incompetency could lead to individuals being committed wrongfully for fringe or unpopular ideas.[13] Finally, a patient's lack of insight may not rise to the level of anosognosia or be sufficiently pervasive to warrant a finding of incompetency. Without a documented history of patients' behavior, it may be difficult to determine whether a patient is in denial or living with anosognosia.[19]

If a patient denies obvious symptoms or holds erroneous beliefs, they are incompetent

According to one prominent theorist, anosognosia, coupled with absurd beliefs or denials of verifiable symptoms of schizophrenia, warrants a finding of incompetency.[20] For example, when an individual denies an objectively apparent symptom of schizophrenia (e.g., insomnia), a finding of incompetency would be justified because denial of a quantifiable symptom demonstrates that the individual's mental processing is so broken down that such an individual is incompetent.[13] Likewise, a patient who denies their illness because they believe the symptoms of schizophrenia arise as a result of an infestation of evil spirits (as opposed to a brain disorder) should be found incompetent.[13] In either circumstance, there is clear evidence that the patient has delusions and symptoms of schizophrenia; coupled with a lack of insight, there is cause for a finding of incompetency.[13] When a patient's denial of illness is caused by delusions or the patient denies visible symptoms, there may be less cause for concern that a court is wrongfully taking away a patient's right to refuse treatment. Requiring gross denial of symptoms or plainly false beliefs *and* denial of objectively apparent symptoms of the illness may help mitigate concerns that a patient is in denial, misdiagnosed with a psychiatric condition, or wrongfully persecuted for his or her beliefs.[13] Denial of an apparent symptom demonstrates that a patient cannot understand a diagnosis or appreciate its impact – requirements of many informed consent statutes. Separately, this view may encourage patients and doctors to thoroughly explore the individual's reasoning.[21]

A patient with anosognosia is incompetent

In 2017, in *People v. D.A.*, a California appellate court held that an individual with schizophrenia and severe anosognosia was incompetent and could not give informed consent.[22] As a result, the court upheld the involuntary administration of antipsychotic medication, emphasizing testimony from the patient's doctor, who stated that the patient did not understand he had schizophrenia and refused to take his medication. The doctor testified that as a result of the lack of medication, the individual had experienced worsening symptoms and felt persecuted by those trying to treat him.[22] The court considered the patient's ignorance of his symptoms and diagnosis and found that he was unable to weigh the pros and cons of medication and could not productively participate in his treatment decision due to his lack of insight.

The doctrine of informed consent aims to protect patient free will.[23] To effectuate autonomy, competency tests ensure that patients who are able to make their own decisions are, in fact, permitted to have that choice.[23] Scientific evidence arguably supports a finding of incompetency on the basis of anosognosia, as it indicates anosognosia interferes with the ability of a patient to make decisions about their treatment.[12] Psychiatric conditions directly affect parts of the brain that allow individuals to think, make decisions rationally, and understand the likelihood of events happening in the future.[24] Arguably, without proper insight into their conditions, individuals cannot make a free choice.[24] Instead, the choice has been made by the disease because it has infiltrated their decision-making capacity. Allowing patients with poor insight to decline medication does not necessarily affect their free choice, which is the goal of informed consent, because the disease dictates the choice.[24] A finding of incompetency on the basis of anosognosia, then, may help doctors best determine and effectuate a patient's autonomous choice.

Separately, finding patients incompetent on the basis of anosognosia may help retain patients' ability to choose in the long term.[24] When patients with anosognosia refuse treatment in the present, they may be making a decision *never* to treat because their lack of insight will likely worsen without treatment over time. With treatment, in contrast, symptoms of anosognosia may lessen, potentially allowing patients to *gain* insight over time.[24] Some argue that if the goal of informed consent is to effectuate autonomy, ensuring patients' long-term autonomy is best accomplished by finding patients with anosognosia incompetent in the present.[24]

Charting a compassionate path forward: Documented anosognosia warrants legal incompetency

Appreciation of illness is fundamental to the goals of informed consent and necessary for a finding of competency

Effectuating and respecting an individual's autonomous choice is, ultimately, the goal of informed consent. As explained above, schizophrenia may have direct impacts on the parts of the brain responsible for an individual's decision-making. Anosognosia impacts an individual's ability to think rationally and directly affects the brain's ability to accurately process information. If an illness, like schizophrenia, or symptom, like anosognosia, directly affects the part of the brain that contributes to a person's ability to freely make choices, the illness or symptom must be considered in the competency determination.[24] Under those circumstances, it cannot be said that the patient is actually acting with autonomy, cutting against a central tenet of informed consent.

Although traditional notions of informed consent focus on a patient's current state of mind, when a patient's decision in the present will effectively serve as the only meaningful opportunity to decide, considering future implications of the decision are warranted. Accordingly, if the goal of informed consent is to effectuate a patient choice, informed consent must consider whether a patient can appreciate the illness, particularly where an illness can obfuscate a patient's actual decision-making.[24]

A balance between patient autonomy and modern science

Despite some jurisdictions already requiring patients to "appreciate" their illness to exercise their right to refuse treatment, statutory language varies. For example, in Alaska, the statutory definition of competency explicitly requires, *inter alia*, patients to appreciate that they have an impairment.[15] In contrast, Tennessee's statute is less specific.[16]

Alaska's statutory language provides the clarity necessary to ensure that anosognosia is considered in a judge's competency determination, and provides a starting point for model statutory language.

This article, however, contends that the statutory language must go further to both protect individuals and reflect modern science. Concrete statutory language would protect patient autonomy, by ensuring those who have insight into their condition but, for their own reasons, do not want to undergo treatment, are found competent to refuse treatment. Separately, detailed language would ensure that only those who have medically documented anosognosia and not mere denial are found incompetent. Explicit language safeguards against judges reading their own beliefs about denial into their statutory interpretation. And, most importantly, tailored language ensures that the statute reflects the best science available to test for anosognosia. In sum, the article proposes a model statute incorporating Alaska's language and includes additional components that aim to protect an individual's right to choose treatment. This proposed statute moves the conversation toward a humane approach to effectuating autonomy for people with anosognosia.

"Competent" means that the person:

a) Has the ability to assimilate relevant facts and to appreciate and understand their situation with regard to those facts[15];

b) Appreciates that they have a mental illness or impairment, if the evidence so indicates[15]

   a. A person's denial of his or her mental illness is evidence that the person lacks the capability to make treatment decisions when the person's denial is a result of anosognosia, a significant deficit in insight.[19] Denial is evidence of anosognosia when it has lasted over a period of at least six months, the denial does not change even if the individual is presented with evidence, and the individual offers alternative absurd explanations to persuade others that he or she does not have an illness.[19]

      i. The lack of insight must be documented during a period of at least six months, and a doctor must be willing to testify to the patient's lack of insight as a symptom of his or her disease, not mere denial.[19]

c) If a person is found incompetent under Section b, he or she may be administered antipsychotic medication involuntarily, if a doctor has determined it is appropriate.[22] When and if the person obtains insight into his or her medical condition (or in one year, whichever time period is sooner) the person's capacity must be reassessed by a medical professional and the person's competency must be reassessed by a judge.

Author Biography

Nina M. Labovich is an attorney. Previously, she was a judicial law clerk at the US District Court for the District of Massachusetts. She is a graduate of Boston College Law School and Wesleyan University. This article is an abbreviated version of her Note, published in the Boston College Law Review in 2021, during her third year of law school. Opinions expressed in this article are the author's own and do not reflect the views of her employer.

References

1. Powers R. *No One Cares About Crazy People: The Chaos and Heartbreak of Mental Health in America.* Hachette Books; 2017.

2. National Alliance on Mental Illness. Anosognosia. NAMI. www.nami.org/about-mental-illness/common-with-mental-illness/anosognosia/. Accessed July 1, 2024.

3. Moldoff WM. Malpractice: physician's duty to inform patient of nature and hazards of disease or treatment. 79 A.L.R. 2d 1028. *Am Law Rep.* 1961.

4. Consent GB. *Black's Law Dictionary.* 11th ed. Thomson Reuters; 2019.

5. Pegalis S. *American Law of Medical Malpractice.* 3rd ed. Thomson Reuters; 2024.

6. *Natanson* v. *Kline*, 350 P.2d 1093 (Kan. 1960).

7. *Canterbury* v. *Spence*, 464 F.2d 772 (D.C. Cir. 1972).

8. Schuck P. Rethinking informed consent. *Yale Law J.* 1994;**103**:919.

9. Wolff K. NOTE: determining patient competency in treatment refusal cases. *Georgia Law Rev.* 1990;**24**:743–745.

10. Berg J, Appelbaum P, Grisso T. Constructing competence: formulating standards of legal competence to make medical decisions. *Rutgers Law Rev.* 1996;**48**:348–358.

11. Dastidar J, Odden A, Dastidar JG. How do I determine if my patient has decision-making capacity? *The Hospitalist.* Published August 3, 2011. www.the-hospitalist.org/hospitalist/article/124731/how-do-i-determine-if-my-patient-has-decision-making-capacity. Accessed July 1, 2024.

12. Knepper K. The importance of establishing competence in cases involving the involuntary administration of psychotropic medications. *Law Psychol Rev.* 1996;**20**:103–105.

13. Saks E. Competency to refuse treatment. *North Carolina Law Rev.* 1991;**69**:952–957; 990–992.

14. Idaho CODE § 66–402(9) (2020).

15. Alaska Stat. § 47.30.837(d)(1).

16. Tenn. Code Ann. § 32–11-103(1).

17. ALA. CODE § 26-2A-20(8).

18. *In re Virgil D.*, 524 N.W.2d 894 (Wis. 1994).

19. Amador X. *I Am Not Sick I Do not Need Help! How to Help Someone with Mental Illness Accept Treatment.* 10 ed. Vida Press; 2012.

20. Saks E. Competency to refuse medication: revisiting the role of denial of mental illness in capacity determinations. *South Calif Rev Law Soc Justice.* 2013;**22**:181–182.

21. Saks E. Some thoughts on denial of mental illness. *Am J Psychiatry.* 2009;**166**:973.

22. *People* v. *D.A.*, No. B278615, 2017 WL 3614096, at *1–2 (Cal. Ct. App. Aug. 23, 2017).

23. Winick B. *The Right to Refuse Mental Health Treatment.* American Psychological Association; 1997.

24. Epright M. Symposium: conundrums and controversies in mental health and illness: coercing future freedom: consent and capacities for autonomous choice. *J Law Med Ethics.* 2010;**38**:803–805.

Chapter

33 Evidence-Based Treatment for Schizophrenia
A Personal Perspective

Bethany Yeiser

My name is Bethany Yeiser, and I am an individual living with schizophrenia. My schizophrenia has been in full remission since 2008, thanks to treatment with clozapine, the vastly underutilized medication for refractory schizophrenia.

My journey through schizophrenia and finding my way back was not easy.

I was born in 1981 to a loving family. My childhood was wholesome and happy. At age 7, I began studying violin, which quickly became my passion. I began practicing for 4 hours a day at age 13 and was accepted as a student of a violin professor at the Cleveland Institute of Music that same year.

I also excelled academically. At age 15, I discovered Ohio's Post-Secondary Educational Options Program, allowing high school students to take classes at local colleges and universities for dual high school and college credit. After attending Lakeland Community College for 2 years, I graduated from high school with 2 years of college credits and a 4.0 GPA.

My dream school was the University of Southern California, as I was attracted to their music program. However, after visiting USC, I realized how many other exciting academic options were available to me and soon settled on a bachelor's degree in biochemistry and molecular biology.

In 1999, at age 17, I traveled from Ohio to USC. I would live in the honor's dormitory, having been awarded a half-tuition scholarship. From the beginning, I was extremely busy with difficult classes including organic chemistry. I was happy to land a position in a research laboratory during my first semester, studying enzymes that replicate DNA (which had important implications in certain human cancers). I also auditioned to become concertmaster of USC's community orchestra and won.

But something was wrong. I remember wanting nothing to do with the other students, usually eating alone and never going to social functions or outings.

I committed to attending a local church but rarely mingled. I would arrive late and leave the minute it was over to rush back to the lab.

During my junior year of college, I began to develop a deep-seated urge to change the world, leaving a great legacy and impact. At this time, my church was sponsoring a small group of young women to visit a remote and impoverished community in China.

I left for China during the winter break of my junior year of college. While there I remember thinking: Can I change the lives of a million people in China? Or millions? Something inside of me said yes, this was possible, and that it would happen immediately.

Looking back, I understand this was delusional thinking. If I wanted to impact a large number of impoverished Chinese people, there was the need to pursue higher education, perhaps a PhD in economics or political science. I would have needed to study Chinese for years and live in China for some time to establish relationships and credibility. Instead, I believed my next step forward was to visit Africa, to live among a different culture of people in need. During the summer of 2002, prior to the start of my senior year at USC, I spent 2 months living in Nairobi. The church in Cleveland where I had grown up sponsored me and paid nearly all my expenses.

About this time, I developed a symptom of schizophrenia I had never heard of, dromomania. This is an uncontrollable urge to travel.

Upon my return from Africa, I began planning a trip to Thailand to visit an American family I knew there. But suddenly, I was unable to focus, even struggling to pass my classes. My parents were at a loss to understand what was happening in my life. But they knew who I was, and how much my degree meant to me. They were entirely certain that if they told me they might withdraw their funding if I continued with my travel plans, I would cancel my trip. However, my psychiatric physician looks back on this time as the onset of my first psychotic break. Convinced that traveling to Thailand was more important to my future than my college degree, I told my parents I was going to Thailand. Then, I refused all contact with them for the next four and a half years, during which I descended into a life of psychosis and homelessness. I believed that my parents would try to prevent me from making a worldwide impact. I thought my travel around the world was commanded by God and saw my parents as adversaries.

I soon dropped out of USC officially and lost my dorm room, refusing all help from friends and family, paranoid they would stop me from making my worldwide impact. I had maxed out my credit cards in Thailand and rapidly ran out of money.

In March 2003, I became homeless. Nonetheless, I quickly became an expert at washing up in public bathrooms and carrying only light changes of clothing to appear like a student with a backpack. I would stay most nights and sleep in the USC library. I actually made some friends in the library with engineering students who regularly wrote code late into the night.

I prevaricated about my status as a student, telling acquaintances that I was a part-time graduate student. Had I been in my right mind, I very likely would have been a part-time graduate student with an interest in international affairs on the side. I told myself my lies were acceptable since, once I became a successful billionaire, no one would care.

In my free time, I started studying ancient Hebrew at a library every day and, after a few months, I developed a basic proficiency. I also made friends with a computer engineer and his wife from mainland China who taught me how to chat in Mandarin Chinese, until my paranoia surfaced, and I became too afraid of them to continue free lessons. To this day, in 2024, I retain my ancient Hebrew proficiency and have basic conversational skills in Chinese.

But about 3 years later, on January 28, 2006, again, everything changed. I was sitting on a park bench on the university campus in the early afternoon when I heard voices in my head for the first time, insulting me, yelling at me, and then changing to a positive tone and complimenting me. I immediately realized something was not right. However, I thought through mental illness and decided that I was too strong, too smart, and too normal to ever be mentally ill. I concluded that what I was experiencing must be normal and, since no one else was talking about it, I should not either.

About that time, I gave up hiding in libraries and lounges on the USC campus, afraid I would be caught.

My backup plan was a local churchyard. I would stay there for the next 13 months.

With time, my hallucinations became more problematic. I heard voices in my mind which I knew no one else could hear, as well as voices and noise (such as cars passing by or birds chirping) in my reality. When hearing noise in my reality, I was entirely unaware if these were real sounds or hallucinations. One day I looked in a mirror, but my face resembled the face of the character Lisa from the show The Simpsons.

My hygiene plummeted as I stopped washing up in public restrooms. It was hard to do it quickly, and I always was afraid someone would walk in on me while I had one of my feet in the sink. At this time, I also became shameless about rummaging for food to eat in garbage cans on the streets of LA, even when other people noticed, because I was so hungry.

On October 14, 2006, my twenty-fifth birthday, the voices pressured me relentlessly to go back to the campus and spend the night in a lounge where I had stayed several times and never been caught. I went there again 2 days later, dirty, and clearly not belonging on the campus. I remember looking out the window and seeing Los Angeles Police Department officers, which I had never seen on campus before. They were there to pick me up, and I was taken to jail for about 3 days.

In the back seat of the police car, I asked the officers if they would take me home afterward (which to me was the campus area). They said yes, of course. I did not know they were being sarcastic. When I entered the jail, they asked me if I needed medical attention. I saw a large room with women getting shots. Since they needed medical attention, I wondered why they were in jail.

My jail cell was a tight fit for 2, but there were 4 of us in it. When they took my fingerprints, I was terrified the ink would give me a terrible disease. Soon, I was transferred to a big room that was literally as dark as a cave. During my life I had never been afraid of the dark before but in jail, I was. We had a 15-minute break later with some translucent light coming in from the roof and then were returned to the darkness. I recall one good thing about the jail – I greatly appreciated the hot food they served us.

The morning of the third day, I was taken to a courthouse where I signed paperwork declaring I would return for my day in court, though I had no way of getting there and was embarrassed to show up dirty and with shoes that had almost completely fallen apart.

You would think that my traumatic experience in jail would have changed my life – that I would have finally called family or friends and asked for help. But I did not. I believed God wanted me to wait in the churchyard. I believed a billionaire was coming and could enter my life at any time. I resolved to wait for him. The judicial and social service systems had failed me. I resumed sleeping outside, homeless, and in need of medical assessment and treatment.

In November 2006, the day before Thanksgiving, I was unable to read a newspaper and decipher the date but guessed it was a week before Thanksgiving. I always left the churchyard early in the morning and never returned until evening, but that day, because my hallucinations were so intense and bothersome, I went to the churchyard in the afternoon.

A couple of police officers called out to me asking where I lived. When they did not believe the lie everyone else seemed to believe, they picked me up and took me to jail a second time. Many people stayed at that churchyard. To this day, I do not know what my crime was that afternoon.

My second experience in jail was much different than the first. We had clean uniforms, and there was more natural light. At times, I was in intensely crowded spaces for hours, as we were shuttled to different parts of the building. But after 5 days, one morning, I woke up thankful for the jail. I was released a few hours later. Looking back, again, I see the failure of the systems of judicial and social services. My life outside, homeless, had become so difficult, jail did not seem so bad.

March 3, 2007, was my fourth-year anniversary of becoming homeless, though I did not know the date. The voices were severe, the most irritating stimulus I could ever imagine, forcing me to scream profanity, though I had never used profanity in my life prior to hearing the voices. Suddenly, a police officer I had not seen snuck up to me and pulled my hands behind my back. When I was told I was being taken to a psychiatric ward, I was actually happy to hear it. I expected to be released immediately.

Being involuntarily hospitalized was a terrible experience. I resented my doctor and was absolutely certain I was not sick. But on my first medication, which I was mandated to take, the visual hallucinations, delusions, and paranoia disappeared. When my parents visited, still interested in a relationship,

I wondered why we were not already in touch. They had never done anything wrong, and after the medication had cleared my mind, I understood that.

I left the hospital with no paranoia, no delusions, and no visual hallucinations, but the voices I heard inside my mind were still there, which led me to believe the medication was not helping at all. What I needed was an education about my illness and medication. I needed someone to point out to me the changes in my behavior and clarify that these changes were directly due to the antipsychotic medication. However, instead, I was discharged from the hospital without knowing my diagnosis, what it meant, or what the pills were for. I also was unaware that my psychiatrist had told my parents that I was permanently and totally disabled, which meant that I would never work or attend college again, or live independently.

I flew to Cincinnati with my parents, as they had moved there from Cleveland while I was in California. They gave me a beautiful room, invited me to meet their friends, and encouraged me to walk through their vibrant community.

My antipsychotic side effects soon became unbearable. I had akathisia, an extreme restlessness that never went away, as well as a flat affect. I found myself sleeping 16–18 hours a night, and developed a ravenous appetite, quickly gaining over 15 pounds. Because I did not believe I needed this medication, and thought it was ruining my life, I did the logical thing, and discontinued my pills. At first, as the side effects went away, I felt great. However, within about 2 weeks, my command hallucinations were back, causing me to scream and shout profanity. I was soon hospitalized for a second time.

During my first Ohio hospitalization, I still did not receive information about my diagnosis and symptoms, or how my medication worked. However, a physician sat down with me and told me what I believe was the most important thing I needed to know: if you go off your antipsychotic and on it again, it can be less effective, even at higher dosages. He explained to me that this is what leads to disability. That day, I was convinced to always take my medication, and I have taken my antipsychotic now without interruption for 17 years.

The next 12 months were the hardest of my life, as I was given 5 different atypical antipsychotics, and sometimes combinations of 2 of these antipsychotics. I thought my first 3 doctors were correct, that I would be permanently and totally disabled. But just when everything seemed hopeless, I was referred to a new psychiatrist, Professor Henry Nasrallah, MD, a renowned schizophrenia expert who started me on clozapine, the only antipsychotic approved by the FDA for treatment-resistant schizophrenia. Within 4 to 6 months, the auditory hallucinations disappeared, and I fully recovered.

Following my recovery, in 2009, I enrolled at the University of Cincinnati and graduated with honors in molecular biology (3.84 GPA). Over the following 2 years, I wrote and published a memoir called *Mind Estranged: My Journey from Schizophrenia and Homelessness to Recovery*, about the journey of my recovery. Today I work both as President of the CURESZ Foundation and as a national motivational speaker, frequently traveling around the United States. I share my story of full recovery, though I was repeatedly told my recovery would be impossible. Some people have told me I am the exception to the rule. This is what led me recently to publish another book, together with Dr. Henry Nasrallah, that we called *Awakenings: Stories of Recovery and Emergence from Schizophrenia*, featuring 28 recovery stories of individuals who have made remarkable recoveries after being diagnosed with schizophrenia.

There are many changes we need to see in the mental health-care system of the United States. The most urgent in my opinion is the creation of a new standard of commitment for involuntary hospitalization, and it needs to be easier to require psychiatric evaluations. Looking back, I should never have been allowed to struggle on the streets outside for 13 months before I was taken to a hospital for evaluation. Months before I was committed, had I seen a doctor, he probably would have recommended an involuntary hospitalization. But I was neglected, and no one took me to see a physician for evaluation and treatment. And because of the high standard for involuntary commitment, my parents were powerless.

In our country, in order to be involuntarily hospitalized, a person must be a danger to self or others or gravely disabled (which I finally became in 2007). Many families have loved ones who are desperately sick but do not meet these difficult criteria. Some parents will take their acutely psychotic son or daughter to a hospital, but because they are not "sick enough," they are turned away. The parents have to simply wait for their loved one to get worse in order to qualify for admission to a psychiatric hospital, unless they get arrested and end up in jail as a criminal.

It is absolutely essential to give people as much autonomy as possible, but those who are paranoid, delusional, and experiencing hallucinations often are totally unaware they are sick and will refuse help that could treat their psychotic symptoms and greatly improve their lives. Many of these people with serious psychiatric brain disorders descend into homelessness, as I did, and their quality of life becomes very poor. Unfortunately, many more of these people, like me, will end up in jails or prisons, though psychosis influences their behavior and their real need is for a hospital where they can receive medical treatment. In the United States, it is much easier to become homeless or be jailed than it is to be involuntarily hospitalized for psychiatric and medical assessment and treatment.

Perhaps I was one of the lucky ones, only incarcerated twice for about 8 days in total. Looking back, I realize how easy it is for a psychotic individual to commit a petty crime. I also realize that I would never have consented to a life-changing involuntary hospitalization, but because of it, I was able to redeem my life. It placed me on the path to the functional success I enjoy today.

Education is vitally important. People struggling with conditions such as breast cancer or diabetes are given pamphlets, stuffed animals, other gifts, information for support groups, and told what to do if they have medication side effects. People with schizophrenia, on the other hand, are often left with very little information, or none at all, and a bottle of pills they can choose to take or discard. It is rare to offer first-episode patients, or any patients, long-acting injectables. This is unfortunate because those formulations are highly effective at preventing relapse due to poor adherence to pills.

In our society, we do not see children or elderly persons with dementia living on the streets. If a child is facing homelessness, social services come to their rescue and bring them to a place where they have housing, clothing, food, and education. A person struggling with Parkinson's disease cannot simply refuse medication and choose to live underneath a bridge. Our legal system is set up such that many of the neediest among us, who cannot make rational choices on their own, or choose to get help, are not simply left to suffer. But when it comes to schizophrenia, severely psychotic persons are largely unprotected and forgotten, or end up jailed, homeless, or prematurely dead.

Recently, in Cincinnati where I live, a social worker saw a woman at a church event whom he had previously met when she was homeless. She looked groomed and well, and he approached her to ask what had happened. She looked at him and said, "Why? Why did you leave me outside for such a long time?" Following her involuntary hospitalization, she was able to begin a new life, and today, she does not understand why no one brought her to a hospital much sooner.

I wish I had never dropped out of USC and that my homelessness had never happened. I also wish that I had never been driven by insanity to hide on the campus in libraries and lounges for years, waiting for an imaginary person. I wish I had never been taken to jail for trespassing on a campus where I was once so excited about attending classes and scoring A's. But today, through sharing my story, I hope to be instrumental in helping more needy Americans get the treatment they need. We need to get them off the streets and keep those who need treatment out of our jails and prisons. Most importantly, we need to offer the most vulnerable among us the hope and potential recovery that comes with effective treatment for psychiatric brain disorders.

Due to my experiences, as well as my desire to prevent others from having to go through something similar, I serve as President of the CURESZ Foundation, which I founded in 2016 with the psychiatrist who brought me to full recovery, Henry Nasrallah, MD. CURESZ stands for Comprehensive Understanding via Research and Education into SchiZophrenia. The CURESZ Foundation provides education, advocacy, and information about cutting-edge and underutilized treatments for schizophrenia such as clozapine for treatment resistance, long-acting injectable medications for relapse prevention due to nonadherence, and new medications for movement disorder tardive dyskinesia. We offer support for families including a caregivers' mentoring program, student-based clubs, a support group, and a wide range of educational videos.

Inmate Mental Health Assistants

An Emerging Best Practice for Carceral Settings

Craigen Armstrong, Kerry Morrison, David Nelson, Dain Sanderson, Anthony Matzke, and Bernardo Martinez

Introduction

At Los Angeles County Jail, considered by some to be the largest mental health treatment facility in the USA, an innovative program that started in 2016 has demonstrated that compassionate care, provided by peers and supported by clinical and custody staff, can have a transformative impact on incarcerated patients with serious mental illness. The rapport and trust that result from the relationships created between inmate mental health assistants (MHAs) and the patients under their care are grounded upon a posture of radical hospitality where patients are seen and heard, feel safe, and can exercise choice.

The inmate MHAs at the Twin Towers Correctional Facility (TTCF) work daily with incarcerated patients who have severe, complex, and complicated mental health needs. These MHAs provide patients with "trauma-informed care in a wellness-focused setting so that they can learn self-sufficiency, independence, become medication-compliant, in some cases, with an understanding of self and healing," according to the County of Los Angeles Board of Supervisors. This innovative program is led by the Correctional Health Services (CHS) Department in the Los Angeles County Jail, which is responsible for mental health care. The partnership between the CHS and the Los Angeles Sheriff's Department (LASD), which has jurisdiction over the jail, is an essential ingredient.

The original inmate MHAs developed a vision for a program that would be founded upon education and training, not only for the patients under their care, but also for others who were recruited out of the general population of inmates. These non-mentally ill inmates voluntarily accepted this role as inmate MHAs.

The MHAs describe their philosophy of how they come alongside the patients under their care as peers; the structure of a typical day in a mental health pod, which includes education, chores, purposeful engagement, and socialization; and the goal of the overall program, sharing their vision for how this can be replicated. They freely share their curriculum (including quizzes) that teaches patients about positive lifestyle habits, court competency, and personal goal-setting.

They also describe the training developed to equip the inmate MHAs for this work, which involves living embedded in a mental health pod with up to 24 patients, 24 hours a day. The MHAs learn about the nature and treatment of various mental illnesses, the intricacies of the legal system and the establishment of court competency, how to lead by example and communicate effectively, and the importance of nutrition and hygiene.

What follows is a synopsis of the program, in their own words.

Who we are

MHAs are highly trusted inmate peers who undergo extensive training in trauma-informed care. We live and work within the specialized mental health pod at TTCF, inside Los Angeles County Jail. Our pods house 20–30 individuals, each experiencing a spectrum of mental health disorders.

We are volunteers, but, more than that, we are advocates, mentors, and connectors for those navigating serious mental illness in an environment not designed for healing.

Why we exist

Our role was created to bridge the communication gap between incarcerated patients and clinical staff, especially psychiatrists. We ensure that symptoms, behavioral concerns, and emotional needs are not only observed but heard and responded to.

Many individuals in our care cannot always speak up for themselves. Some are silenced by stigma, fear, confusion, or the weight of their condition. As MHAs, we speak up – for them, with them, and, sometimes, instead of them.

We operate with dignity, empathy, and presence, always rooted in the belief that every person deserves to be seen, heard, and cared for.

As the original MHAs have described, we are in the middle of this crisis every day. There is no one closer to and more intimate with this situation. So, what is the problem? The first issue is the environment of the jail. The sad and true part is that this jail is not closing or going anywhere. This will continue to be the residence for many patients in the future. Most patients have lived most of their lives in one of the most punitive environments in the USA. So that's the first part. Just take out mental disorders for a second and focus on the nature of the environment. We have to have settings in the jail that are truly restorative and offer meaningful services and skills where individuals not only get their mental health needs taken care of, but they also learn to correct faulty thinking patterns and gain real employable skills or an education that furthers and supports their stability on the outside.

The jail plays a huge role: Just having basic needs met like a shower, a roll of toilet paper, and a toothbrush can prevent the frustration that sometimes precipitates decompensation, leading to disciplinary action that helps nothing. There has to be some investment in education and restorative programs in the jails so that people have an environment where they can begin the healing process. We know it can be done because we have managed to do it.

As MHAs, we know what it takes, what will work, and what won't work. We have a model that will change the way incarceration is carried out in the jails, establishing environments that keep patients stabilized, healthy, and educated. The strongest factor here is that this is all operated by justice-impacted individuals who understand this problem better than anyone. We live it every day, and we develop intimate and trusting relationships with those who are under our care. They tell us things they wouldn't tell anyone else.

Core framework: The MHA model

Creating a successful mental health program behind bars begins with understanding the unique needs of the incarcerated population. This is not only a matter of clinical care – it is a matter of dignity, safety, and human rights.

Change in this environment does not happen overnight. Long-standing stereotypes and distrust between incarcerated individuals and correctional staff are deeply rooted. These biases can hinder progress unless we proactively build bridges to communicate between patients and psychiatrists, clinicians, correctional staff, and the department of correctional health. Developing our mission statement was a significant step toward shaping our identity.

Our mission is to advocate, support, and create change for the underserved and marginalized, despite the obstacles. Our push for proper care for every patient and purposeful opportunity for every inmate is unwavering. Knowing the road to effective treatment and self-growth has no finish line, our daily operations are routed in love, unselfishness, integrity, truthfulness, teamwork, and organized effort. This guide offers a practical framework to do exactly that.

The program is a groundbreaking initiative that emphasizes treatment over punishment. It thrives because of the collaboration between correctional health professionals and trained inmate MHAs.

Our motto: Transforming the traditional approach to rehabilitation from the inside out.

The role of MHAs

MHAs are trusted inmate peers trained in:

- Active listening
- Crisis de-escalation
- Confidentiality
- Peer mentorship

Institutional mental health support program step-by-step guide: Institutional recreation model for mental health care

Goal: Building a better tomorrow

This institutional model not only addresses the mental health needs of inmates but also promotes a transformational culture within correctional facilities. With the right foundation, we can create a system that supports healing, reduces recidivism, and uplifts everyone involved – staff, inmates, and society alike.

Our mission statement

To advocate, support, and create change for the underserved and marginalized, despite obstacles. Our push for proper care for every patient and purposeful opportunity for every inmate is unwavering knowing the road to effective treatment and self-growth has no finish line.

Our core values

We anchor our daily operations in:

- Love – unconditional, patient, and nonjudgmental
- Unselfishness – service over self, always
- Integrity – doing what's right, especially when it's hard
- Truthfulness – honest reporting, honest feedback
- Teamwork – one unit, many voices, shared mission
- Organized effort – disciplined consistency to serve others

Our impact

MHAs are essential to the well-being of one of the most vulnerable populations in the jail system. We are trusted by staff, respected by our peers, and valued by patients. Our presence reduces crisis incidents, improves psychiatric outcomes, and fosters a culture of healing from within.

Step 1: Safe and secure housing environment

- Establish designated pods or units exclusively for inmates with mental health disorders (e.g., schizophrenia, mood disorders, anxiety, delusions).
- Ensure the space is physically and emotionally safe, separate from the general population, and designed to reduce overstimulation.

Step 2: Assign inmate MHAs

- Recruit and train peer inmates as daily assistants who live embedded in the pods with the patients they serve.
- Responsibilities include:
  - Supporting meals, recreation, hygiene, and group activities.
  - Facilitating communication between staff and inmates.
  - Promoting positivity through mentorship and support.

Step 3: Facility enhancement

- Redesign pods with uplifting elements:
  - Murals, motivational quotes, and educational posters.
  - Mission statements focused on healing and growth.
  - Contributions from cartoon artists or creative therapy organizations.
- Introduce pictures, plants, and pets:
  - Use therapy animals for weekly visits.
  - Add plants and nature-themed elements to create a calming atmosphere.

Step 4: Recreation and creative expression

- Provide access to safe games (table tennis, cards, foosball).
- Introduce musical instruments (guitar, piano) and art supplies.
- Promote creative expression as part of therapy and personal growth.

Step 5: Cleanliness and upkeep

- Ensure the facility maintains a hospital-grade level of cleanliness.
- Assign MHAs to:
  - Sweep daily.
  - Mop weekly.
  - Wax and polish floors every 1–3 months.
- Clean, orderly spaces help foster pride, professionalism, and dignity.

Step 6: Dedicated correctional care staff

- Appoint an additional correctional officer specifically for this program.
- This officer oversees mental health-focused care staff, ensuring:
  - Staff are aligned with trauma-informed care values.
  - Operations reflect rehabilitative rather than punitive models.

Step 7: Select purpose-driven staff

- Assign staff who are:

- Committed to rehabilitation and human dignity.
- Open to collaboration with mental health professionals.

- Conduct collaborative interviews with staff and inmates to identify:

- Those suited for therapeutic roles.
- Inmates open to personal growth and change.

We may wear the same clothing, but we walk with a different purpose – one rooted in compassion and guided by the belief that rehabilitation begins with connection.

Remarks of Father Alberto Carrara to the American Psychiatric Association – May 2025

Alberto Carrara

As we gather here today under the theme of optimizing interventions for schizophrenia to avoid dire outcomes, I invite you to zoom out – not to lose focus, but to gain depth. The failure to treat people with schizophrenia, the persistence of homelessness, untreated psychosis, and premature death are not simply lapses in clinical delivery. They are signs of a deeper ethical misalignment. As a neuroethicist and member of ICONN – the International College of Neuroethics and Neuroscience – I believe we need a new lens, one that reframes our approach to human persons with schizophrenia from within the interior logic of the human person.

Neuroethics, at its core, is not merely ethics applied to brain data. It is a systematic and informed reflection on both neuroscientific findings and their interpretations – especially the models we construct of the brain, the mind, and the person. These models matter. They shape how we diagnose, treat, and legislate. They determine whether our interventions liberate or limit, whether they dignify or dehumanize.

Let us be clear: Schizophrenia, especially in its most severe forms, impairs not only perception and reasoning – it fractures the very unity of consciousness, disrupting the person's capacity for coherent self-representation and deliberate freedom.

To illuminate this, I propose a biosystemic model – a stratified understanding of human consciousness and free will – that allows us to locate, with precision, where and how schizophrenia erodes freedom, and therefore where ethics and policy must respond.

Stratifying consciousness, calibrating freedom

Human consciousness is not a monolith. It is a dynamic, bottom-up system structured across at least six dimensions: interoception, exteroception, integrative perception, awareness, proprioception, and phenomenal self-awareness. Each layer is not only a level of conscious experience – it is the foundation of a corresponding form of freedom:

- *Intero-freedom:* The ability to respond to internal bodily states.
- *Extero-freedom:* The capacity to react meaningfully to external stimuli.
- *Integrative-freedom:* The power to synthesize sensory input into coherent perception.
- *Aware-freedom:* Reflective insight into one's own condition and choices.
- *Proprio-freedom:* Control over bodily movement and spatial agency.
- *Self-freedom:* The highest tier – phenomenal consciousness and the capacity for self-directed, value-based choice.

Now consider what happens in schizophrenia.

The disease does not destroy the nervous system like amyotrophic lateral sclerosis (ALS) or Parkinson's. Rather, it scrambles the layered architecture of consciousness. Delusions distort integrative-freedom. Hallucinations override extero-freedom. Anosognosia erases aware-freedom. And in its most severe forms, self-freedom – the freedom that makes us fully human – is silenced.

This is not mere impairment. This is a disintegration of freedom from within. And yet, tragically, our policies too often wait until the patient can "choose" help – assuming a level of freedom that the condition has already dismantled.

What neuroethics demands

Neuroethics demands that we stop asking the wrong questions. We should not be asking, "Is this person refusing care?" but rather: "At what

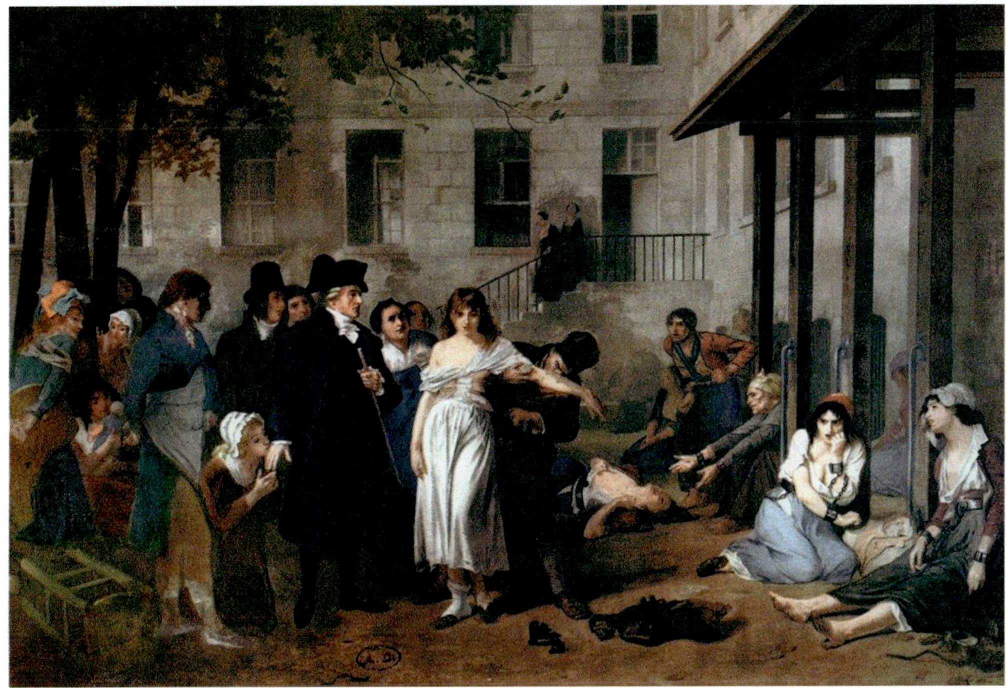

level of consciousness – and thus freedom – is this person operating?"

If the answer is that self-freedom is compromised, then our ethical responsibility is not inaction, but intervention.

This is where we must distinguish between paternalism – which seeks control – and *parens patriae* – which recognizes responsibility for those who cannot exercise full autonomy. People with schizophrenia, especially those with anosognosia, are not merely resistant. They are structurally incapable – at least temporarily – of self-rescuing from a collapsing conscious order.

And so, we must speak clearly: Treatment is not coercion. It is restoration. The stratification of freedom tells us where intervention is not only justified, but ethically imperative. To withhold care until "consent" reemerges is to abandon the patient to disintegration. That is not ethics. That is abandonment dressed up in autonomy.

Policy implications: Restoring autonomy, not violating it

From this perspective, early and assertive treatment is not a violation of rights, but a precondition for their

recovery. The person with schizophrenia is not a problem to manage. They are a subject whose freedom must be scaffolded – reconstructed – from within.

When we apply this layered model of consciousness, we can:

- Target interventions where integration breaks down (e.g., perceptual therapies for hallucinations, cognitive remediation for integrative deficits).
- Justify legal mechanisms for urgent care based not on subjective distress, but on measurable collapse in freedom.
- Redefine psychiatric recovery not merely as symptom reduction, but as the restoration of layered autonomy.

This is a profound shift: from compliance to dignity. From documentation to discernment.

A neuroethical call to action

Let me end where I began: with dignity.

Schizophrenia is not just a clinical challenge. It is a mirror held up to our ethical systems. Neuroethics, as I understand it, is the discipline that forces us to look into that mirror – not to despair, but to reconstruct the moral architecture of care.

Let us no longer be complicit in a system that calls neglect autonomy and calls abandonment compassion. Let us instead build neuroethically informed pathways of care – where neuroscience guides us not only toward what is possible, but toward what is just.

In the layered ruins of disintegrated consciousness, we must place not blame, but bridges – bridges back to autonomy, to relationality, to dignity.

Because every person with schizophrenia is not a broken machine. They are a stratified, wounded freedom calling out – quietly, incoherently, perhaps even violently – for a chance to be restored.

That is our task. That is our responsibility. That is our human obligation.

Index

Printed in the United Kingdom by TJ Clays Ltd.